HEALTH AND HEALTH CARE IN BRITAIN

Second Edition

Rob Baggott

First edition 1994
Reprinted three times
Second edition 1998

Published by
MACMILLAN PRESS LTD
Houndmills, Basingstoke, Hampshire RG21 6XS
and London
Companies and representatives
throughout the world

ISBN 0–333–69476–7

A catalogue record for this book is available
from the British Library.

This book is printed on paper suitable for recycling and
made from fully managed and sustained forest sources.

Copy-edited and typeset by Povey–Edmondson
Tavistock and Rochdale, England

Printed and bound in Great Britain by
Creative Print & Design (Wales), Ebbw Vale

10   9   8   7   6   5   4   3
06   05   04   03   02   01

Contents

List of Tables, Figures and Exhibits

■ **Table**

■ **Figures**

■ Exhibits

Preface to the Second Edition

The main objectives of the second edition of this book remain the same as for the first: to help the reader understand the workings of the British health care system while giving an insight into contemporary health issues and debates. The very fact that a comprehensive revision is necessary so soon indicates the pace of change in this field. Indeed, almost every aspect of health care has been affected to some extent by new policy developments, structural reforms, technological change, managerial and professional initiatives. Moreover, further changes can be expected. In May 1997, a Labour government took office – the first in almost two decades. Although the new government accepted several aspects of the reforms introduced by the Conservatives in the 1980s and 1990s, it declared its intention to make further changes and to develop fresh proposals.

Given the extent of change in recent years and the probability of further reform in the future, the task of revising the book has not been an easy one. However, I am grateful for the opportunity to produce a second edition, for two main reasons. First, it has enabled me to ensure that the book remains a useful resource to those requiring a broad, informative guide to the contemporary health care system and the key debates surrounding it. It is perhaps appropriate at this point to record my thanks to the many readers, tutors and reviewers who kindly expressed positive sentiments about the first edition. Secondly, the revision has enabled me to respond to various constructive comments and suggestions. Indeed, the new chapter on health service users (Chapter 11) is a direct response to comments made by some reviewers.

Apart from this new chapter, the structure of the book remains much the same. The first three chapters set out the broad context of health care: trends in health and illness, the professions, and the main critiques of health care. Chapters 4 and 5 examine the evolution of the British health care system and its present structure. Chapters 6, 7 and 8 of the book focus on the development and implementation of health policies in relation to NHS management, the funding and the provision of health services. Chapter 9 and 10 examine primary care and community care respectively, and Chapter 12 focuses upon public health. Finally, Chapter 13 assesses the broad impact of the Conservatives' health policies and examines the approach taken so far by the Blair administration.

I would like to thank a large number of people for their help and support, although ultimate responsibility for the book remains mine. First of all, as always, I would like to thank my wife Debbie and my children Mark, Danny and Melissa for their love and support. Many of my colleagues at De Montfort University, along with researchers at other universities, have also been extremely supportive and helpful and deserve my thanks. Lack of space prevents me from mentioning everyone; but the following includes those who have been particularly helpful in relation to this project: Helen Bentley, Ellen Carter, Merrill Clarke, Holly Crossen-White, Alison Hann, Mike Hart, Jackie Leatham, Victoria McGregor-Riley, Fred Mear, Pat Mounfield, Sally Ruane, Professor Mike Saks, Professor Mel Chevannes and Professor Andrew Watterson. In addition, I would like to thank Sue Dewing, Julie Conroy and Sue Smith of the PPMS Resources Centre, librarians Elizabeth O'Neill and Olwyn Reynard, and Carole Shaw and her staff. Thanks also to Professor David Wilson and Professor John Coyne for their continued encouragement and support. Finally, I must record my appreciation to Keith Povey, my copy-editor, and to my publisher, Steven Kennedy, for his invaluable help and advice.

ROB BAGGOTT

List of Abbreviations

AIDS	Acquired Immune Deficiency Syndrome
AHA	Area Health Authority
BMA	British Medical Association
BPA	Basic Practice Allowance
BSE	Bovine Spongiform Encephalopathy
CHC	Community Health Council
CJD	Creutzfeldt–Jakob Disease
CIP	Cost Improvement Programme
CMO	Chief Medical Officer
CNO	Chief Nursing Officer
COMA	Committee on Medical Aspects of Food
DGH	District General Hospital
DGM	District General Manager
DoH	Department of Health
DHA	District Health Authority
DHSS	Department of Health and Social Security
DMT	District Management Team
DMU	Directly Managed Units
EBM	Evidence-based Medicine
ECR	Extra Contractual Referral
EHS	Emergency Hospital Service
FHSA	Family Health Services Authority
FPC	Family Practitioner Committee
FPS	Family Practitioner Services
GHS	General Household Survey
GMC	General Medical Council
GP	General Practitioner
GPA	Good Practice Allowance
GPF	General Practitioner Fundholders
HAI	Hospital Acquired Infection
HAZ	Health Action Zone
HCHS	Hospital and Community Health Services
HISS	Hospital Information Support Systems
HIV	Human Immunodeficiency Virus
HMC	Hospital Management Committee
HMO	Health Maintenance Organisation
HRT	Hormone Replacement Therapy

HSSB	Health Services Supervisory Board
JCB	Joint Commissioning Board
LPG	Local Planning Group
ME	Myalgic Encephalomyelitis
MHCO	Managed Health Care Organisations
MIT	Minimally Invasive Therapy
MoH	Ministry of Health
MOH	Medical Officer of Health
MRI	Magnetic Resonance Imaging
NAHAT	National Association of Health Authorities and Trusts
NAO	National Audit Office
NCT	National Childbirth Trust
NCEPOD	National Confidential Enquiry into Peri-operative Deaths
NCVO	National Council for Voluntary Organisations
NHI	National Health Insurance
NHS	National Health Service
NHSE	National Health Service Executive
NHSME	National Health Service Management Executive
NNS	Neighbourhood Nursing Service
OECD	Organisation for Economic Cooperation and Development
OPCS	Office for Population, Census and Surveys
PAC	Public Account Committee
PCG	Primary Care Group
PET	Positron Emission Tomography
PHCT	Primary Health Care Team
PVS	Persistent Vegetative State
QALY	Quality Adjusted Life Year
RAWP	Resource Allocation Working Party
RCN	Royal College of Nursing
RCT	Randomised Controlled Trial
RGM	Regional General Manager
RHA	Regional Health Authority
RHB	Regional Hospital Board
RMI	Resource Management Initiative
SGT	Self-Governing Trust
SHA	Special Health Authority
SMR	Standardised Mortality Ratio
STD	Sexually Transmitted Diseases
STG	Special Transitional Grant
TQM	Total Quality Management
VFMU	Value for Money Unit
WHO	World Health Organisation
WRVS	Women's Royal Voluntary Service

To Mark, Danny and Melissa

■ *Chapter 1* ■

Health and Illness

Let us begin on a note of optimism. In terms of surviving to adulthood, life expectancy, and the chances of a living a life relatively free from the threat of fatal disease, the British people have perhaps never had it so good. Present standards of health are relatively high, not only in comparison with past generations, but also internationally. Britain in the 1990s is a comparatively healthy place in which to be born and to live.

However, this broad assessment is in many respects misleading. The focus upon overall standards of health can disguise important variations between different sections of the population. Any judgement about health standards must therefore be based on a careful analysis of health and illness trends. This introductory chapter attempts to provide such an analysis, beginning with the concept of health. This is followed by a discussion of important variations in health and illness in Britain, within an historical and global context.

■ Defining health

There are two main ways of defining health; the positive approach, where health is viewed as a capacity or an asset to be possessed, and the negative approach, which emphasises the absence of specific illnesses, diseases or disorders (Aggleton, 1990, p. 5).

□ *Positive health*

The World Health Organisation (WHO) has defined health as 'a state of complete physical, mental and social well-being and not merely the absence of disease or infirmity' (WHO, 1946). As well as emphasising health in a positive sense, this definition is significant in stressing mental as well as physical aspects of health, and social as well as individual well-being. This definition also has been criticised for being utopian, though it is perhaps more appropriately viewed as an ideal towards which health care and other social actions may be orientated (Twaddle, 1974). Even so, there are problems with the definition and measurement of well-being – a rather woolly notion – which raise further questions about the utility of the definition as a policy goal.

1

The WHO definition is an abstraction. The health of individuals and groups has to be seen in relation to their environments, expectations, and capacities. A ninety-year-old would not expect, and would not be expected by others, to have the capacity to run a marathon. Yet he or she may well be healthy, relatively speaking, given society's expectations about nonagenarians. In addition, seriously disabled people may live a full and fulfilling life, and in this sense may be regarded as healthy.

Related to this is the idea that health is a form of strength. In a rather narrow sense, strength can be seen as being synonymous with physical fitness. Yet it has a wider meaning which goes beyond the simple ability to exert oneself physically. One can conceive of health as an inner strength which people may develop in order to deal with the problems and stresses of life. Almost paradoxically, health may involve suffering as a creative way of dealing with destructive feelings (Wilson, 1975). Illich, in his critique of medicine (to be discussed further in Chapter 3), argues that health designates the intensity with which individuals cope with their internal states and environmental conditions. According to this view, a healthy environment is presumably one which encourages personal responsibility and the ability to cope with life's many problems.

To summarise, health in a positive sense can be seen as a feeling of general well-being on an individual and social level. More specifically it can also be seen as a process of adaptation to the environment, a capacity to function, and a strength to cope both with specific illnesses and with life in general.

□ *The negative concept of health*

In terms of the negative concept of health, an individual is regarded as being healthy when not suffering from a particular illness or disease. The terms 'illness' and 'disease', although often used interchangeably, can be distinguished. Disease relates to a biological malfunctioning, diagnosed by doctors, while illness refers both to the personal experience of disease and its wider social implications (Kleinman, 1978). The negative concept of health is closely associated with orthodox medicine, which is focused mainly on disease. It is often argued that doctors are not particularly interested in health in a positive sense and that the negative approach to health has tended to predominate (Gould, 1987). This is discussed further in Chapter 3.

□ *The measurement of health, disease and illness*

The predominance of the negative approach, coupled with the difficulties of interpreting concepts such as 'social well-being', has implications for the measurement of health. Rather than indicating standards of health in a positive sense, official health statistics tend to measure how unhealthy we are. The emphasis is very much on mortality (death), morbidity (disease) and treatment or service statistics. Analysis of health trends is also usually confined to the changing prevalence of disease.

Yet it is possible to measure health in a positive sense. For example, life expectancy and infant mortality statistics (the latter is usually expressed as the number of deaths in children under one year of age per thousand live births) are often used as indicators of the resistance of the population to disease. Certain treatment statistics may also help build up a picture of the positive aspects of health. Immunisation rates, which indicate a community's potential resistance to certain diseases, can be viewed as an indicator of positive health. The growing use of mental health services and antidepressants, on the other hand, indicates the poor level of mental well-being in society, though it also reflects the greater willingness of sufferers to seek help and the wider availability of such therapies.

Finally, there are social surveys – such as the General Household Survey (GHS) – which ask individuals about their own attitudes to health, fitness and lifestyles as well as their experiences of ill-health. These can serve as indicators of positive health, making it possible to construct a less one-sided analysis of health trends.

■ Health trends and variations

The experience of health and illness can vary in several ways. There is often a variation over time, certain diseases being more prevalent in some historical periods than in others. Health and illness can vary over one's lifetime, with individuals being more prone to particular illnesses at certain stages in their lives. There are also significant geographical variations in health and illness. Such variations can be found at the regional and local, as well as the international level. Finally, health and illness may vary according to the location of individuals in the social structure. There are differences in health between social classes, between the sexes, and between ethnic groups in the population.

□ *Historical trends*

In 1901, average life expectancy at birth in the United Kingdom (UK) was only 45.5 years for men and 49 years for women. In 1996 a new-born male could expect to live 74.4 years on average; a new-born female, 79.7 years. Over the same period, infant mortality fell from 142 to 6.2 per 1000 live births. These figures suggest a significant improvement in the overall health of the population. But at the same time there has been an equally significant change in the burden of ill-health.

Perhaps the most marked trend this century has been the decline of the major infectious diseases widespread in the Victorian period: cholera, typhoid, measles, whooping cough and tuberculosis. Although medical interventions in the form of drug therapies and vaccination programmes were important in reducing morbidity and mortality related to these diseases, their decline was already underway due mainly to improved standards of living. However, medical intervention certainly played a much more significant role in the decline of many other infectious diseases, such as diphtheria and poliomyelitis. The contribution of medicine to the reduction of infectious disease is discussed further in Chapter 2.

The decline of the major infectious diseases has been offset to a considerable extent by a growth in the incidence of other, chronic, diseases. In the post-Second World War period, for example, the number of measles cases in the UK declined from over 600 000 in 1950 to just over 20 000 in the mid-1990s. Over the same period the number of deaths from lung cancer increased from just over 13 000 to almost 40 000. This illustrates the way in which lifestyle-related diseases have superseded the old infectious epidemics. Deaths caused by infectious diseases represent less than 1 per cent of the total number of deaths in England and Wales, compared with 13 per cent only sixty years ago. Currently, almost half of the mortality in England and Wales is due to circulatory diseases such as heart disease and stroke, with a further quarter of deaths attributed to cancers.

Much of the burden of ill health today can be associated with modern lifestyles and environments. For example, a considerable proportion of circulatory diseases and cancers have been linked to lifestyle factors such as smoking, alcohol abuse, poor diet, stress and lack of exercise (Jacobson, Smith and Whitehead, 1991). It is now widely believed that action to promote healthy lifestyles and environments is needed to tackle the modern epidemics. These efforts are discussed in more detail in Chapter 12 in the context of the British government's national health strategy.

A broader indication of the nation's health is given by large-scale surveys of health and fitness. According to the *Health Survey for England*, less than half the British population regularly indulge in active sports, games and physical activities: 47 per cent of men and 36 per cent of women are active at moderate levels or above – defined as twelve or more occasions of moderate activity in the previous month (DoH and OPCS, 1995). This survey also found that a fifth of adults had not taken any moderate exercise (which includes gardening, brisk walking, heavy housework) in the month prior to interview.

Surveys also yield information about individual self-reported illness and disability. It is estimated that there are over six million adults in Great Britain – approximately 15 per cent of the adult population – with at least one form of disability (OPCS, 1988). 32 per cent of respondents reported long-term illness in the 1994 GHS survey (OPCS, 1996), and almost one in five claimed to have a long-standing illness which limited their activities; 14 per cent of respondents claimed that illness had restricted their activities in the two weeks prior to the interview. The most common self-reported long-term illnesses are diseases and disorders of the musculoskeletal system (reported by 151 per thousand of the population), the heart and circulatory system (93 per thousand), and the respiratory system (71 per thousand) (OPCS, 1996). It is clear from successive surveys that the proportion reporting a long-standing illness has increased significantly in all age and sex categories in recent years. In 1976, for example, only a quarter of respondents reported such illness, with 16 per cent reporting limiting long-term conditions and less than one in ten claiming to have restricted activity.

The focus on chronic illness and disability should not produce complacency about the relatively low levels of infectious disease today. Older infectious diseases such as tuberculosis have returned. Food-borne infectious diseases appear to be increasing – food poisoning notifications quadrupled between 1985 and 1995. There is also anxiety about new infectious diseases – such as Legionnaires' disease and new forms of infection which may be able to cross the species barrier, such as BSE (Bovine Spongiform Encephalopathy). Furthermore the growing resistance of microbes to antibiotics is an alarming trend raising the prospect of a new era of infectious disease (Garrett, 1995; Krause, 1981; Morse, 1993).

Reported cases of sexually-transmitted diseases (STD) have risen dramatically during the post-Second World War period. In 1951, less than 100 000 cases of STD were reported in the UK. By 1990 this figure had risen to well over half a million. Forecasts of a world AIDS (Acquired Immune Deficiency Syndrome) epidemic did much to stimulate concern about STD. By the mid-1990s there were over 11 000 reported cases of AIDS in the UK, of which more than two-thirds had died. Yet the number of people diagnosed as HIV (human immunodeficiency virus)-positive, who may develop AIDS, was set to rise to around 30 000 by the turn of the century. Moreover, the actual number of HIV-positive people is thought to be significantly higher than the number of reported cases.

The extent of mental illness is a further cause for concern. Trends are very difficult to establish, however, as the interpretation of mental illness has varied considerably between different historical periods (Scull, 1979). In recent years the growing use of mental health services and antidepressant drugs is believed to indicate a deterioration in mental health. But, as suggested earlier, such statistics reflect the availability of such therapies as well as changing perceptions of need.

Certainly, the level of mental illness represents an enormous social problem today: 15 per cent of general practitioner (GP) consultations relate to mental health problems. Around 70 per cent of women and 50 per cent of men at some time during their lives consult their GP regarding their mental health. In one large-scale survey, one in seven adults reported experiencing a neurotic disorder within the previous week (Meltzer *et al.*, 1995).

Mental and physical illness are often related, though in ways which are poorly understood. Serious physical illnesses, such as cancer, can have wide-ranging psychological implications, not only for the sufferer but also for their relatives. Mental health problems can lead to physical illness, injury and even death. Addictions, such as smoking, alcohol misuse and drug abuse, are linked to a range of physical diseases and disorders. Suicide deaths (over 3000 a year in England and Wales in the 1990s), and injuries resulting from suicide attempts, are closely associated with mental health problems (see Royal College of Psychiatrists, 1995).

□ Life cycles and demographic change

Not only does health (and ill-health) vary over time, it also varies over an individual's lifetime. There is a kind of life cycle in operation, with people being prone to certain illnesses at particular times in their lives. Figure 1.1 illustrates the main causes of death in different age groups for men and women, showing that the main causes of mortality in younger people are quite different from those which kill the middle-aged and elderly. Violent death, accidents and injury (both external and self-inflicted) are major causes of death in younger people. Around 20 000 people a year die from accidents or violent incidents every year in Britain. A third of these deaths are road-traffic-related, 40 per cent of these involving the under-25s. Circulatory diseases, cancers and respiratory diseases are the most common causes of death in the older age groups.

Studies of self-reported illness confirm the chronic nature of disease in older age groups. The GHS survey found that in the oldest age groups, those reporting such illness are a majority. Figure 1.2 illustrates the differences in self-reported chronic illness between the various age and sex groups. Although total life expectancy has increased, the prevalence of chronic illness and disability in old age remains at a high level, so that those additional years of life are often extra years with a disability, not of healthy life (Bone *et al.*, 1995; Dunnell, 1995). Almost two-thirds of disabled men, and nearly three-quarters of disabled women, are over sixty years of age (OPCS, 1988).

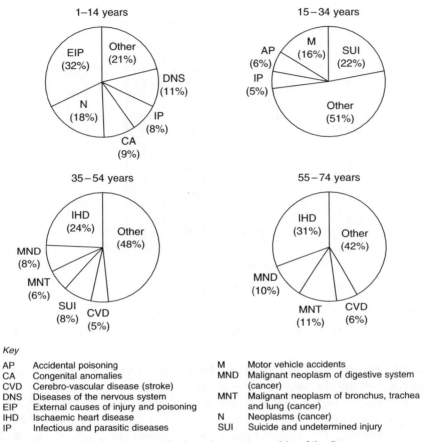

1–14 years

EIP
(32%)

Other
(21%)

DNS
(11%)

N
(18%)

IP
(8%)

CA
(9%)

15–34 years

AP
(6%)

M
(16%)

SUI
(22%)

IP
(5%)

Other
(51%)

35–54 years

IHD
(24%)

Other
(48%)

MND
(8%)

MNT
(6%)

SUI
(8%)

CVD
(5%)

55–74 years

IHD
(31%)

Other
(42%)

MND
(10%)

MNT
(11%)

CVD
(6%)

Key

AP	Accidental poisoning	M	Motor vehicle accidents
CA	Congenital anomalies	MND	Malignant neoplasm of digestive system
CVD	Cerebro-vascular disease (stroke)		(cancer)
DNS	Diseases of the nervous system	MNT	Malignant neoplasm of bronchus, trachea
EIP	External causes of injury and poisoning		and lung (cancer)
IHD	Ischaemic heart disease	N	Neoplasms (cancer)
IP	Infectious and parasitic diseases	SUI	Suicide and undetermined injury

Note: Percentages indicate the proportion in each age category dying of the disease.

Source: Chief Medical Officer, *On the State of the Public Health 1995* (HMSO, 1996).

Figure 1.1   *The main causes of death in selected age groups, males (England), 1995*

There are also some important variations in mental illness between the different age groups. In general the elderly have higher levels of mental illness. Depression is common in the elderly, affecting about one in five of the over-65s. Dementia is also a major form of mental illness among the elderly with one in twenty of the over-65s, and one in five of the over-80s suffering from it. Severe mental illness is also found in younger age groups. Around 150 000 people in the UK suffer from schizophrenia, a mental illness which develops mainly in young adults. Suicide, which as noted earlier is associated with mental illness, is a significant cause of death among both old and the young. In the past suicide rates have been highest

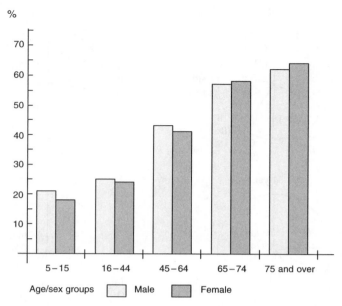

Source of data: OPCS, *General Household Survey 1994* (HMSO, 1996).

Figure 1.2   *Respondents reporting long-standing illness (Great Britain), 1994*

among the elderly, but during the 1980s and 1990s there was a marked increase in suicide rates in younger age groups.

The discovery that older people are more likely to die from chronic disease and to have long-standing conditions and disabilities should come as no surprise. Yet it does raise questions about the implications of an increasing elderly population – a trend which is being faced by most developed countries today. The projected growth of the elderly population in the UK is shown in Figures 1.3 and 1.4. This shows that, following a sharp rise in the elderly population in the 1960s and 1970s, something of a plateau has now been reached. This situation is expected to persist until the early years of the twenty-first century when there will be a further significant rise in the proportion of elderly people in the UK, reaching almost a fifth of the total population by the year 2030. Figure 1.4 illustrates the growth in the 'very elderly' population over the same period. By 2030 one in twenty of the population will be aged over eighty.

The predicted growth of the elderly population is more spectacular in other countries. It is estimated that by the year 2030 Switzerland will have the highest proportion of over-65s – 29 per cent of its population. In the same year it is likely that the elderly will account for over a fifth of the populations of Sweden, Germany, Italy, Austria, Norway, France, Finland, The Netherlands and Canada. The increasing elderly population, while

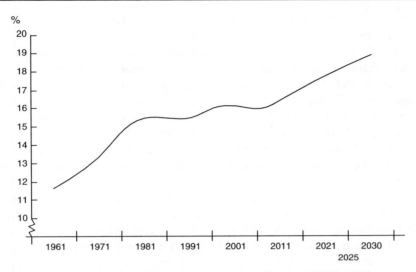

Source of data: Calculated from Central Statistical Office, *Social Trends 22* (HMSO, 1992).

Figure 1.3 *The increase in the elderly population (UK), percentage of total population over 65 years old*

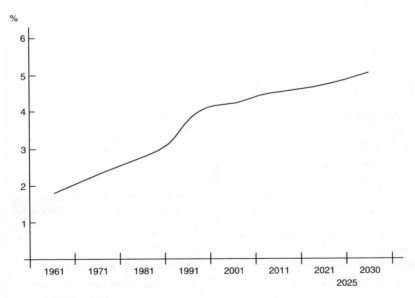

Note: Projections from 1996.

Source of data: Calculated from Central Statistical Office, *Social Trends 22* (HMSO, 1992).

Figure 1.4 *The increase in the elderly population (UK), percentage of total population over 80 years old*

affecting all the main industrialised countries, is therefore likely to have a greater impact on some than on others.

The growing proportion of elderly people in society is not a problem in itself. Rather, it is the likely consequences of this growth for health care provision and other social services which causes concern. Relative to other age groups, the elderly, and particularly those over the age of 75, are heavy users of health care. Figure 1.5 illustrates the relatively high levels of health care expenditure accounted for by the elderly, and in particular by the very elderly. The implication is that the growth of the elderly population, all other things being equal, will produce an escalation in the costs of health care.

The rising cost of caring for the elderly is only a problem if society cannot afford it. Yet there is a fear that the growth in the elderly population will not only add to the cost of care but will prevent society from generating the necessary resources (Johnson, Conrad and Thomson, 1989). In 1961 there were almost six people of working age for every person aged over 65. By the year 2011 this ratio will be less than four to one. This implies that the working population will face an increasingly heavy burden of providing the resources necessary for the care of the elderly.

This gloomy scenario has been challenged. Some have pointed out that the dependency ratio (the ratio between those of working age and the rest

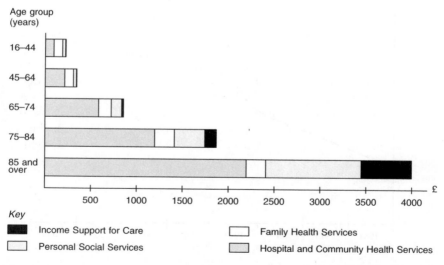

Source of data: A. Robins and R. Wittenberg, *The Health of Elderly People – An Epidemiological Overview* (HMSO, 1993).

Figure 1.5 *Per capita health and social care costs by age group (England), 1989/90*

of the population, that is the elderly and children) is remarkably stable over time (Thane, 1987). So the growth in the elderly population is to some extent offset by changes at the other end of the age structure. It has been estimated that the dependency ratio will not begin to rise much above today's level until the second decade of the next century (Ermisch, 1990). A continuation of low birth-rates therefore could produce savings on spending programmes such as education, releasing resources for services such as social care needed by the larger elderly population. It is further claimed that estimates of the rise in the elderly population have been exaggerated; indeed there has already been a downward revision of projections in recent years.

Another criticism is that the cost of the growing elderly population has been over-estimated (House of Commons, 1996a; Abel-Smith, 1996). Ermisch (1990) has discovered that the ageing population will not place much pressure on resources until 2011. According to this study, by the middle of the next century, expenditures on health and social care will only need to be 12 per cent higher than today providing that resources per person in each age group remains the same (this increase compares with a 14 per cent increase in real resources during the 1980s). Robins and Wittenberg (1993) estimate that an annual increase of 0.7 per cent in resources will meet the demographic pressures, though they warn that other factors such as rising health care costs should also be taken into account. However, as Abel-Smith (1996) noted, most health care costs are devoted to people in their last year of life. The predicted rising costs of an ageing population are heavily based on the assumption that more people will survive to the stage at which they will incur high health care costs. But a recent study (Scitovsky, 1988, cited by Abel-Smith, 1996) found that those who die in their 80s consume 20 per cent less in their last year of life than those who die aged 65–79. The implication of this is that greater longevity does not necessarily increase (and may even help to curb) health care costs in the longer-term. A further point is that in spite of the higher than average levels of disability in old age, elderly people are fitter than is commonly supposed (Jarvis *et al.*, 1996). The vast majority of over-60s are capable of looking after themselves (and others – the elderly making up one-third of the ranks of informal carers). Even among the over-80s, the majority are fairly mobile. It is also possible that the future elderly population may be even healthier and will not therefore need current levels of service provision (Bosanquet, 1975). Studies in the United States, for example, found that levels of chronic disability among the elderly declined in recent years, even among the very old (Manton *et al.*, 1995).

Despite these counter-arguments, and the recent evidence upon which they are based, concern about the growth of the elderly population remains. Even if people live healthier lives for longer periods, they will inevitably at some stage require health care and social support. The increase in overall costs may not be so great as earlier predictions implied. Nevertheless, health care systems will face an enormous challenge in accommodating the new and varied needs brought by future demographic trends.

☐ *International variations*

Countries such as Britain have had considerable success in reducing disease and increasing life expectancy. But some countries, particularly those in the Third World, are still fighting battles which were won in the developed world long ago. When studying health and illness one cannot ignore the global context.

It is a tragic fact that out of the 50 million deaths that occur in the world each year, almost a quarter (12.2 million) are of children below the age of five (WHO, 1995). Most of these child deaths are due to infectious diseases. Each year four million children aged under five die from respiratory diseases, mostly pneumonia. Diarrhoea-related diseases are associated with over three million deaths of children in this age group. Other major killers include poliomyelitis, tetanus, measles, diphtheria, whooping cough and tuberculosis, which together kill a further two and a half million children.

Infant mortality is high in the developing world. But poor standards of health are found among adults as well as children. The average life expectancy in the least developed countries is two-thirds that found in the developed market economies (WHO, 1995). There are several reasons why the health of less-developed countries is worse. First, the climate of many developing countries produces an environment which can be damaging to health. Over two-fifths of the world's population live in areas threatened by malaria and around 100 million actually suffer from the disease. Other tropical diseases, such as schistosomiasis (a water-borne parasitic disease), affect twice this number.

High levels of infectious disease in Third-World countries are not simply due to the environment. Poverty and deprivation, which can be attributed to wider economic and political factors, undermine the health of many people in these countries (George, 1976; Sen, 1981). As the WHO (1995, p. v) has itself observed 'Poverty . . . is the world's deadliest disease'. Children are particularly affected, with more than 30 per cent of under-fives worldwide being undernourished (WHO, 1995, p. 6). In some cases the economic situation is made worse by unstable political and economic conditions, leading to civil war and famine. Such a combination of circumstances can lead to public health disasters, as in Ethiopia, Rwanda and Somalia to name only a few examples.

A further problem is poor health services. About a million people worldwide do not have regular access to health care services (WHO, 1995). The least developed countries have rudimentary health care systems. Expenditure on health care per capita in the poorest nations is less than 1 per cent of the amount spent in developed market economies. Moreover, in many cases even these limited resources have been mis-spent on inappropriate secondary care services, when good quality, accessible primary care was really required. An added problem in recent years has been the burden on poorer countries to repay international debts, which has reduced their ability to fund public health projects (Abel-Smith, 1994, pp. 155–9).

Nevertheless, there have been significant improvements in health in many Third-World countries during the post-Second World War period. Death rates in virtually all of these countries fell significantly (Phillips, 1990). This was due in part to better medical facilities and public health programmes in these countries, and in particular to efforts to improve basic health services (see Mills and Zwi, 1995). But general improvements in living standards have played a major (and some would say the main) role.

Economic development, however, often brings new problems. There is increasing evidence that Third-World countries are now having to bear a much heavier burden of chronic and degenerative diseases than before. This is partly due to the adoption of lifestyles found in the developed world. Take tobacco smoking, for example, which is associated with a range of cancers and circulatory diseases. Rates of smoking are growing faster than the population in Asia, Latin America, and Africa. Developing countries are now responsible for over half of tobacco consumption. Some countries – notably China and India – have experienced a considerable rise in tobacco-related diseases in recent years. It is not surprising, therefore, that tobacco is recognised as one of the most serious threats to the health of the Third World (Nath, 1986).

Diseases of poverty and affluence coexist in Third-World countries, along with diseases of climate and those which are 'man-made'. Furthermore, as if this is not enough, AIDS has disproportionately affected many of these countries. The majority of HIV-infected adults – over eight million out of a global total of 13–15 million in 1994 – are in Africa (WHO, 1995). However, it is expected that in the future Asia will take over as the centre of the AIDS epidemic, given the rapidly rising rates of HIV infection there, particularly in Southern and South-East Asia (Mann, 1993).

Although the picture looks bleak for many developing countries, one must be careful to avoid over-simple generalisations. The Third World is not as uniform in terms of health and health care as is often assumed.

Indeed there are many different 'worlds', consisting of groups of countries in particular regions (Latin America, Africa and so on), or at similar levels of economic development. Notably, the least developed countries in 1993 had much lower life expectancy rates at birth (51 years) than other non-industrialised countries (66 years). In the same year the least developed nations also had a much higher average infant mortality rate (110 per 1000) than the rest (59 per 1000). A similar difference occurs with health expenditure: in 1991 an average of $11 per head per annum was spent by the least developed nations, compared with $39 in other developing countries (WHO, 1995).

☐   *The industrialised countries*

In comparison with the Third World, the industrialised countries suffer relatively less from infectious diseases and more from chronic and degenerative diseases. Over three quarters (78 per cent) of deaths in the developed world each year are attributed to heart disease, strokes and cancer (WHO, 1995). Moreover, the trend towards chronic disease in these countries will continue as their populations age.

These broad trends mask a considerable variation in health and illness within industrialised countries (WHO, 1996). Infant mortality rates vary considerably, even among European countries, from under 6 (per 1000 live births) in Finland in the mid-1990s to just under 15 in Poland. Life expectancy at birth also varies significantly, from 64 years in the case of Hungarian males to almost 75 in Greece and Sweden. Mortality rates from specific categories of disease vary substantially within Europe. During the 1990s, death rates from infectious disease in Italy and Austria were less than half the rate found in France, Switzerland and Poland. Standardised death rates from cancer were roughly 50 per cent higher in Hungary and Denmark compared with Greece and Portugal. Mortality rates from circulatory disease are considerably lower in France, Switzerland and The Netherlands than in Finland, the Irish Republic and most of the former 'Eastern bloc' countries.

Compared with other European countries, the UK has a low mortality rate from infectious diseases. However, it has suffered from a higher than average mortality rate from cancer. In the case of circulatory disease, UK mortality is about average. However, it has one of the highest mortality rates from coronary heart disease among European countries. One should also bear in mind that the overall statistics for the UK (and for other countries too) tend to obscure important variations between sections of the population and different parts of the country. The nature of these variations will be explored later in this chapter.

Differences in general and specific mortality rates and in rates of illn between industrialised countries may be interesting, but are they significant? Some variations undoubtedly reflect specific local conditions such as differences in climate, demography, physical geography, and social and economic conditions. They may also relate to differences in the diagnosis of disease by the medical profession in each country, as we shall see in the next chapter. To some extent variations are due to differences in the accuracy of information systems which record illness and death. Variations in health and illness between countries can reflect other factors, such as the method of organising health services, the funding of the health care system, and wider health and social policies. Used with caution, however, such variations can provide a basis for judging both the comparative effectiveness of health care systems and national health strategies. This in turn raises the possibility of countries learning from those which have achieved most success in improving the health of their populations.

☐ *Regional and local variations*

As suggested earlier, there are important variations in health and illness within industrialised nations. Scotland, Wales and Northern Ireland have higher infant mortality rates than England. Scotland has a much higher death rate from cancers and strokes than other parts of the UK. Scotland and Northern Ireland have high rates of heart and circulatory disease compared with England and Wales. Coronary heart disease mortality rates in Scotland and Northern Ireland were 25 per cent higher than in England and Wales in the mid-1990s (WHO, 1996).

Within England many areas also have relatively poor levels of health, with the northern regions being as bad in many respects as Scotland and Northern Ireland. A general North–South gradient has been identified with the northern regions having a higher death rate for men and married women (adjusted for the age of the population) than the southern regions (Townsend, Davidson and Whitehead, 1992). Also, the general health of the population is worse in the North and Midlands than in the South.

However, the immediate local environment is regarded as a more important determinant of health than the region in which one resides. Urban areas, particularly purpose-built inner city estates and deprived industrial areas, are the least healthy; rural and prosperous areas the most healthy (Charlton, 1996). Hence in the North one can find areas where the population's health is good, while some localities in the South have very poor levels of health (Drever and Whitehead, 1995).

Finally, regional, local and indeed other forms of social inequality are not confined to the UK (Fox, 1989; Power, 1994). In the United States, for example, the infant mortality rate for non-whites in Washington DC is more than double the national average. Many other developed countries, such as Italy for example, have considerable regional inequalties in health. In the Third World the problem of geographical inequalities is even more striking, with wide differences in health between rural and urban environments (Phillips, 1990).

■ Social structure and health

□ *Social class, deprivation and health*

Interest in the relationship between social class and health in the UK was stimulated by the Black report of 1980 which found considerable inequalities in health status between different socio-economic groups (DHSS, 1980; Townsend, Davidson and Whitehead, 1992). Although an official report, this document was disowned by the government of the day, for reasons which will be discussed in later chapters. Further studies of health inequalities have confirmed many of the findings identified in the Black report and have provided additional evidence of widening health inequalities since its publication (Drever, Whitehead and Roden, 1996: Goldblatt, 1989; McLoone and Boddy, 1994; Marmot and McDowall, 1986; Phillimore *et al.*, 1994; Smith, Bartley and Blane, 1990; Townsend, Davidson and Whitehead, 1992; Whitehead, 1987).

There are considerable differences in mortality between the social classes (Delamothe, 1991), illustrated by the fact that 62 of the 66 major causes of death in men are more common in social classes IV and V (unskilled and semi-skilled manual workers) than in other social classes. Also, of the 70 major causes of female deaths, 64 were more common in women married to men in social classes IV and V than in the other social classes. Life expectancy for someone born into social class I is seven years higher than for a person born into social class V. Stillbirths, infant mortality and deaths of children are all more likely in social classes IV and V. A child born into a family where the father is an unskilled worker has twice the risk of being stillborn or of dying in infancy compared with one born into a professional family (OPCS, 1992).

Class differences can be expressed in the form of Standardised Mortality Ratios (SMRs). These are useful when comparing the health of populations with different age and sex structures (see Exhibit 1.1). SMRs are expressed as index numbers. If a population subgroup has an SMR over 100 this means that it has a higher than average mortality, even after taking into account age and sex differences. An SMR of under 100 reflects a lower than average level of mortality. Figure 1.6 illustrates that in the case of men, the 'non-manual' social classes have a lower than average SMR, and the 'manual' social classes have higher SMRs. Indeed, the SMR for unskilled men (social class V) is more than twice that for professional men (social class I).

Exhibit 1.1 *Standardised mortality ratios*

The Standardised Mortality Ratio (SMR) is a useful technique for comparing the health of different sections of the population. It represents the actual number of deaths in a particular section of the population (e.g. professional men) over a given period as a proportion of the number of expected deaths. This is then multiplied by 100 to give an index number.

$$SMR = \frac{\text{Actual deaths}}{\text{Expected deaths}} \times 100$$

The number of expected deaths is calculated by multiplying the number of people in each age category within the population subgroup by the overall death rate for that age category in the population as a whole. The expected number of deaths for each age group are then added together.

A simplified worked example is shown below:

Age	*(a)* Social Class I Number of Males *(1 000s)*	*(b)* Male death rate per 1 000 *(general population)*	Expected Deaths *(a × b)*
16–44	500	4	2 000
45–64	260	40	10 400
65–74	100	62	6 200
75 and over	50	120	6 000
Total expected deaths			24 600
Actual deaths among males in social class I			16 236

$$SMR = \frac{16\,236}{24\,600} \times 100 = 66$$

If the SMR is less than 100 (as above) then this section of the population has a low death rate and is regarded as being relatively healthy. An SMR greater than 100 indicates it is less healthy than the general population.

SMRs can be used to compare the relative mortality of social classes (as in the worked example). They can also be used to compare other population subgroups, such as those living in different localities and ethnic groups.

Social class differences for males are considerably wider when mortality is expressed in terms of number of years of potential life lost due to premature death (Blane, Smith and Bartley, 1990). In 1981 mortality among males in the 20–64 age group led to the loss of 114 years of potential life per 1000 population in social class V. This was almost three times the number of years lost by the population in social class I (39 years per 1000). The same study found that for women aged 20–59, those in social class V lost just over twice as many years of potential life (34 per 1000 population) compared with social class I (16 per 1000).

There is a significant variation in morbidity between the classes, based on self-reported illness statistics (OPCS, 1996). Rates of self-reported long-standing illness in men and women vary considerably with social class. This is most evident in middle-aged people. For example, 21 per cent of middle-aged men (aged 45–64) in non-manual occupations (social classes I, II and IIIN) reported a limiting long-standing illness in 1994 compared with 32 per cent of manual workers (social classes IIIM, IV and V). The figures for women in the same age group were 24 per cent (in households headed by a non-manual worker) and 29 per cent (in households headed by a manual worker).

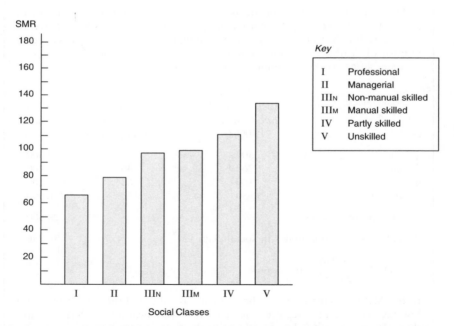

Source of data: OPCS Longitudinal Study (S. Harding, 'Social Class Differences in Mortality of Men: Recent Evidence from the OPCS Longitudinal Study', *Population Trends*, 80, Summer 1995, pp. 31–7).

Figure 1.6 *Standardised mortality ratios (SMRs) of social classes, males (15–64), Great Britain, 1976–89*

Further evidence of social class differences has been found in occupational studies such as that undertaken by Balarajan (1989) into the mortality rates of male NHS workers, which found significantly higher rates among lower paid 'manual' occupations. Research into the health of civil servants at different grades also revealed that employment grade and salary were strongly related to both objectively measured and self-reported health status (Marmot *et al.*, 1991).

Variations in morbidity by social class are consistent with data from lifestyle surveys, which focus on health as well as illness. The survey reported by Blaxter (1990) found that at all ages and in each aspect of health measured, health experience was poorer as social class declined. Differences between social classes did exist at the start of adult life but were small and not always quite regular. However, the effect of social circumstances was more noticeable as people grew older. By middle age, class differences in health had become wider, particularly among men. Among people aged over 60 (and especially among those over 70) social class differences became even greater in terms of the individual's subjective assessment of their own health. Yet, paradoxically, in terms of actual disease the health of classes appeared to converge in old age. This was partly due to the 'healthy survivor' effect, the least healthy among the manual classes dying before old age, leaving those who were more healthy by the very fact of their survival. However, more recent research by Marmot and Shipley (1996) suggests that socio-economic differences in mortality persist into old age. Although occupational grade, as one might expect, appears to play a smaller role in mortality after retirement, other 'non-work' based measures of socio-economic status (such as car ownership) seem to become more important.

A number of factors have been associated with socio-economic variations in health and illness. Unemployed people have worse health than the employed population (Bethune, 1996; Fox and Shewry, 1988; Morris, Cook and Shaper, 1994). This is true of mental as well as physical health. The unemployed have twice the level of neurotic symptoms compared with employed people (Meltzer *et al.*, 1995). Differences between those in work and the unemployed population cannot be explained simply in terms of their previous health status or pre-existing social circumstances (Moser *et al.*, 1990). Moreover, the fear of unemployment and job insecurity is known to have an adverse effect on health (Bartley *et al.*, 1996; Bartley and Owen, 1996; Ferrie *et al.*, 1995).

Other circumstances are believed to have a damaging effect on health – including poor housing and homelessness for example (Arblaster and Hawtin, 1993; Lowry, 1991). The local economic and social environment is also a key factor, as noted earlier, interacting with individual circumstances in ways which adversely affect health. Finally, poverty is known to have an impact on child health and development in particular (Wilkinson, 1994; Spencer, 1996)

A brief review of the evidence on health inequalities indicates a clear class gradient and a link between deprivation and health status. Yet the underlying causes of these variations in health, morbidity and mortality have been the subject of much political controversy. The precise nature of these arguments will be explored in Chapter 12, alongside the strategies which have been suggested as a means of tackling health inequalities.

□ *Other social inequalities*

Ethnicity

Generally speaking, individuals born abroad are no less healthy than the rest of the British population. Indeed, if mortality rates are taken as an indicator some ethnic groups are healthier than the average: Caribbean men, young Asian women, elderly Asian men and elderly Africans and Caribbean people all have lower SMRs when compared with the respective age/sex group in the general population (Balarajan and Bulusu, 1990). In addition, most ill-health suffered by ethnic groups in Britain is common to the rest of the population. The biggest threats to health – circulatory diseases and cancer – are the same irrespective of ethnic background.

However, it appears that certain diseases occur more frequently among some ethnic groups than in the general population (Balarajan and Raleigh, 1993; Hopkins and Bahl, 1993; Smaje, 1995). For example, the Asian community is more likely to suffer from coronary heart disease. The coronary heart disease mortality rate for those originating from the Indian subcontinent is 36 per cent higher for men and 46 per cent higher for women when compared with the national average (Balarajan, 1991). Asian people are also more at risk from other circulatory diseases such as strokes, as indeed are those born in the Caribbean and in Africa.

Those originating from the Indian subcontinent have a much higher than average rate of tuberculosis infection. The same is true, though to a lesser extent, of people of Caribbean origin (Balarajan and Bulusu, 1990). Certain cancers (such as liver cancer) are more common in ethnic groups, although cancer mortality overall is lower than the general population. There is a disproportionately high incidence of diabetes in West Indian and Asian communities (Nikolaides *et al.*, 1981). In addition, there are higher reported rates of mental illness in the Caribbean community, the incidence of schizophrenia, for example, being higher than among the general population. Caribbean people have higher than average (and Asian people below average) rates of admission to mental hospitals and are up to three times more likely to be detained under the Mental Health Act (Cochrane and Bal, 1989; Cope, 1989).

In addition, there are a number of diseases which are rarely found in Britain outside certain ethnic groups, such as rickets (in Asian people) and the blood disorders, sickle-cell anaemia and thalassaemia (in people originating from Africa, including Afro-Caribbeans, Asia, the Middle-East and the Mediterranean). Finally, stillbirths are more common in the Asian, African and West Indian communities. Neonatal death rates (that is, deaths under 28 days) are generally higher for ethnic groups with the exception of the Bangladeshi community, while postneonatal death rates (between 28 days and a year) are higher than average among the Caribbean and Pakistani population, but lower than average among the Bangladeshi, Indian and African communities (OPCS, 1992).

How can these variations be explained? Smaje (1995) offers a number of potential explanations. First, artefactual explanations: that variations are due at least in part to biases in research and problems of definition and measurement. Others, too, have identified problems in the study of 'race' and health (Ahmad, 1993), arguing that research often reflects the interests of health professionals rather than the ethnic minority communities. Particular criticism has focused on the evidence relating to mental health where apparent higher rates of mental illness for certain ethnic groups have been attributed to racial stereotyping, misdiagnosis based on a lack of understanding of cultural differences, and attempts by professionals to 'pathologise' ethnic communities (see Smaje, 1995, p. 67; and Sashidaran and Francis, 1993).

Material explanations, relating race to other inequalities such as social class and income, may have some validity, though it is not easy to separate the influence of these other factors. Cultural explanations – attributing variations to different beliefs about health and to different lifestyles – are superficially attractive, but are often residual and underdeveloped. Other explanations are couched in terms of the process of migration itself. For example, this process may involve social selection, so that the health of those who move to another country may not be typical. Unfortunately this hypothesis is ambiguous. It is possible that the migrant population could have been selected on the basis of its healthy attributes (that is, mobility and survival of the fittest) or because it was less healthy than average (that is, those who are sicker have fewer life opportunities and are forced to look elsewhere in order to survive). A further explanation is that the actual process of migrating to another country and settling there may itself have health implications, even for future generations.

Two other explanations are highly controversial. First, that ethnic populations are genetically predisposed to certain types of ill-health. Apart from diseases such as sickle-cell anaemia, there is little to suggest that genetic factors play a key role. However, as genetic science moves apace it is possible that new links may be discovered which have an ethnic dimension, raising the prospect of a highly-charged debate.

Secondly, variations can be explained in terms of racism. The argument here is that racism has a direct impact upon the health of ethnic groups. This may happen in a number of ways. Overt and implicit racism can contribute to illness through stress and physical violence. Racial discrimination can affect material conditions which in turn can have implications for health. Finally, insensitivity to race and ethnicity in service delivery may also affect the health of these groups. Undoubtedly, all these factors play a part, but it is difficult to directly link ill-health to racism, in view of its various manifestations. A more practical approach is to focus on the specific factors linked to illness, such as material conditions and poor access to services and then to tackle these directly.

This raises a number of important questions. How should the special needs of ethnic groups be identified? How should services be more responsive to these needs? Attempts have been made over the years to formulate health strategies for the ethnic minorities at national and local level, but these efforts have been piecemeal and tentative (Bahl, 1993; Johnson, 1993; Smaje, 1995). Examples from the 1980s include the *Stop Rickets Campaign*, the *Asian Mother and Baby Campaign*, and Department of Health funding for project work on health of ethnic groups. During the 1990s the central bureau of information on health and race issues known as SHARE was established, and NHS Executive guidelines were issued on the spiritual needs of patients with different faiths. More recently, however, policy has begun to focus more systematically on the health needs of ethnic groups. In 1993 the Department of Health introduced an eight point plan to achieve equitable representation of ethnic minorities at all levels in the NHS to reflect the ethnic composition of local populations. In an effort to gather more information about ethnic groups, the NHS introduced ethnic monitoring of in-patients with effect from April 1995. In addition, government policies such as the *Health of the Nation* (Chapter 12) and *The Patient's Charter* (Chapter 11) have demonstrated some awareness of the ethnic dimension, though much, as ever, depends upon implementation at the local level. The purchaser–provider split (see Chapter 9) also created the potential for a service more geared to the needs of ethnic groups, providing of course their requirements could be built into the contracting process (Jamdagni, 1996).

Gender

The gender gap in health is neatly summarised by Miles (1991): 'Women live longer but suffer from more health problems in their lifetime and many of these problems are specific to the female gender.' In 1996 the life expectancy of a woman at birth was over five years longer than for a man. The death rates for women are lower than for men in every age group, and for most disease categories. The rates of self-reported long-standing illness for women have usually been slightly higher for women than men, though the 1994 General Household Survey (GHS) (OPCS, 1996) shows these rates to be exactly the same at 32 per cent. More elderly women than men report long-standing illness, perhaps reflecting their survival to ages where such levels of illness are likely to be experienced. Finally, women are more likely than men to use health services: according to the 1994 GHS 17 per cent of females consulted GPs in the two weeks prior to interview compared with only 12 per cent of men (OPCS, 1996). Women are also more likely to report having outpatient appointments (15 per cent in a three-month period compared with 14 per cent among men), but the proportion of men and women reporting inpatient stays during this period was the same at 18 per cent (OPCS, 1996).

Breast cancer and cancers of the genito-urinary system are major causes of death in women. Every year, around 15 000 women in the UK die from breast cancer, the biggest cause of death from cancer among women. A further 2000 women in the UK die from cervical cancer. Other diseases are found more commonly in the female population, such as osteoporosis and cystitis. Women also appear to suffer disproportionately from mental illness. According to one large-scale survey, almost one in five women (18 per cent) reported experiencing a neurotic disorder in the week prior to interview compared with 12 per cent of men (Meltzer *et al.*, 1995). Married women and women living in urban areas seem to suffer above-average levels of anxiety and depression, while working-class women are far more likely to suffer from depression than middle-class women (Brown and Harris, 1982). The mental health of men also varies with regard to marital status (married men generally have better mental health) and socio-economic status (employed men and males in social classes I and II have better than average mental health).

Social circumstances also affect other aspects of women's health. Women in social class V are more likely to experience chronic illness and to report limiting illness than those in other social classes (Doyal, 1995, p. 13). Material conditions are also a significant factor, and it is argued that the nature of women's lives, involving caring, secondary employment and a lack of economic independence, makes them particularly vulnerable to deprivation and its health implications (Payne, 1991). The combination of the caring role in the context of hardship can have a particularly adverse impact on women's health (Graham, 1993).

During the twentieth century the role of women has undergone dramatic change, particularly in relation to the world of work (Bullock, 1994). Over two-thirds of women now have jobs outside the home (Central Statistical Office, 1995). Given that surveys have consistently found that economically inactive women have more mental and physical health problems than women in paid employment, one would expect this trend to have a beneficial impact upon women's health (Meltzer *et al.*, 1995, Warr and Parry, 1982). In reality it has had a differential effect depending on other social circumstances. Paid employment is generally associated with more illness for working-class women with children, but less for middle-class women having the same family responsibilities (Blaxter, 1990, p. 101). Much of the impact on women's health seems to depend on the extent to which women have to combine the responsibilities of work and home. As Doyal (1995, p. 24) observes 'because they usually retain responsibility for domestic labour, many women workers become physically and emotionally exhausted'.

Much also seems to depend upon different aspects of health and the type of work undertaken. The association between paid work and better health is less apparent for physical than mental health and applies less to women in full-time work, and those in professional and managerial posts (Bartley, Popay and Plewis, 1992). Interestingly, this study found no relationship between employment status and domestic conditions, suggesting that the impact of paid work in terms of improved income may offset the negative effects of combining a high domestic workload with employment.

It is apparent that social changes are leading many women to adopt what have traditionally been regarded as male lifestyles and habits. Around a third of women under the age of 50 smoke, the same proportion as men in this age group. The increase in smoking among women has been associated with the recent growth in female lung cancer rates. Lung cancer is now the second largest cancer killer of women (it remains the largest cause of death by cancer in men). Alcohol consumption among young women is also increasing and this has been paralleled by an increase in drink-related problems (DoH, 1992a). At the same time, women are particularly at risk from other 'lifestyle' diseases associated with female culture and image in western society, such as anorexia and bulimia (Lawrence, 1987).

■ Conclusion

Minimising health inequalities in terms of gender, ethnicity, class and region is the key to further improvements in general levels of health. In addition, health services must be appropriately geared to the needs of the various sections of the population. This is particularly important in the case of women and ethnic minorities, who have specific health needs different in some ways from those of the general population.

Yet health inequalities represent only one category within a range of challenges facing contemporary health care. As we have seen, the increasing elderly population has wide ramifications. This development will require some increased expenditure on health and welfare services, though there is debate about exactly how much. At the very least a redirection of health care will be required to meet the new pattern of needs generated by demographic change.

The focus on the burden of chronic illness should not distract attention from other major causes of ill-health and mortality, such as accidents in the home, on the road and in the workplace. Nor should there be complacency about the threat of infectious disease, even in the UK which has a comparatively good record in this area. Finally, one should not concentrate exclusively on physical illness: mental illness, as has been shown, is a major challenge that requires an appropriate response.

Later chapters explore the extent to which the British health care system has sought to meet these various challenges. Before this, however, it is important to discuss further the context of these changes by exploring the crucial role of the medical profession in contemporary health care.

■ *Chapter 2* ■

Medicine and the Medical Profession

Medicine, both as a profession and as a body of scientific knowledge, exerts so much influence over health care that observers often speak of medical hegemony – a domination of health care by medical ideas, concepts and practices. This chapter investigates medical hegemony, beginning with a discussion of the nature of orthodox medicine. This is followed by an examination of alternative medical approaches and perspectives. The status of the medical profession and the roots of its power are then explored, both in relation to health care and with regard to the wider social context. Finally, the challenges to medical hegemony are discussed.

■ Medicine

Modern medicine is a subtle combination of art and science. Medicine is an art in the sense that its practice involves a wide range of mental and physical skills. These run from the dexterity of the surgeon to the ability to communicate with patients in a sensitive way. Medicine is also regarded as an art because it requires personal capacities for judgement and under-standing. When doctors actually diagnose and treat patients such capacities are at least as important as scientific knowledge.

Modern medicine is strongly underpinned by scientific methods, principles and disciplines. It is heavily based on what has become known as the biomedical model or biomedicine (Engel, 1977). The main features of this model and its development are discussed below.

□ *Medicine as a science: the development of biomedicine*

Biomedicine is based on a belief that the only satisfactory basis for medical practice is scientific experimentation, observation and discovery. From this perspective, medicine is the accumulation of a body of scientific knowledge and its subsequent application to the diagnosis and treatment of disease.

Important discoveries in anatomy and human physiology during the seventeenth and eighteenth centuries laid the foundation for the development of biomedicine. These discoveries included the circulation of the blood, the functions of organs, and the impact of external agents upon these organs. Scientific experimentation gradually became accepted during the nineteenth century as the legitimate source of medical knowledge. Experiments became more sophisticated and important discoveries were made about disease processes. In particular, there were great advances in the understanding of the bacterial causes of disease. Experiments by scientists, such as Louis Pasteur and Robert Koch, led to the identification of the infectious agents which caused major diseases such as cholera and tuberculosis. Medicine increasingly focused on germ theory – the idea that diseases were largely caused by specific infectious agents in the environment.

Medical knowledge of the body's structure and composition also improved a great deal during the nineteenth century. Advances in microscope technology enabled the study of cell biology. This in turn led to the work of Rudolf Virchow on cellular pathology, the study of cell changes associated with disease.

A further area of medical advance came from better understanding of body chemistry. It was discovered that chemical processes were responsible for regulating a wide range of the body's activities, and that diseases could be attributed to deficiencies in these processes. This was to lead to the discovery of hormones and vitamins, which have a crucial role in the maintenance of health.

Advances in medical knowledge led ultimately to the development of new techniques and interventions. Diagnosis benefited from the development of instruments to measure blood pressure, blood flow and heartbeat. Surgery improved with the advent of antiseptics, pioneered by Joseph Lister. The emergence of effective anaesthetics not only made surgery more bearable for patients, it also gave surgeons extra time to perform operations, thereby facilitating the development of more complex surgical techniques. Furthermore, the increasing institutionalisation of health care in hospitals provided doctors with improved conditions, both for observing disease processes and for applying new medical technologies.

Meanwhile, the growing knowledge of bacterial causes of disease led to the development of vaccines to prevent these diseases, and so-called 'magic bullets' to cure them. An example of the latter was the discovery by Paul Ehrlich in 1910 of Salvarsan as a treatment for syphilis. This was followed by the development of antibiotics, beginning with the discovery of penicillin by Alexander Fleming in 1928. The early part of the century also

---

Exhibit 2.1   Diabetes mellitus

■ **Aetiology**

This disease occurs as a result of a deficiency in the production of insulin, a hormone secreted in the pancreas, which regulates glucose levels in the body. The deficiency leads to an accumulation of glucose in the blood and sugar in the urine, which in turn produces a range of symptoms (see below). The relationship between these symptoms and insulin deficiency was discovered by empirical observation and scientific experimentation. Particularly important were experiments conducted by Frederick Banting and Charles Best in the 1920s. The pancreatic ducts of dogs were blocked in order to reproduce the symptoms of diabetes. When the accumulated pancreatic secretions were subsequently injected back into the animals (and later into humans), the symptoms were alleviated.

■ **Diagnosis**

The common presenting symptoms of diabetes mellitus are increased thirst, excessive passing of urine, weight loss and a propensity to infections. The longer-term complications include nerve damage, producing a loss of sensation in the limbs, and damage to other organs including the kidneys and the eyes. Tests for excess glucose in the blood and sugar in the urine will confirm the diagnosis.

■ **Treatment**

The patient may be given insulin to counteract the deficiency. He or she may have to observe certain dietary restrictions.

---

saw attempts to treat diseases caused by hormone deficiencies, such as diabetes (see Exhibit 2.1), and those caused by vitamin deficiencies, such as rickets.

These medical interventions were based on scientific knowledge and methods. In exploring the disease process, medicine increasingly focused upon specific aetiology, the attribution of disease to specific biological causes and processes. The aim was to reveal through scientific means the nature of the disease process, then, on the basis of this understanding, to discover how this process could be reversed or limited.

Scientific methods and observations often demonstrate only a statistical association between events. Yet there are many examples where the suggestion of a causal relationship has led to a particular course of action. The classic example is Edward Jenner's experiment with inoculation in the eighteenth century. Jenner was able to prevent smallpox by inoculating people with material taken from cowpox sufferers. Yet the disease process which led to this outcome was not fully understood until the following century. Similarly, the identification by John Snow in 1854 of contaminated water supplies as the factor responsible for outbreaks of cholera preceded the identification of the cholera organism by almost thirty years. By the time Koch had made this discovery, efforts to improve water supplies and sanitation were well under way. Intervention on the basis of partial and circumstantial evidence of disease processes is a particular feature of the public health model of medicine discussed later.

☐ *The features of biomedicine*

The development of medicine as a scientific exercise led to a focus on the disease process. Biomedicine concentrates mainly on biological changes which can be defined, measured and isolated. It is directed towards the dysfunction of the various organs and tissues of the body rather than the condition of the patient as a whole. Indeed, biomedicine can be regarded as a negative perspective on health (see Chapter 1) because it views health more in terms of the absence of disease than the possession of healthy attributes. Finally, it emphasises the value of advancing technology, both in the diagnosis and treatment of disease.

Biomedicine has undoubtedly added to our knowledge and understanding of many diseases. It has also produced valuable practical improvements in the treatment of patients, which have led to improvements in both length and quality of life for many individuals. Yet in spite of these achievements, biomedicine has been subjected to considerable criticism in recent years. Some feel that its domination is in many respects inappropriate to modern health problems (Inglis, 1981), while others cast doubt on the extent to which the rational scientific principles are actually employed in medical practice today (Payer, 1989).

☐ *Is modern medicine scientific?*

The history of medicine contains many examples which indicate that the biomedical model, with its emphasis on rational scientific principles, is not always applied in practice. There are many cases where good evidence based on scientific methods has been hotly contested or simply ignored by other practitioners. Take for example, the fate of Semmelweiss, a nineteenth-century Viennese obstetrician, who was concerned about the high mortality rates of mothers following childbirth. He observed that the mortality rates from puerperal sepsis (postnatal infection of the genital tract) was much higher in wards attended by medical students than in those where midwives only attended. Guessing that this was due to the cross-contamination of medical students at postmortems (which midwives did not attend), he ordered students to thoroughly disinfect themselves between attending cases. The death rate dropped dramatically. Yet

Semmelweiss' study was received with hostility by the leading lights of the profession, who questioned the validity of his study and scorned his life-saving recommendations (Inglis, 1965). Such a shocking example may be seen as interesting merely for its historical value, to illustrate how far medicine has come. But one should not be too complacent. One can find examples in the modern context where practice is being conducted either in the absence of scientific knowledge or at variance with it (see Exhibit 3.2).

The idea that doctors operate within the narrow confines of the biomedical model has been rejected by some supporters as well as critics of modern medicine. Some doctors openly reject the strict application of the biomedical model, claiming it to be an abstraction which has limited application in practice (Black, 1984). Others argue that modern medicine is not wholly focused on disease but is eclectic, taking into account wider influences on health such as lifestyle and emotional factors (Brewin, 1985). Some also believe medical practice is less dominated by the biomedical model than in the past. According to Tudor-Hart (1981), doctors are increasingly concerned about health promotion, the environment and public health, and as a result are more likely to intervene at a social and political level in order to promote health in a broader and more positive sense.

Certainly, the biomedical model does not describe the approach of every medical practitioner in every single situation. It perhaps applies less to general practitioners and community-based doctors than to their hospital colleagues. The model is probably more applicable to the older rather than to the younger generation of doctors.

It is also the case that the biomedical model cannot be entirely insulated from the culture in which it is being applied. Doctors are influenced by non-medical models of health. After all, both medical and lay models are shaped to some extent by the culture in which they operate (Helman, 1990; Herzlich and Pierret, 1985). Moreover, doctors to some extent retain lay assumptions about illness after clinical training and these assumptions can supplement the orthodox approach in practice (Gaines, 1979).

The extent to which the identification of disease is influenced by culture was explored in a comparative study of medicine and health in West Germany, France, Germany and the USA by Lynn Payer (1989). She claimed that the choice of diagnoses and treatments is not a scientific process, for two main reasons. First, most consultations are about health problems – such as, fatigue or anxiety, for example – for which there are no scientific solutions. Second, cultural factors, which vary from nation to nation, have a great impact on the treatment of disease and upon the diagnosis of illness. Payer gives a number of examples to back up her case. She notes, for example, that blood pressure considered high in the USA might be considered normal in the UK. While low blood pressure, considered to be a problem by German doctors, is not regarded as such by their British and American counterparts.

☐ *Subjectivity*

So modern medicine may not be as scientific as many doctors claim. It has been pointed out that doctors cannot even agree on the meaning of a fundamental term such as 'disease' (Campbell, Scadding and Roberts, 1979). Confusion within the medical profession surrounding the concept of disease, and variations in the application of disease concepts, means that medicine is far more subjective than has been commonly supposed. Doctors operate within a framework of medical knowledge which focuses upon specific diseases. They may be tempted to pigeonhole patients' illnesses into convenient categories in order to make the situation more manageable. Indeed, according to Payer (1989) doctors sometimes use so-called 'wastebasket diagnoses', when patients are presenting ambiguous symptoms. For example, a patient complaining of fatigue actually may be suffering from one of a number of possible diseases. Yet it may be convenient for the doctor simply to tell the patient that he or she has a 'virus', 'anaemia' or even 'depression' without further elaboration.

Diseases are deviations from normality. Yet, with the exception of extreme cases, deviations from normality are inherently ambiguous (Twaddle, 1974). Health status changes do not therefore follow automatically from biological changes. Instead, the latter are events requiring interpretation, based on medical judgement, which is in turn influenced by a variety of cultural and social factors.

Kennedy (1981) claims that doctors make two sets of judgements when diagnosing patients. First, they must assess whether the patient's problem or condition represents a deviation from what would be considered normal. Second, they have to make a judgement about the deviation itself, and whether this constitutes an illness. According to Kennedy such judgements are subjective and related to social and cultural values. Kennedy gives as an example the American Psychiatric Association's debate over the definition of homosexuality as an illness. From this point of view, medical practice is a political enterprise with medical judgements reflecting doctors' beliefs about social order.

The case of obesity further illustrates the subjectivity of medicine. Obesity is seen by many doctors as a major public health problem (Garrow, 1991; Royal College of Physicians, 1983a). It is defined objectively – in terms of a Body Mass Index (calculated from an individual's weight and height ratio). Yet the extent to which an individual's body weight is judged to deviate excessively from the norm is in turn related to cultural values and expectations. Dutch doctors, for example, are far more likely to diagnose obesity than their British counterparts (Payer, 1989).

This is not to deny that extreme obesity is linked with chronic illness. Individuals should pursue a recommended balanced diet, provided there is a sound empirical foundation for these recommendations. The point is that the identification of obesity as a medical condition may be as much the result of social and cultural values as objective, scientific fact and that the same reasoning may apply to other conditions with an overt social dimension.

☐ *Difficulties of diagnosis*

The scientific basis of medicine may be undermined by the fact that some diseases are difficult and in some cases impossible to diagnose. Initial signs and symptoms may be highly ambiguous. Furthermore, many illnesses do not have objective symptoms or signs. This often leads to disputes about whether disease is present at all.

Such controversy has surrounded myalgic encephalomyelitis (ME), an illness with influenza-like symptoms followed by chronic physical and mental fatigue. ME sufferers are in no doubt that they are ill, but doctors have been reluctant to accept their condition as a genuine illness, largely because there is no objective way of testing for the disease (see Exhibit 2.2).

An additional problem for the traditional biomedical model is that a disease may have multiple causes. Alzheimer's disease, for example, is now thought to be caused by environmental as well as genetic factors. Many cancers result from an interaction of multiple factors. Doctors accept that the causes of illness are increasingly complex. However, the acceptance of a number of possible causes for a particular illness does leave much more scope for doubt, ambiguity and subjectivity.

Critics argue that the kinds of factors discussed above render the biomedical approach inappropriate in the present context (Kennedy, 1981; Inglis, 1981). They claim that the biomedical emphasis of modern medicine is misdirected, and that doctors are hiding their subjective judgements behind a smokescreen of pseudo-science. Some doctors react defensively by upholding the sanctity of the biomedical model. Others, as we have seen, argue that although modern medicine remains scientifically based, medical practice is far more eclectic and is able to incorporate new theories and concepts which improve our understanding of the causes of illness.

Modern medicine, however, remains strongly wedded to the guiding principles of the biomedical model. This is reflected by the failure of alternative models to displace this orthodoxy.

Exhibit 2.2   Myalgic encephalomyelitis

ME is a syndrome which involves chronic physical and mental fatigue. Other symptoms include vertigo, ringing in the ears, blurred vision, muscle spasms, memory impairment, excessive sweating and an inability to concentrate. The illness can be long-term, lasting over ten years in a quarter of sufferers.

Those suffering from ME feel stigmatised. They have difficulty in obtaining the social support and understanding which the sick normally expect. Moreover, they find that many doctors cannot offer much help in the way of advice, care or treatment. Some are less than sympathetic to sufferers, preferring to believe that they are neurotic. Indeed the medical profession has been reluctant to acknowledge ME as a genuine illness, opinion being strongly influenced by a study of an outbreak at the Royal Free Hospital in 1955 which identified the incident as a form of mass hysteria. One of the main difficulties in obtaining recognition for ME is that there is no clear test to confirm diagnosis, as in the case of diabetes mellitus for example. Although some research has identified the presence of a virus in a minority of sufferers, an objective test for ME does not exist at present.

However, more recently a combination of media coverage, pressure from patients and increasingly from doctors (some of whom have themselves been victims of the illness), has prompted a more considered response from the profession as a whole. In 1996 a combined report from the Royal Colleges of General Practitioners, Physicians and Psychiatrists examined the evidence regarding ME. It argued that chronic fatigue syndrome (CFS), which the authors believed to be a more appropriate term for the symptoms of ME, was a recognisable illness and deserved to be taken seriously. The report also noted that although psychological and social factors were present in many cases the illness should not be regarded as purely and simply as a psychiatric illness (Mulube, 1996).

☐ *Other medical models: public health medicine*

Public health has been defined as 'the science and art of preventing disease, prolonging life, and promoting health through the organised efforts of society' (Cm 289, 1988). McKeown's work (1979), the definitive statement of the revitalised public health perspective, argued that modern medicine focuses primarily upon the disease process within the individual and ignores the wider social, economic and environmental factors relevant to health.

Much of McKeown's argument is based on historical evidence that challenges the conventional view of the contribution of modern medicine. Diseases such as measles, whooping cough and tuberculosis were in decline well before the introduction of immunisation and effective medical treatment. McKeown identified better nutrition and rising standards of living as the key factors in the reduction of morbidity and mortality since the late nineteenth century. Improvements in health are partly attributed to better hygiene during the Victorian era (Wohl, 1984). The limited contribution of medical science to the health of patients in this period has also been acknowledged by others (Bynum, 1994).

McKeown pointed out that the major causes of ill-health and death – cancer, heart disease and circulatory disease – are largely the result of individual behaviour and the environment. Orthodox medicine is viewed as providing an inappropriate response to these problems. It is reactive, waiting for illness to happen, and requires conclusive evidence of a specific disease process. Modern health problems – as suggested earlier – frequently involve a complex combination of factors and action is often needed to protect and promote health when evidence is less than complete (McKeown, 1979).

While many of McKeown's conclusions have been supported by others (Fuchs, 1974; McKinlay, 1979; Powles, 1973), some have challenged aspects of his thesis. Szreter (1988) accepted that modern medicine cannot be credited with the decline in mortality over the past century, but disputed that rising nutritional and living standards were the main reasons for falling mortality rates. He argued that the medical profession played a key role in improvement of health through their involvement in the Victorian public health movement. They were also active in promoting local preventive measures, including the establishment of community health services.

Sagan (1987), while sharing McKeown's cynicism about the impact of medical care, rejects the argument that public health measures or nutrition were primarily responsible for declining mortality. Sagan identifies the reduction in family size and modern parenting behaviour as the main reasons for the improvements in health. He identifies the social support function of the family unit as being particularly significant in the maintenance of mental and physical health.

Finally, McKeown's thesis has been attacked for not appreciating the full contribution of modern medicine. The Victorian period brought important innovations, such as chloroform anaesthesia. But more importantly it laid the foundations for later discoveries and made possible the development of new forms of treatment which were effective. In addition many of the subsequent improvements in medical treatment not only saved lives but improved the quality of life for many. Improvements in the quality of life do not always show up in mortality and morbidity indicators. Hip replacements are a commonly cited example (Morris, 1980). Furthermore, it has recently been shown that medical treatment does add years to life. Bunker, Frazier and Mostelle (1994), examining the impact of medical care in the USA, found that curative medicine added between 44 and 45 months to life expectancy. Preventive measures added a further 18–19 months.

In the nineteenth century the public health model was highly regarded and provided much of the rationale for such interventions as sanitary improvements, housing reforms and vaccination. For most of the twentieth century it has been very much the junior partner to the biomedical model. There are, however, signs that this may be changing. As noted earlier, some doctors are paying more attention to the wider causes of ill-health. Furthermore, during the late 1980s the Chief Medical Officer in the Department of Health signalled his concern by undertaking the first review of public health in England for over a hundred years. Subsequently, national health strategies directed at tackling some of the main causes of illness and death were introduced throughout the UK (see Chapter 12).

☐ *Alternative medicine*

In addition to the public health model there are alternative medical approaches based on different theories of health and illness (Micozzi, 1995; Saks, 1992; Sharma, 1995). The main forms of alternative medicine are shown in Exhibit 2.3.

The distinguishing feature of alternative therapies is their marginal standing in relation to the medical establishment and the health care system rather than any common approach. Alternative medicine covers an enormous range of therapies based on a variety of theories and methods. Moreover, some alternative therapies have features which are not radically different from some aspects of the biomedical approach. Osteopathy and chiropractic, for example, are aimed at correcting the body's mechanical functions just as (by different methods and using different theories) the biomedical approach has tended to emphasise physical dysfunction. Homoeopathy uses drugs aimed at specific disorders, though it takes a different view of the causal processes at work. Also, many of the plants used in herbalism have been exploited by orthodox medicine as remedies for specific diseases.

In addition to these similarities and overlaps there are a number of more general points to make about the relationship between alternative and orthodox medicine. First, most of the alternative therapies are, in fact, interventionist – they involve some form of treatment for specific disorders. Second, they are often focused on the individual, though some take into account relevant background factors in a more systematic and comprehensive manner.

A further point is that alternative therapies are not necessarily in competition with conventional medicine. Patients using them do not necessarily lose confidence in orthodox medicine. Furthermore, many

---

Exhibit 2.3　*Alternative medicine*

■ **Acupuncture**

This practice, developed in ancient China, is based on the theory that there is a connection between body organs and body surface. Acupuncture involves using needles to stimulate acupuncture points under the skin in an attempt to influence the related organs. It is claimed that acupuncture has a more general effect in promoting relaxation and relieving pain.

■ **Homoeopathy**

A system of medicine based on the principle that agents which produce certain signs and symptoms in healthy people cure the same signs and symptoms of disease. The more a drug is diluted, the more potent it will be as a cure. Furthermore, the treatment given will be tailored to the individual, rather than to the characteristics of the disease as is generally the case in mainstream biomedicine.

■ **Chiropractic**

This is a manipulative therapy designed to maintain the spinal column in a good state of health, without the use of drugs. The therapy is aimed at dealing with specific disorders such as back and neck pain, headaches and other disorders of the nervous system.

■ **Osteopathy**

This is similar to chiropractic in that it involves the manipulation of the spine in order to remedy disease and dysfunction of the musculo-skeletal system. However, osteopaths' manipulative techniques are based on different theories of the causes of illness from those adopted by chiropractors.

■ **Herbal medicine**

The use of plants and herbs to deal with specific illnesses and to maintain health. A related therapy – aromatherapy – involves body massage using oils extracted from plants.

■ **Hypnotherapy**

The inducement of trance has been used to combat a variety of psychological disorders such as anxiety, phobias and insomnia. Hypnotherapy is sometimes used by individuals who are trying to change unhealthy lifestyles such as smoking. Hypnotherapy has also been used in the treatment of conditions with physical symptoms where there may be an underlying psychological cause.

■ **Reflexology**

This therapy is based on a belief that different areas of the feet are internally linked to other parts of the body. Manifestations of illness are treated by massaging the relevant area of the foot which corresponds to the parts of the body affected.

qualified doctors are now taking a greater interest in alternative therapies. Osteopathy is practised by a small but growing number of doctors in this country. Around fifty British medical practitioners are qualified osteopaths and 700 doctors are members of the British Medical Acupuncture Society (Saks, 1992). One in twelve of all general practitioners (GPs) in the UK are members of complementary medical bodies (Fulder, 1992, p. 169).

Given this level of participation, some now believe alternative medicine is a misleading term, preferring instead 'complementary medicine'. If more orthodox doctors adopt these therapies in future, one may see greater incorporation of alternative techniques into mainstream medicine. However, alternative therapies have in the past been viewed with considerably hostility by the orthodox medical establishment (see Saks, 1995). Although there is evidence of a change of attitudes, it is important not to exaggerate the degree to which these therapies have been accepted and incorporated by the mainstream.

Take, for example, the British Medical Association (BMA) working party report of the 1980s which strongly criticised the lack of a rational scientific base for many of the alternative therapies and rejected the theories which underpinned them (BMA, 1986b). It argued that unconventional techniques could be incorporated within mainstream medicine if they were properly subjected to evaluation. It also maintained that where alternative therapies were of value, they should only be undertaken by suitably qualified persons operating within an approved system of qualification and registration and under the direction of the medical profession. More recently, however, the BMA position on alternative medicine has shifted. In 1993 it produced a further report which was far more positive about the role of alternative medicine while continuing to stress the importance of evaluation and the need for statutory regulation of alternative practitioners (BMA, 1993).

Alternative therapies have already begun to move in this direction. Some therapists now operate under the auspices of a national regulatory body, licensed by the state. The General Osteopathic Council (GOC), created by legislation in 1993, regulates professional standards, ethics, discipline and qualifications for these practitioners. The GOC also maintains a register of practitioners and in future only those included on the register will be legally permitted to call themselves osteopaths. Chiropractors have followed osteopaths in seeking statutory regulation and a similar regulatory structure for these practitioners will shortly be in place. Alternative therapies are also seeking ways of demonstrating their effectiveness. For example, one recent study found a greater improvement among patients with low back pain who were treated by chiropractors compared with those receiving conventional outpatient management in hospital (Meade *et al.*, 1995). However, studies of the impact of alternative therapies are often challenged because they rarely adopt the randomised controlled trial (RCT) method of evaluation favoured by conventional medical researchers (see Chapter 3).

Alternative therapies continue to flourish. It has been estimated that there are over 10 000 alternative therapists in the UK (Fulder, 1992, p. 168). This figure excludes faith healers, of which there are a further 20 000. The number of therapists has increased rapidly in recent years as more people have turned to alternative medicine, with the biggest growth being in acupuncture and homoeopathy.

Surveys reveal a high level of public interest in alternative therapies. In 1996 a survey by the Research Council for Complementary Medicine (*British Medical Journal*, 1996) found that in the previous year 10 per cent of the British public had consulted a practitioner of complementary medicine, with acupuncture, chiropractic, osteopathy, homoeopathy, herbal medicine and hypnotherapy being the most popular, accounting for three-quarters of those therapies used (over 150 other therapies were identified). Meanwhile, in other countries the public are even more enthusiastic about alternative medicine. In France, Australia and the USA around a third of the public use such therapies in any one year. In Russia, half of the population use alternative therapies, while in Japan the figure is 60 per cent.

In the UK it appears that alternative medicine is being boosted by the recent changes in the NHS. Many GPs now have greater control over budgets and have a greater incentive to refer patients to alternative therapists because of their relatively low cost and increasing popularity. Studies reveal that around 45 per cent of GPs are commissioning or providing complementary medicine (Thomas *et al.*, 1995) while more than two-thirds of health authorities are purchasing such therapies (Adams, J., 1995).

However, there are factors likely to constrain the growth of this sector of care, not least the continued opposition of the orthodox medical establishment. Another is the emphasis on evidence-based medicine, which given the problems of demonstrating the effectiveness of complementary therapies in scientific terms, could lead to more restrictions on their use by public sector budget holders. Finally, a serious threat is posed by moves towards further European integration which has created pressures for uniformity in the standards of health care qualifications. As a consequence, the rights of alternative therapists to practise may be restricted.

□ Lay models of health and illness

There is a rich and growing literature exploring the different ways in which ordinary people view health and illness. Orthodox medicine does seem to exert a considerable influence upon lay views (Calnan, 1987). However, the latter are notoriously complex and have a certain independence (Fitzpatrick, 1984; Williams and Calnan, 1996). Moreover, while orthodox medicine is supreme in terms of its formal domination of health care, lay health beliefs, knowledge and behaviour regarding illness can have an impact on health care in practice. This can occur in a number of ways.

First, the individual's health beliefs may influence the decision to seek treatment. If individuals do not perceive themselves to be ill, their symptoms are unlikely to be presented to doctors. As a result, their illness will probably remain hidden and the condition will not come to the attention of the doctor (Mechanic, 1961; Robinson, 1971). Second, even if the individual sees a doctor and is diagnosed as having a particular disease, this does not guarantee that the patient will agree with the diagnosis. Neither does it ensure that he or she will comply with the prescribed course of treatment (Ley, 1982; Thompson, 1984).

There are ways in which the medical profession can circumvent such attitudes and behaviour. Screening programmes, for example, can be used to detect illness. Compulsory treatment has been used in the past, particularly in the areas of mental illness and immunisation. But at the end of the day, lay perspectives still retain a character of their own, influenced in part by the medical profession itself but also by the deeper cultural and ideological influences within society.

■ The medical profession

□ *Medicine as a profession*

There is much disagreement between sociologists over the precise meaning of the term 'profession' (see Johnson, 1972; Wilding 1982). However, most would agree that medicine has the key features commonly associated with a profession, primarily the application of a body of expertise, knowledge and skills. It operates within a framework of licensing, where only those sufficiently qualified can practise legitimately following a considerable period of approved education and training (see Exhibit 2.4). There is a long-standing system of self-regulation in medicine and a well-developed sense of service standards. Furthermore, as with other professions, those who practise medicine tend to be drawn from middle-class or upper-middle-class backgrounds. Finally, medicine is organised by a range of bodies which take responsibility for education, licensing, the maintenance of standards and the representation of interests.

Exhibit 2.4　Medical education and training

Medical education and training can be divided into three stages: undergraduate medical education, postgraduate training and continuing medical education and training. *Undergraduate medical education* is provided by the university medical schools. Having successfully completed the five year course, students obtain provisional registration from the General Medical Council for their pre-registration year working as a house officer in a hospital setting, leading to full registration. Specialisation then takes place as doctors choose which branch of the profession they will follow: hospital medicine or general practice (some may choose to specialise in public health medicine at a later stage). Trainee General Practitioners undertake a three year course which includes two years of working in hospitals and a vocational year attached to a training practice. Those focusing on hospital or public health medicine proceed through a succession of training posts with a view to eventually securing the post of consultant. Once qualified, it is important that doctors are aware of new developments in medicine and that they are willing to learn new skills and techniques. Hence the importance of continuing medical education.

For many years, there has been much concern about the quality of medical education at each of these stages. The General Medical Council (GMC), which is responsible for the quality and assessment of undergraduate medical education (and has a broader remit for the coordination of medical education at all levels), has urged medical schools to modify their courses, in particular to reduce factual content and to increase the development of vocational skills. The GMC has the power to close a medical school and may undertake formal visits to institutions. In practice, however, it relies mainly on persuasion to improve standards and bring about change.

Postgraduate medical training is in flux following the Calman report (DoH, 1993a). This report was prompted by the European Union's concern that the existing system of specialist medical registration inhibited the free movement of doctors, discriminating against those qualifying in Europe. But at the same there were long-standing complaints about the informality and unsystematic nature of medical training in the UK. The Calman report proposed the following changes. First, a reduction in the length (and increase in intensity) of the postgraduate training period from an average of 12 years to 7. Second, the creation of a unified training grade for higher specialist training, the Specialist Registrar Grade. Third, a new Certificate of Completion of Specialist Training (CCST), to define the end-point of specialist training, making the holder eligible for a consultant appointment.

⟶

According to Freidson (1988, p. xv) 'it is useful to think of a profession as an occupation which has assumed a dominant position in a division of labour so that it gains control over the determination of the substance of its own work'. Over the years the medical profession has successfully monopolised important areas of work and demonstrated an ability to insulate itself to a large degree from outside interference relative to other health care workers.

Exhibit 2.4 continued

The acceptance of the Calman recommendations by government marked another step in the direction of a consultant-provided service, rather than a consultant-led service. This policy was reflected in previous initiatives – such as *Achieving a Balance* (DHSS, 1987) which sought to increase the number of consultants by 2 per cent a year, and the 'New Deal' for junior doctors which attempted to reduce their hours of work. Both these initiatives had some effect, but fell some way short of their objectives. *Achieving a Balance* exceeded the target 2 per cent annual increase in the number of consultants, but the number of juniors also increased, making the balance difficult to achieve in practice. The New Deal limited junior doctors' hours to 83 a week by April 1993, and then to 72 by the end of 1994 (no more than 56 of which should be spent actually working). However, in reality many junior doctors still work longer than these official limits.

Most observers agree that the number of consultants must expand in order to deal with the increased workload. Expansion, however, depends upon the availability of funding. Furthermore, many consultants remain opposed to the Calman programme (Mather and Elkeles, 1995). But other factors will assist reform. Particularly important are changes in the funding of clinical education and training. Medical school deans (for undergraduate education) and postgraduate deans (for the training of specialists) now have budgets for commissioning training from trusts (or GPs). Resources are allocated on the basis of explicit contracts drawn up between the regional offices of the NHS, the medical schools (or the postgraduate dean in the case of specialist training) and trusts/GPs. In theory this could make the providers far more responsive to the training needs as identified by the commissioning bodies. In addition, the commissioners of education and training have a greater incentive to monitor the quality of services and can reduce funding or remove students and trainees if the contract is not being fulfilled.

Efforts have been made in recent years to strengthen *continuing medical education*. The Royal Colleges have been heavily involved. For example, in 1994 the Royal College of Obstetricians and Gynaecologists announced that continuing education would become compulsory for all the members of this speciality. It proposed that qualified specialists would have to undertake at least 200 hours a year of education in order to remain on its register of trained specialists. Furthermore, under new regulations introduced in 1997, the GMC was given powers to require practitioners to undertake retraining when their performance falls demonstrably below the standards expected.

Within health care, doctors enjoy superior status. The way in which alternative therapists have been successfully marginalised by the orthodox medical profession has already been noted. Other health care professions act for the most part under medical direction and instruction. They have less autonomy and are weaker in terms of their political organisation and leverage. Nurses, for example, have much less control over health care than doctors (Salvage, 1985). Much of their workload is routine and, according to many nurses, their contribution to the care of patients is not maximised (see Exhibit 3.7). Politically, nurses are less well organised than the medical profession (Hayward and Fee, 1992).

Tension between the medical and nursing professions, though common enough within the everyday working environment (Walby and Greenwell, 1994), has tended to be implicit rather than overt. Even when there has been open conflict between the nursing and paramedical professions on the one hand and the medical profession on the other, the latter has invariably dominated. An often-cited example is the struggle between doctors and midwives over childbirth and maternity care (Donnison, 1988), a conflict which continues today (see Exhibit 3.7).

According to Armstrong (1990) the status of nursing and paramedical professions has improved during the twentieth century, through registration, education, self-discipline and licensing. While paramedical skills have achieved professional recognition, however, the core of medical power has not been eroded and indeed this has been due in no small measure to the ability of the medical profession to shape the development of these other health professions (Larkin, 1983). The rising status of nursing and other health professions, reflected in improvements in education, training and research, has in some cases led to the transfer of routine medical tasks (see Exhibit 3.7). Even so, this does not appear to have as yet undermined the doctor's dominant position within the division of labour in health care, although there are other pressures, discussed later, which provide more of a challenge to medical hegemony.

☐ *Doctors, patients and the public*

Another aspect of medical hegemony lies in the doctor–patient relationship. Most studies have emphasised the power of the former over the latter (see Byrne and Long, 1976; Tuckett *et al.*, 1985), though this relationship does vary according to the type of illness. In chronic and longer-term cases there appear to be more opportunities for patients to participate in decision-making (Szasz and Hollender, 1956). Moreover, lay views can influence health care in practice and doctors cannot divorce themselves entirely from broader cultural influences regarding health and illness

Nevertheless, on an individual level doctors tend to dominate the relationship. Patients are traditionally passive in the UK. This may be due to the long history of charitable health care in this country, which placed most patients in a highly dependent position. An alternative explanation is that the absence of a health care market in the UK in the post-Second World War period inhibited the kind of health care consumerism found in the United States. Yet even in the USA only a minority of patients indulge in consumerist behaviour (Hibbard and Weekes, 1987). Moreover, simple consumer models are not necessarily the best way of enhancing patient participation, as we shall see in Chapter 11. The passivity of patients in the UK could be related to our deferential culture. It is conventional wisdom that the British have a traditional respect for authority, and that it is alien to the British culture to complain. But even those patients wishing to complain about the standards of service have faced difficulties. Complaints procedures are complicated and intimidating (although a new procedure has recently been introduced in an effort to remedy some of the problems – see Chapter 11). Compensation and redress are difficult to obtain. Furthermore, patients have a general disadvantage in terms of knowledge and information (Association of Community Health Councils, 1992).

There are signs that patients may be becoming less passive. There has been a greater focus on the importance of patients' views, particularly in general practice. Some doctors have attempted to alter the style of consultation in order to improve communication with their patients (Savage and Armstrong, 1990). In addition, the 1980s and 1990s produced a number of health care reforms such as *The Patient's Charter*, for example, which attempted to instil a consumerist philosophy into British health care. Furthermore, there is evidence of a greater willingness to resort to legal action as a means of redress for medical errors and shortcomings in service standards. In the UK the amount paid out annually in medical negligence claims by the NHS doubled between 1990 and 1994 and is expected to rise even higher in the years ahead.

The medical profession enjoys considerable social status beyond its dominant position in relation to patients and other health professions. Public opinion surveys point to a high degree of satisfaction with the work of doctors (Jowell *et al.*, 1989; Bosanquet, 1994). There is evidence of a high level of respect for doctors, compared with other occupations and professions. This is universal and is not confined to the UK. Even in the United States, where one might expect the high financial rewards of doctors to create an atmosphere of envy and hostility towards the profession, doctors are nevertheless held in relatively high esteem by the public (Ginzberg, 1990).

☐ *Internal hierarchies and specialisation*

Medicine itself is an arena for professional conflict and endless battles over status. Such conflict has a long history, Inglis (1965, p. 33) observes that 'from medieval times, the different clinical groupings and factions had fought each other with remarkable consistent ferocity and malice'. The status of doctors varies considerably. Compare, for example, the prestige enjoyed by the consultant with the relatively humble position of the junior doctor. Traditionally, hospital doctors have enjoyed higher status than those working in the community and in general practice (Honigsbaum, 1979) though this is much less the case today.

Stars can rise and fall. Surgery, for example, has greatly improved in status during this century, due partly to the development of new surgical technology. In previous centuries the physicians were the most prestigious wing of the profession (Parry and Parry, 1976). General practice, which at the turn of the century was regarded with great inferiority, has gradually shaken off its lowly image. Its status is likely to continue to rise in view of the contemporary emphasis on primary care and the development of GP-focused commissioning, both of which have given important new responsibilities and roles to general practitioners (see Chapters 8 and 9).

☐ Explaining medical hegemony

Four factors appear to be associated with the status of medicine. These are: the social composition of the medical profession; its role in legitimising health and illness; the autonomy doctors have in relation to their work; and the political organisation of the profession.

☐ Social composition

The social status of the medical profession can be attributed in part to the exclusive social background of its individual members. There are three common beliefs about the composition of the medical profession. First, that it is male-dominated. Second, that doctors tend to come from 'medical families', where at least one parent has a medical background. Third, that it is largely restricted to those from upper-middle class backgrounds.

It is true that women are in a minority in the medical profession. Just under 30 per cent of doctors in the UK are female (compare this with 10 per cent in the USA, and 70 per cent in Russia). Women are in an even smaller minority in the higher clinical grades – less than one in five of UK consultants are female (Allen, 1994). Women are particularly under-represented in the more prestigious specialties. They are, however, more strongly represented in those branches of the profession that are increasing in importance, such as general practice. Women have also made greater inroads into hospital medicine, with the proportion of female hospital doctors more than doubling over the past 20 years. Furthermore, the proportion of women studying medicine has doubled over the same period. Half of new medical students are now female.

Turning to the second point, it is not true to say that most doctors come from 'medical families', though a proportion do. A study of a sample of doctors by Allen (1994) discovered that 16 per cent had followed either one or both parents into the profession. The same study confirmed that doctors are drawn mainly from the upper middle classes. At the time of application to medical school, three-quarters had fathers whose occupation placed them in social classes I or II. This proportion has not varied significantly in recent years. The evidence appears to support the view that medicine is to a large extent a socially exclusive profession, though it is not impossible for those from working-class backgrounds to break into the profession. Indeed, the proportion of newly-qualified female doctors coming from skilled manual worker family backgrounds has doubled in recent years.

□ *Legitimation of health and illness*

Medical knowledge is regarded as an important source of power in itself (Foucault, 1973; Turner, 1987). Doctors have the power to define and redefine the social meaning of various conditions and states. According to Parsons (1951), the function of medicine in legitimising illness is particularly important. Parsons regarded illness as a form of social deviance that could undermine the social system. It therefore had to be controlled, the instrument of control being the medical profession. Hence, doctors certify who is genuinely ill and who is not. The genuinely sick (as certified by the medical profession) are absolved of responsibility to fulfil social obligations, while those whose sickness is not legitimised are labelled as malingerers and subjected to social disapproval and sanction. In this way the extent of deviance is controlled through the 'sick role', and social order is preserved.

Parsons' analysis has been challenged on a number of grounds (see Turner, 1987). It has been argued that exemption from social obligations varies according to particular types of illness and with the social position of sufferers. Even when an illness is recognised by the medical profession as being genuine, sufferers may continue to be stigmatised if their condition is seen as a continuing threat to the social order (Goffman, 1968). Hence the consequences of social disapproval are not confined to malingerers. Indeed, individuals suffering from genuine illnesses may be deprived of privileges and rights. Mentally-ill people, for example, may be deprived of their liberty while individuals diagnosed as being HIV-positive may be discriminated against in the markets for jobs and housing. Moreover, the assumption that the sick role removes responsibility from the individual is in some circumstances incorrect. For example, drug addicts and alcoholics are often blamed for their particular illnesses.

In spite of these flaws, Parsons' focus on the function of medicine in legitimising illness provided at least a partial explanation of the role of the medical profession in modern societies. It also stimulated others to further explore and clarify this important role. Recent work in this field has sought to reach a deeper understanding of the role of the professions, including medicine. Johnson (1995), adopting a Foucauldian perspective (Foucault, 1979) and building on work by Starr and Immergut (1987), Larson, (1977) and Abbott (1988), perceives the professions as socio-technical devices through which the means and ends of government are articulated. Hence in the realm of health care the medical profession can be seen as a resource of governing. In other words its expertise, technologies, practical activities and social authority can make modern, complex society amenable to governing by, for example, overseeing established definitions of illness. As we shall see later, in the context of the debate about the decline of medical power, this approach also implies a departure from the conventional view of the state–profession relationship.

☐ Autonomy and self-regulation

Self-regulation and clinical autonomy are traditionally seen as important symbols of medical power and status. Yet they are more than just symbolic, giving doctors an advantage over both patients and other health professionals in clinical settings.

The autonomy of the medical profession takes two main forms: clinical autonomy and self-discipline. Doctors are resistant to direction in clinical matters. As professionals they believe in their own judgement to guide diagnosis and treatment. Yet there is often disagreement on what constitutes a clinical decision. Williams (1988) has noted the difficulties in distinguishing between strictly clinical factors and other factors such as the availability and use of resources. Doctors agree that clinical decisions cannot be taken in a vacuum, detached from personal, moral, ethical, legal and economic constraints (Hoffenberg, 1987). Johnson (1995) too points out that autonomy of technique is not solely determined by doctors themselves but is the product of a discourse involving doctors, officials and the public.

Despite the difficulties in defining clinical autonomy, it is broadly true that doctors resent interference in matters concerning the admission and treatment of patients. Even peer review (the monitoring of medical work by the profession itself in an attempt to maintain and promote good practice) though increasingly accepted by doctors is still viewed with suspicion by some, while the thought of supervision and direction being undertaken by people with a non-medical background is anathema to them.

Doctors in the UK have enjoyed a high level of clinical autonomy compared with their counterparts in the USA, for example (Harrison and Schulz, 1989). However, in recent years there has been pressure for greater accountability and control of medical work in the UK (see Chapter 6).

In addition to clinical autonomy the medical profession treasures the power of self-discipline. In the UK the body responsible for regulating the profession is the General Medical Council (GMC). This body maintains a register of doctors and regulates the fitness of doctors to practise. It investigates complaints about doctors from the public, the police, the NHS and from other doctors. Ultimately, doctors found guilty of serious professional misconduct can be suspended or removed from the register, but only about two dozen doctors a year are actually subjected to such a fate.

The GMC is dominated by doctors, with only a quarter of its members being lay people. Pressure for reforming the GMC has often come from within the profession itself (Stacey, 1992). In the 1970s such pressure led to an inquiry into the regulation of the medical profession (Cmnd 6018, 1975) and subsequently a number of new measures were introduced, including a new procedure to deal with doctors whose performance was impaired by illness. Changes were also made to the composition of the GMC: members elected by the medical profession (as opposed to those appointed by the medical establishment) were given a majority of seats on the GMC.

Over the years the profession has resisted radical change despite Parliamentary and public pressure for new procedures to investigate cases of medical incompetence and unacceptable behaviour by doctors. However, in 1997 new legislation came into force to enable the GMC to deal more effectively with doctors whose performance is seriously deficient (as well as those who are accused of serious professional misconduct such as sexual misdemeanours). Under the new system, complaints about doctors alleging serious deficiency will be screened by the GMC. If substantiated, the doctor's performance will then be professionally assessed and remedial action (such as counselling or retraining) undertaken where necessary. In addition, special registration conditions can be imposed upon the doctor found to be seriously deficient, restricting or regulating his or her practice (for example, preventing the doctor from performing a particular operation). Ultimately the doctor can be prevented from practising until the remedial requirements have been met.

These changes have been broadly welcomed, but there are two outstanding concerns. First that the new powers only deal with serious deficiencies in performance. Secondly, much depends on the screening process which, though necessary to filter out frivolous and malicious complaints, may also screen out cases which from the point of view of the complainant constitute serious deficiencies. However, it should be noted that there are alternative routes for such complainants. In 1996 the NHS complaints procedure was reformed and extended to cover complaints about clinical matters. These changes are discussed in Chapter 11.

☐ *Political power, politics and the state*

The medical profession has established its pre-eminence largely through its political clout (Freidson, 1988; Moran and Wood, 1992). The major landmark was the Medical Act of 1858 which established the GMC and a register of qualified medical practitioners. Since then the profession has been able to maintain its position through effective political organisation. The role of the GMC has already been discussed. The other principal medical organisations are the British Medical Association (BMA) and the Royal Colleges of Medicine (see Watkins, 1987).

☐ *The British Medical Association (BMA)*

The BMA is the main representative organisation for British doctors. Over three-quarters of practising doctors are members, and it has a long-established reputation as an effective pressure group (Bartrip, 1996; Eckstein, 1960; Grey-Turner and Sutherland, 1982). The BMA lobbies on public health issues such as smoking and road safety, and has even campaigned in recent years against boxing on health grounds. But most of its activity is concerned with sectional issues such as doctors' pay and conditions of work. The craft committees, which operate under the auspices of the BMA, are recognised by the Department of Health as negotiating bodies acting on behalf of each branch of the profession: hospital consultants, junior doctors, doctors specialising in public health, and general practitioners.

During the postwar period, the BMA has been regarded as a powerful group, accepted by the government and possessing extensive political contacts. Over the years it has enjoyed the privilege of being consulted by government on a wide range of health policy matters. However, the BMA's relationship with the Conservative governments of the 1980s and 1990s was less than harmonious. The BMA openly opposed a range of government policies, such as the NHS internal market. Moreover, when introducing these policies the Conservative government often failed to consult the BMA to the same extent as in the past. Even when discussions took place, its advice was often ignored.

☐ *The Royal Colleges of Medicine*

The Royal Colleges (such as the Royal College of Physicians, the Royal College of Surgeons and so on) proclaim themselves to be non-political. Their main responsibility lies in the accreditation and training of specialists. They are, however, consulted by the government on a wide range of health issues.

The Royal Colleges usually operate with a much lower public profile than the BMA. Yet they are in regular contact with the Department of Health, putting forward their views on a range of issues. The Royal Colleges have representation alongside the BMA on the Joint Consultants' Committee, which since its creation in 1949 has met regularly with officials at the Department of Health. The Royal Colleges are also represented on the Standing Medical Advisory Committee, which advises the Department of Health on a wide range of medical matters.

Over the past few decades, the Royal Colleges have raised their public profile to some extent. In the 1960s, for example, the Royal College of Physicians began to publicise the health dangers of tobacco and called for action to reduce smoking. Along with the Royal Colleges of Psychiatrists and General Practitioners, it has called for action on alcohol abuse. The Royal Colleges of medicine have been involved in the creation of anti-alcohol and anti-tobacco pressure groups in recent years, while in 1987, three Royal College presidents became further involved in public controversy, this time over the funding of the NHS.

☐ *Medical power in decline?*

The medical profession is certainly well-organised. Although there are a number of groups representing the profession, they tend to complement rather than conflict with each other and present a relatively united front. This has not always been the case, as illustrated by the divisions between the Royal Colleges and the BMA at the time of the creation of the NHS. But generally there appears to have been less overt conflict and rivalry between the main medical organisations than between, say, the nursing unions, which are very fragmented. The overall solidarity of the medical organisations has been a considerable source of strength.

The past two decades have been challenging for the medical profession. As suggested earlier, its relationship with the government deteriorated considerably. Public exchanges between ministers and representatives of the profession became vitriolic on occasion. The privileges of medical advice and consultation, while not totally withdrawn, became more limited. For example, the BMA and the Royal Colleges were not consulted on major issues such as the NHS White Paper of 1989 (Klein and Day, 1992).

These developments must be seen in perspective. Hostility between the government and the doctors has broken out on a number of occasions in the postwar period. During a contractual dispute in 1965 general practitioners threatened mass resignation from the NHS. In the 1970s there was an enormous dispute between the government and the medical profession over the phasing-out of pay beds in the NHS.

Klein and Day (1992) argue that the disputes of the 1980s were of a different order from those of the 1960s and 1970s. Yet they also point out that they are not unprecedented. Similar structural upheavals in health care took place in 1911 (the introduction of National Health Insurance) and again in 1945 (the creation of the NHS). In both cases, the government of the day confronted the profession and introduced structural change in spite of opposition. Klein and Day also note that the period following such reforms has tended to be more constructive, with the government working once again with the profession in an atmosphere of cooperation.

The re-establishment of what Klein (1990a) has elsewhere called 'the politics of the double bed' has occurred to some extent. Following the departure of Prime Minister Margaret Thatcher, the protagonist of the internal market reforms, the medical organisations reported an improvement in their relations with government. Even so, tensions remained and complaints from doctor's organisations about inadequate consultation continued under the Major government (Baggott, 1995). It remains to be seen how this relationship will fare under a Labour administration.

Elsewhere, beyond the political sphere, some commentators identify a long-term decline of medical power (Armstrong, 1990). It has been argued that doctors have suffered greater blows to their autonomy in recent years compared with other professions such as the legal profession (Brazier *et al.*, 1993). Certainly, the fortunes of the medical profession compare adversely with predominantly private sector professions in an era when the public sector has been under attack (Perkin, 1989), though doctors have perhaps suffered less than many other public sector professions in this period (Deakin, 1991).

Doctors in the UK now face greater restrictions on their freedom, particularly when speaking to the media about the condition of the NHS (*British Medical Journal*, 1994). The emergence of NHS trusts has undoubtedly encouraged such restrictions on grounds of commercial secrecy. There also appears to be an increasing use of NHS disciplinary procedures to remove and suspend doctors from their posts, which undermines the tradition of self-regulation.

Furthermore, doctors in the UK have since the early 1980s been subjected to a barrage of reforms designed to make them more accountable (Moore, 1995). These included the introduction of general management, which led to the creation of a professional management hierarchy (Loveridge and Starkey, 1992) to counterbalance the power of the medical profession. Other specific reforms have included measures to monitor and evaluate clinical activity and resource-use, such as medical audit and resource management. Finally, the creation of an internal market in health care represented a further challenge to which doctors had to respond (Flynn, 1992).

The challenge to the medical profession appears to be fairly universal (Godt, 1987; Freddi and Bjorkman, 1989; Moran and Wood, 1992; Wilsford, 1991). Indeed, in some countries, notably the USA, the challenge has perhaps been even greater with some claiming that medical autonomy has been seriously eroded (Armstrong, 1990; Ginzberg, 1990; McKinlay, 1988). Alford (1975), in attempting to make sense of power relations in the US health care system, devised a model of structural interests with wider significance in the debate about medical power. According to Alford, the health care system comprises three structural interests. The dominant interest is the *professional* monopoly of the medical profession. The subsidiary interest is that of the *corporate rationalisers*. These are the politicians and managers of health care (and, in the American context, the private funders of health care). These interests seek to challenge the professional monopoly by introducing planning and cost control, with the aim of limiting medical autonomy. As spending on health increases, these challenging interests become more influential. Finally, there is the *community interest*. This is the repressed interest, which lacks coherence and a power base, and which as a result exerts little influence over health care.

North (1995) has re-applied Alford's model to the present-day NHS. She notes that the original classification of interests is not always appropriate. For example GP-led commissioning bodies are a combination of professional monopolist and corporate rationaliser. Even so, she observes that the values of the corporate rationaliser are becoming ever more influential. Although professional monopolists – such as hospital consultants – remain powerful, they are increasingly subject to the discipline and ethos of the corporate rationalisers. These issues are discussed further in Chapter 6.

Others emphasise that medicine can still draw on many sources of power to prevent or divert pressures for change (Coburn, 1992). Indeed, observers of the US health care scene indicate that the medical profession can, when under pressure, retain sufficient professional power to enable it to dominate, if not control, the health sector and that at the very least reports of its decline are exaggerated (Bjorkman, 1989; Mechanic, 1991).

Indeed, there are great difficulties in evaluating the impact of change upon the medical profession. As Elston (1991, p. 61) has observed, 'too often different theories about the present and future status of medicine seize on one aspect of change and draw general conclusions about overall rise or fall, ignoring other, countervailing tendencies'. A great deal depends upon the way in which medical domination has been conceived in the past. The traditional focus on the technical autonomy of the medical profession, however, is only one of several aspects which we need to consider (see Light, 1991). Moreover, as Johnson (1995) argues, the benchmarks of medical autonomy and state intervention taken in isolation are too narrow to provide a basis for evaluating the power of the profession. One should instead look at the role of the medical profession in the broader context of the state and with regard to the institutionalisation of expertise. According to this perspective, it is not inevitable that increasing restrictions on aspects of medical autonomy will necessarily undermine the profession; it may well be strengthened provided that its expertise continues to be valued (although it should be noted that Johnson himself believes there is a likelihood that professionalism as a characteristic institutional form might be undermined by the emergent expertise in appraisal and performance monitoring). Similarly, Salter (1996) notes that pressures (such as the desire for greater accountability and cost control) increasingly require a redefinition of the relationship between the profession and the organs of government. This may require a loss of autonomy among individual practitioners but does not mean that the medical profession is collectively weaker as a result.

■ Conclusion

During the twentieth century the medical profession consolidated its dominant position within the health care system. Recently, however, this medical hegemony has been under pressure on several fronts. The domination of health care by orthodox medicine has been increasingly criticised, and interest in complementary therapies has grown. Nursing and paramedical professions have seen an improvement in their status, and alternative medicine has grown in popularity. Orthodox medicine's 'poor relation', the public health approach, has experienced a revival. There has been a greater interest in lay perspectives of health and illness. Moreover, during the 1980s medical organisations began to lose influence over important policy developments and their relationship with government became less harmonious. Doctors voiced fears that their independence and autonomy were at risk because of government reforms.

However, these developments, and the challenges they pose for the profession, must be seen in relation to the pre-existing medical hegemony and within the broader context of the modern state. Despite the dire predictions of doctors' organisations, those factors which underpin the power of orthodox medicine remain. As a result 'the acquiescence to medical ways of thinking', which Walby and Greenwell (1994, p. 74) rightly identify as the basis of medical authority, persists. Consequently, the medical profession both collectively and individually continues to exert a powerful influence within the health care system.

■ *Chapter 3* ■

Critical Perspectives on Health Care

As shown in the previous chapter there has been criticism of orthodox medicine from alternative practitioners, other health care professions and even from within the medical profession itself. To these one may add a number of broader critical perspectives of contemporary health care. These include the economic critique, the views of the technological pessimists, the Marxist perspective, the feminist critique, and, finally, the medicalisation thesis. This chapter explores the problems they identify, and their proposals for change.

■ The economic critique

The ever-rising cost of health care has prompted a growing interest in the use and management of resources. Economists and other business-related professions, such as accountants and management consultants, have played a major role in promoting a greater emphasis on efficiency. This economic perspective has attracted wider support: from among the new breed of NHS managers, from some doctors, and from politicians. The emphasis on the efficient use of resources has also raised broader concerns relating to the effectiveness of health care interventions, the accountability of the health care system, and the quality of care provided.

□ *Efficiency and effectiveness*

At its simplest, an effective procedure is one which produces a desirable health outcome. For example, the successful recovery of a patient following an operation. In practice, however, the judgement of effectiveness is rarely as simple as this. According to some, the medical profession judges the effectiveness of a treatment too much in terms of its success in saving lives (Kennedy, 1981; Illich, 1975). It is increasingly argued that the effectiveness of treatment which saves lives but which severely reduces the quality of life is highly questionable, and that the quality of life should be regarded as an equally important standard of effectiveness when judging the value of health care.

Exhibit 3.1   *Types of efficiency*

1. Providing only services that are effective (i.e. where there is clear evidence that patients enjoy better health as a result of care).
2. Providing effective services at minimum cost.
3. Concentrating resources on effective services, provided at minimum cost, that offer the most benefits in terms of health.
4. Providing a mix of effective services at minimum cost and on such a scale that the benefits to society of providing more services are outweighed by the additional costs.

Source: Culyer (1991).

Efficiency can be distinguished from effectiveness. In simple terms, efficiency is achieved where output is maximised from a given input of resources. In reality, the concept is far more complex (Culyer, 1991). There are at least four types of efficiency in relation to health care. These are shown in Exhibit 3.1.

It is possible for a medical procedure to be effective but not efficient. This could happen for a number of reasons. Patients may be cured following medical intervention, but at an unjustifiably high cost relative to the benefits of the treatment. Or there may be an alternative treatment which could have cured at least the same number of patients at a lower cost. From an economic point of view it is not sufficient that health care is effective: it must also be efficient.

☐ Inefficiency in health care

Cochrane (1971), a strong advocate of evaluation within medicine, identified four main aspects of inefficiency in health care: the use of ineffective therapies; the inappropriate use of effective therapies; the inappropriate use of health care settings; and incorrect lengths of stay in treatment facilities.

Later in this chapter, discussion of Illich's (1975) concept of clinical iatrogenesis reveals evidence of harmful treatments and practices. Yet there are therapies which although not positively harmful to patients, may simply be ineffective and therefore represent a waste of resources. To remedy this, Cochrane urged the use of the Randomised Controlled Trial (RCT). The RCT randomly allocates patients to one of two groups. The first receives the treatment that is under evaluation. The second (the control group) is either given a placebo (in the case of a drug trial, a pill without an active ingredient); or is left untreated; or given an alternative treatment. The outcomes for the two groups are then compared.

RCTs provide the basis for recent efforts to promote evidence-based medicine (see Exhibit 3.2). However, there are problems associated with their use, the most important of which are ethical. For example, it is difficult to justify entering patients in a trial, if as a result they are refused treatment which is likely to improve their health or save their lives. Indeed, doctors are reluctant to evaluate by RCT when there is a strong likelihood that the treatment will be effective, when there is no alternative treatment available, or where the known side-effects of treatment are minimal.

Other criticisms of the RCT approach are that it discriminates unfairly against some interventions, notably public health interventions and alternative therapies, which are difficult if not impossible to evaluate by RCT. In addition, as Black (1996) argues, there are situations where RCTs may be inappropriate: where infrequent yet serious adverse outcomes occur as a result of treatment (such as extreme adverse reactions to a drug); when evaluating inventions designed to prevent comparatively rare events (such as cot death, for example), when the outcomes of intervention are in the distant future; and finally where the effectiveness of the intervention depends upon the patient's active participation (this is undermined by the random allocation to treatment under RCT).

☐ *Inappropriate use of effective therapies*

What about the inefficiency associated with the inappropriate use of effective therapies? There is much evidence that medical services are over-produced and over-supplied. Diagnostic tests are a common target for criticism. The Audit Commission (1995a) found that one in five X-rays was unnecessary, costing the NHS as much as £60m a year. Routine tests also involve considerable waste, with blood and urine tests and microbiological tests contributing little to diagnosis in the vast majority of cases (Sandler, 1979; Hashemi and Merlin, 1987).

A tendency to over-diagnose illness has been observed. This is not new, as demonstrated by a classic study in the USA during the 1930s which revealed that doctors tended to recommend tonsillectomies in about half the children they examined, even where they had been previously diagnosed as not requiring the operation (Bakwin, 1945). Modern studies have revealed a similar tendency to recommend unnecessary treatment. In the US, one study found that the proportion of coronary artery bypass surgery deemed either 'inappropriate' or 'equivocal' varied between 23 per cent and 63 per cent (Winslow *et al.*, 1988). In the UK, a study in the Trent region found that almost half of coronary angiography and bypass surgery was performed for inappropriate or unequivocal reasons (Gray *et al.*, 1990).

Exhibit 3.2   Evidence-based medicine

The growing interest in evidence-based medicine (EBM) springs from a number of concerns. First, that clinical practice is not currently informed by accurate and up-to-date research findings. Secondly, as a result of ineffective and inappropriate interventions, resources are being wasted that could be reallocated to other, more effective uses. Third, because the most effective treatments are often not being employed, the quality of care is lower than it should be. Fourth, that variations in the use of effective treatments create unacceptable inequities.

Doctors and medical researchers see EBM as a means of preserving the scientific credibility of medicine. Politicians and health service managers see it as a way of making the health budget go further and giving them a greater influence over how resources are utilised. Patients' representatives welcome EBM as a means of improving and universalising the quality of care.

Nevertheless, specific moves to promote EBM have been controversial, particularly when viewed as efforts to limit the availability of treatments, or where they threaten the doctor's jealously-guarded independence to decide what is best for the individual patient. It is also pointed out that EBM can be expensive; the commissioning of research, improvements in dissemination and the setting of guidelines are not costless. Finally, although some initiatives based on EBM have produced results – an example being the Royal College of Radiologists' (1992) efforts to reduce radiological examinations – there is often a gulf between the aims of EBM and clinical practice (Grol, 1990).

In the UK, a number of EBM initiatives have been introduced. These include:

1. A new approach to *Research and Development* (R&D) funding in the NHS which will be in place by 1998 in England. Following the Culyer report (DoH, 1994a), which recommended greater clarity and account-ability in research and development funding, the new system creates a single budget for R&D for specific activities identified as national or regional research priorities. The strategic framework is set by the NHS Executive with advice from a central research and development committee (in turn advised by regional committees), and a new National Forum (where national sponsors of research can discuss their strategies). One of the key priorities already established is the evaluation of new technologies.

$\longrightarrow$

There is a considerable variation in diagnosis and treatment between countries. Overall, surgical rates in the USA are twice those of the UK (Vayda, Mindell and Rutkow, 1982). Differences in surgical rates are even higher for some operations. For example, one study showed that three times as many hysterectomies were performed on average in the USA compared with England and Wales (McPherson, Strong and Epstein, 1981). Caesarian sections also show considerable variation ranging from 10 per cent of deliveries in the UK to almost 25 per cent in the USA (OECD, 1994a). There are also variations in the management of illness.

Exhibit 3.2 continued

→

2. *Information dissemination.* Initiatives include efforts to improve continuing medical education (CME) – see Exhibit 2.4. Other important developments are the establishment of the Cochrane Centre, which analyses the results of RCTs, and the NHS Centre for Reviews and Dissemination based at York University. In addition publications such as *Effective Health Care Bulletins* and the availability of systematic reviews on CD ROM are vehicles for communicating research findings to practitioners.

3. *Clinical Guidelines* are nationally-agreed statements (produced by the Royal Colleges of medicine and other professional bodies) setting out the consensus view on the treatment and management of particular conditions. More recently, *National Service Frameworks* have been proposed to set out consensus views on the best way of providing services.

4. *Commissioning.* The NHS Executive requires those commissioning health care to do so on the basis of evidence about effectiveness. It has issued guidance in an effort to promote investment in effective treatments and disinvestment in those of doubtful effectiveness (NHSE, 1996a). Increasingly clinical guidelines (and National Service Frameworks) are being included in the specification of service contracts and agreements.

5. *Performance Indicators and Audit.* Comparative data sets now exist for the purpose of monitoring clinical effectiveness. In addition clinical audit (see Chapter 6) may identify effective and ineffective practice (although so far this potential has not yet been fully exploited). Clinical audit, and the commissioning process, can also be used as a means of developing and implementing clinical guidelines.

6. The Blair Government proposed two new bodies to improve clinical effectiveness and service quality: a *National Institute of Clinical Excellence* to produce guidelines on clinical and cost effectiveness of services; and a *Commission for Health Improvement* to promote improvements in clinical services.

For example, average lengths of stay in hospital vary between countries. In the case of appendicectomy, the length of stay is 9.4 days in Germany, 4.9 days in the UK and only 3.3 days in the USA.

The accuracy of such studies can be challenged on methodological grounds. It is particularly difficult to establish beyond doubt that such variations are unrelated to the prevalence and severity of illness in the general population. The pitfalls of international comparisons should always be remembered when interpreting such data. One should also take note of variation in surgical rates within countries as well as between them.

Nevertheless, there are several possible explanations of why doctors might over-provide medical services, and why this may vary between countries. Some simply believe that doctors simply prefer intervention to inaction (Illich, 1975; Kennedy, 1981). According to Payer (1989), this dominant interventionist philosophy is more deeply ingrained in the profession in some countries (such as the USA) than in others (for example, the UK).

Doctors may over-provide services if they fear the consequences of litigation. Failure to intervene may be construed as negligence and it is easier to prove medical negligence than incompetence or malpractice. Legal factors may partly explain the variation between countries. Litigation by patients is more common and generally more successful in the USA than in the UK, though, as noted in the previous chapter, British patients are becoming increasingly litigious. Over-provision may also reflect patients' demands and expectations in a broader sense. Doctors feel that they are increasingly expected to 'do something' by the patient and that such pressure is at least in part responsible for 'inappropriate' or 'equivocal' referrals and treatment.

The system of remunerating doctors also seems to play a part in encouraging over-supply. In the USA, most doctors traditionally received a fee for each service. In an attempt to restrain health care spending, the Americans have introduced tighter regulation of fees and new forms of health care provision. In the UK, however, as we shall see in later chapters, there have been several attempts in recent years to tie doctors' performance more closely to remuneration.

☐ *Other aspects of inefficiency*

It will be remembered that Cochrane (1971) noted that medical treatment was often given in inappropriate settings and that this could be unnecessarily expensive. He believed that certain conditions could be treated more efficiently outside hospital, perhaps in the GP's surgery, or at home. Cochrane also pointed out that patients were often kept in hospital for much longer periods than necessary, again adding to costs.

Some believe that costs can be reduced by reorganising health care so that patients spend less time in hospital and more time in community settings (Audit Commission, 1990, 1992b). The expansion of day surgery, made possible by new surgical techniques discussed later in this chapter, is an important development in this respect. One should not forget, however, that other significant costs may be incurred in caring for patients outside hospital. Investing in primary care is not a cheap option, though it may be more cost-effective. Notably the burden of cost may fall more heavily upon the family or on social services. These factors should always be taken into account when calculating the balance of costs and benefits of transferring care from hospital into the community (see Chapters 9 and 10).

☐ *Priorities and rationing*

The gap between health needs and the provision of services may be partly satisfied by securing greater efficiency and effectiveness in the provision of services. Other possible ways forward are to prioritise health care or ration it more effectively (see Weale, 1988; Cochrane *et al.*, 1992). Prioritisation and rationing are not new concepts in health care. Waiting lists, a constant feature of the NHS, are a form of rationing. Furthermore, ever since the late 1970s the NHS has set out its main priorities.

Economists have devised techniques to help set priorities and to ration care. One technique, the Quality Adjusted Life Year (QALY), has attracted considerable attention (Williams, 1985; Carr-Hill, 1991). The benefits of health care, measured in QALYs, are calculated from estimates of the length and quality of a patient's life following treatment. The costs of treatment are then expressed in terms of a cost per QALY (see Exhibit 3.3). The QALY can be used to compare the relative cost-effectiveness of different treatments for the same illness. More controversially, the technique can be used as a rationing tool, facilitating the expansion of treatment of certain illnesses (those that achieve QALYs at a lower cost) at the expense of others (those that achieve QALYs at high cost).

There is strong opposition from health care professions to the use of cost–benefit criteria in this way. Doctors claim that QALYs undermine their clinical judgement (Smith, 1987). Williams (1988), a pioneer of QALYs in the UK, denies this, arguing that the technique is intended only to improve accountability for the use of resources. Loewy (1980) has criticised the ethics of QALYs, commenting that optimisation of survival and not optimisation of cost-effectiveness is the only ethical rule to follow. Others have attacked QALYs for their discriminatory impact on vulnerable groups such as the disabled and the elderly (Jones and Higgs, 1990) for whom the benefits of treatment (in terms of survival and externally-assessed quality of life) are lower.

The calculations themselves are rather crude. Reducing the quality of life to a single index is problematic, as individuals differ widely in their judgements. Other, more patient-sensitive measures have been devised (Carr-Hill and Morris, 1991). But these raise further problems of comparability between treatments and across different groups of patients (Cairns, 1996). Other technical problems can be found in the calculation of the costs of health care. Many costs, including those that fall on families, social services and the wider community are difficult to establish and are either underestimated or omitted from the calculations.

Exhibit 3.3   *QALYs (Quality Adjusted Life Years)*

QALYs can be used to compare the relative benefits of different forms of care and treatment. Each year which the patient is expected to survive following a course of treatment is weighted by a factor reflecting quality of life. The quality of life weighting relates to various dimensions of disability and distress (which can be converted into a single index – see Rosser and Watts, 1972; Rosser and Kind 1978). Once the number of QALYs generated by each treatment is calculated, it is then possible to compare the relative costs in order to find out which treatment has the lowest cost per QALY. A simple worked example is shown below:

Treatment A

Cost = £10 000 per patient

Life expectancy after treatment = 20 years

Quality of life: (No Distress;

(Rosser's Index)   Slight Social Disability) = 0.990

Treatment B

Cost = £5000 per patient

Life expectancy = 18 years

Quality of life: (Mild Distress;

(Rosser's Index)   Slight Social Disability) = 0.986

Treatment A

QALY = Life expectancy × Quality of life

= 20 × 0.990

= 19.8

Cost per QALY = 10 000/19.8 = £505 per QALY

Treatment B

QALY = Life expectancy × Quality of life

= 18 × 0.986

= 17.748

Cost per QALY = 5 000/17.748 = £282 per QALY

In the light of this simple calculation, treatment B appears to be more cost-effective than treatment A.

The application of QALYs to health care decision-making is at an early stage in the UK, but interest in their use was stimulated by the introduction of the NHS internal market. A number of health authorities in the UK have since considered withdrawing funding from so-called 'low priority' treatments, as we shall see in later chapters.

In some other countries, notably the USA, explicit rationing has gone a stage further. A number of states have expressed concern about large numbers of people not covered either by state or private health insurance schemes and who have difficulty in obtaining access to care. One state, Oregon, responded by formulating a plan to ration public expenditure on health care. The idea was to expand access to state-funded health care to include the uninsured, while restricting the range of treatments paid for by the state (see Exhibit 3.4).

☐ *Accountability*

Calls for a more explicit approach to rationing have been accompanied by a plea for more accountability in health care (see Weale, 1988). Accountability has a variety of meanings (Day and Klein, 1987). In a narrow sense, better accountability means improved financial management: those who deliver health care – professionals and institutions – being held to account for the financial aspects of their activities. Accountability can also be interpreted more broadly, as a responsibility upon health care providers to answer for the decisions they make. On an individual level, it would be facilitated by a greater openness in the making of clinical judgements. This could be brought about by making explicit the criteria used by health care professions when making decisions about treatment. On an organisational level, accountability would be enhanced by clarifying the responsibilities of institutions within the health care system – hospitals, health authorities and government agencies. Better accountability would also result from greater openness at the organisational level, with decisions being subjected to wider public scrutiny.

It is often claimed that the providers of health care, particularly in the UK, are not accountable to the user – the patient (Green *et al.*, 1990). Patients tend to be passive, have little information, and have few rights of redress. In recent years there has been an emphasis on the patient as a consumer of health services. The extent to which this has actually produced a more responsive service is examined in Chapter 11.

☐ *The management of quality*

Concern about the use of resources, the effectiveness of services, and the accountability of providers has produced a sharper focus upon management processes in health care and in particular on the management

Exhibit 3.4   The Oregon experiment

In the late 1980s Oregon, like many other states in the USA, faced two main health care problems: rising health care costs, and large numbers of uninsured people. The state government therefore decided to try a different approach towards the allocation of health care resources. Plans were set out to alter the coverage of Medicaid, the state-run system for funding the care of poor people (and also blind people, the disabled, and children in foster care). The main idea behind the plan was to extend Medicaid to a larger proportion of those on low incomes without private health insurance, while at the same time restricting the range of treatments funded by the programme.

With this in mind the state began collecting cost–benefit data with respect to the various treatments available. An initial ranking of treatments was produced but it was subsequently withdrawn after criticisms of the data collection process. A second list was then produced and at this stage the public were consulted on their views of the benefits of treatment. The top five conditions listed were:

- Pneumonia;
- Tuberculosis;
- Peritonitis;
- Foreign body in throat; and
- Appendicitis.

Also appearing in the top half of the rankings were treatment for cancer of the uterus, heart bypass operations and treatment for the early stages of HIV-related disease.

In the light of this revised ranking, the Oregon legislature approved the funding for the first 587 treatments listed (out of a total of 709). Had the plan gone ahead at this stage, the Medicaid system would have been extended to an additional 120 000 individuals currently excluded from the programme. At the same time, public funding for the treatment of many 'low-priority conditions', including those listed below, would have ended.

- Varicose veins;
- Bronchitis;
- Cancers where treatment will not result in 10 per cent of patients surviving for 10 years;
- Uncomplicated haemorrhoids;
- AIDS (Terminal Stage HIV); and
- Extremely low birth weight babies.

In order to proceed, the Oregon government required approval from the Federal Government in Washington. This approval was initially withheld following pressure from organisations representing disabled people. Further negotiations between state and federal officials produced a number of concessions (including an agreement that treatment for AIDS patients would not be withdrawn). Subsequently, permission was granted which enabled Oregon to introduce its plan for a five-year trial period.

Source: Honigsbaum, 1992.

of quality. The laudable objective of improving the quality of health services through better management has proved to be a contentious one. One reason being that there are different interpretations of health service quality. Secondly, the difficulties involved in measuring quality have by default led to an emphasis on crude and narrow measures which are often hotly disputed. Third, the approach to managing and improving quality of service has drawn on ideas developed mainly in the context of private enterprise and their importation into the public sector has been challenged.

Management gurus, whose ideas have been so influential in recent years, have emphasised certain features of good management and effective organisation (see Drucker, 1954; Demming, 1982; Peters and Waterman, 1982). These include leadership, the setting of clear objectives, performance measurement, refocusing on the needs of the consumer, and the importance of cultural values which reinforce the objectives and performance of the organisation. As we shall see in Chapter 6, those seeking to reform health care management have adopted these broad principles as well as the specific recommendations of individuals drawn from the business world.

☐ *Markets*

Some believe that many of the shortcomings of health care can be addressed by the application of market forces. Economic theory predicts that greater competition between suppliers will in the longer term drive down prices and improve efficiency.

Yet even among the ranks of economists, few favour unrestrained markets in health care. Health care is not a public good in the economists' strict sense of the term: where one person's consumption does not exclude others from consuming the same good (Alchian and Allen, 1974). Yet it does have certain special characteristics which lead most to believe that it would be inefficiently provided or under-provided if left entirely to the private market (Normand, 1991).

There has been greater support for combining the state's role in health care with market forces in the form of a 'managed market'. Some economists argue that effective competition between providers can take place within a publicly-funded health care system, generating considerable benefits in the form of a downward pressure on costs and greater efficiency (Enthoven, 1985). The enclosure of market forces within a clear framework of regulation is designed to rule out sharp practices while ensuring that the system is in harmony with publicly-stated policy objectives, such as fair access to services.

Markets have been seen by many economists and politicians as an antidote, not only to what they regard as inefficient state health care bureaucracies, but also to the power of the health care professions (Gladstone, 1992). Professional bodies are seen as monopolistic producers, controlling the supply of labour and thereby keeping wages (and costs) high. Markets in health care undermine this monopoly by forcing professionals to compete against each other. At the same time, measures can be taken to reduce the control of professional bodies over the supply of labour – by introducing competition from overseas or from less skilled or less well-qualified practitioners. However, despite the theories of the economists, markets in health care have not always behaved as predicted. This will become clear in later chapters, in the context of privatisation and internal markets in the NHS.

☐ Criticism

Most broadly support the promotion of greater efficiency in health care, evaluation of effectiveness, prioritisation on the basis of need, better management, a focus on improving service quality and a greater emphasis upon financial, professional and political accountability. Yet there is a great deal of suspicion about the means which have been suggested to achieve these laudable aims, not least from within the health care professions.

As we have already seen, there is doubt about some of the techniques suggested to improve health services. There is also concern that the emphasis on efficiency is part of a hidden agenda, in two senses. First, it is seen as a means by which the politicians of the right are seeking to undermine the welfare state. Second, while economists may have a useful supplementary role in the allocation of health care resources, there are worries about them occupying a more strategic role (Klein, 1989). The 'efficiency agenda' is seen as a strategy for professional advancement by economists, and other business and management-related occupations. Indeed, health economists have been characterised as imperialists seeking to colonise the minds of health care practitioners (Ashmore, Mulkay and Pinch, 1989). Along with other professional groups, such as accountants, management consultants and NHS managers, they are seen as aiming to subvert the existing medically-dominated structure of professional power, replacing it with a system influenced by their own expertise.

■ Technological pessimists

A second critical perspective focuses on the dependence of modern health care on high technology. It is difficult to define high technology in a simple way, and its meaning is often taken for granted (Richman, 1987). In the context of health care, high technology essentially means the use of complex machinery and advanced techniques in the diagnosis and treatment of patients. Some examples are shown in Exhibit 3.5.

A number of reasons have been advanced to explain why health care has become more dependent on high technology (Reiser, 1978). First, high technology has been supported by the medical profession largely because most believe it introduces a scientific precision into clinical practice. Second, medical education, training and research have all emphasised technological medicine. Third, particularly in the USA, doctors have often felt compelled to use high technology as a defensive mechanism against claims of negligence. Fourth, the public is fascinated by medical technology and generally supports its use. This is underpinned by the portrayal of medical technology in the media, which is generally positive. A fifth reason may be added to this list. According to Jennett (1986), doctors increasingly see the development of high technologies as a symbol of their own success. Finally, medical technology is a huge and profitable industry dominated by powerful corporate interests – such as pharmaceutical , engineering and electronics firms. These corporations have a vested interest in promoting technological change, even when this is not in the interests of patients. Their role in relation to health care is discussed further in the context of the Marxist critique below.

Despite the general support of the public and the medical profession, high technology has been criticised on a number of specific grounds: that it can be inefficient and ineffective; that it may subjugate and depersonalise the patient; and that it can lead to ever more complicated ethical problems.

☐ *Efficiency and effectiveness*

Critics of high technology often point out the scale of both capital and running costs (Council for Science and Society, 1982). An MRI scanner costs around £750 000 plus maintenance costs of £80 000 a year (Whitehouse, 1995). In addition there are running costs, plus upgrading costs (estimated at around £200 000 every few years). The expense of new technology may be justified if the benefits to patients are great. But the main problem is that many new technologies have not even been evaluated at all, either in terms of their efficiency or their effectiveness (Jennett, 1986; Stocking, 1988).

New technology can, however, be both efficient and effective. Some technologies are relatively cheap and yet effective. Take, for example, hip replacements, which are of enormous benefit in improving the quality of life and which cost around £5000 each. Some technologies raise the possibility of reducing costs as well as improving the quality of care for

---

Exhibit 3.5   New medical technologies

It is impossible to detail all the developments in the fast-moving field of medical technology. Here are some examples of the evolution of new technologies over the last decade or so, and other developments anticipated in the future.

Laser technologies. New techniques have been developed and are being used in a variety of treatments ranging from the vaporisation of tumours to delicate eye surgery. The increasing sophistication of laser technology is likely to lead to an expansion in other areas of treatment. For example, they have been used experimentally in the treatment of coronary heart disease.

Extra corporeal shockwave lithotripsy is used in the treatment of kidney stones. Shock waves are administered which shatter the stone, the patient requiring neither anaesthetic nor pain relief. Conventional surgery entails two hours anaesthesia and a painful five-week period of convalescence, including a 10–14 day stay in hospital.

Keyhole surgery, as it is more popularly known, involves passing miniature surgical instruments through small holes in the skin, or through natural orifices. The instruments are attached to an endoscope, a hand-held, flexible tube. This contains optical fibres which deliver light to the tip (inside the body) while transmitting images back to the eye-piece (or to a larger screen where it can be seen by the surgical team). Other endoscopic instruments have been developed for particular procedures and operations: rigid endoscopes are used to view particular organs such as the kidney; arthroscopes are used in the diagnosis and treatment of diseases, disorders and injuries of the joints; and laparoscopes are used to enter the abdominal wall. Hernia repair and gall bladder removal are examples of procedures using laparoscopic surgery.

Diagnostic tools. New imaging techniques such as MRI (magnetic resonance imaging) can assist diagnosis, particularly in the field of neurological disorders. MRI produces highly detailed cross-sectional images of soft tissues by placing the patient in a magnetic field. Meanwhile PET (positron-emission tomography) scanners have been developed to examine chemical processes in the brain and in other organs. It involves injecting a radioactive-labelled

$\longrightarrow$

---

patients. Minimally invasive therapies (MITs) have been heralded as a great leap forward in both respects. Take, for example, lithotripsy (see Exhibit 3.5), which reduces hospital stays for the patient by around a third compared with conventional surgery. There is also less chance of infection following the procedure. Lower costs associated with convalescence have clear resource implications for providers (Audit Commission, 1990, 1992b). Other techniques, such as keyhole surgery, are also believed to cause less injury to the body than conventional techniques and therefore imply shorter hospital stays, less convalescence and a better chance of a complete recovery for the patient.

Exhibit 3.5 continued

⟶

glucose substance into the blood. The accumulation of this substance at various sites in the body is analysed by computer to build up a picture of biochemical activity that can help to detect abnormalities.

Drugs. Pharmaceutical developments include hormone replacement therapy (HRT) used in the relief of post-menopausal symptoms. However, drug regimes are often expensive. For example, Clozapine, a drug used in the treatment of schizophrenia, costs around £2000 a year. Interferon beta, a new drug developed to combat forms of multiple sclerosis, costs around £10 000 a year per patient treated. Genetic technology (see below) is also likely to bring forth new drug-based therapies.

Genetic technologies. It is now possible in some cases to isolate the genes which predispose individuals to certain diseases. According to Yates (1996), 60 disease genes were identified in 1995 including those involved in the onset of Alzheimer's disease. Once the population can be genetically screened for a particular disease, it is then possible to concentrate resources upon those most at risk. In some cases those who currently suffer from disease may be treated with gene therapy (using specially-engineered genetic material). This has already been used experimentally in the treatment of cystic fibrosis. Other developments include DNA vaccines which may enable the body to defend itself against viruses and other pathogens for longer periods.

Other developments. Computer technology has the potential to bring about a vast range of improvements in health care. Modern systems facilitate the storage and retrieval of enormous amounts of data and allow multiple access and interaction between users. Developments already underway include the sharing of patient information by different agencies within the health care system, networking between professionals, and the speedy dissemination of research about the efficacy of treatment to front-line professionals. Computer-controlled or assisted devices will also play an increasing role in the diagnosis and treatment of disease. Some foresee the development of remote-control 'telerobots' in surgery (Buckingham and Buckingham, 1995). It may well be that in future, operations will be routinely performed by tiny computer-controlled surgical devices under the supervision of doctors.

Despite the potential benefits of MITs and other new techniques, it is important that their use is carefully monitored. In the past doctors themselves have shown a reluctance to evaluate new techniques which they feel are unambiguously beneficial. Now there is a greater awareness of the need to evaluate new techniques, prompted by worries about side-effects. But even when a new technique is evaluated this is rarely the end of the story. Take for example the case of gall bladder removal by keyhole surgery (laparoscopic cholecystectomy). Early evidence suggested that the technique was better for patients (for cosmetic reasons and in terms of recovery) than conventional surgery. A later study (Majeed *et al.*, 1996), however, identified a higher risk of bile duct injuries compared with conventional surgery. There has also been concern about the use of keyhole surgery for hernia repair. More generally, Sculpher (1993) has warned that 'there is no automatic link between the advent and diffusion of new minimal access surgery techniques and an increase in the cost-effectiveness of service provision'.

☐ *Doctor–patient relationship*

Some have identified a technological imperative in medicine, whereby technical skill and progress is seen as being more important than interpersonal skills and the patient's interests (Kennedy, 1981). It is often claimed that although the use of high technology often has public support, it alters the doctor–patient relationship in an adverse way. Reiser (1978) has commented that machines direct the attention of both doctor and patient to the measurable aspects of illness and away from personal and social factors relevant to health. Technology can reinforce the disease orientation of biomedicine, discussed in the previous chapter, and may further weaken the position of the patient.

A further problem is that the use of technology may absolve doctors from blame. Illich (1975), among others, has claimed that the depersonalisation of diagnosis and therapy has transformed malpractice from an ethical into a technical problem. The machine also becomes the carrier of bad news and can take the blame when things go wrong.

High technology can also be regarded as inhumane. As Gould (1987) observes with regard to organ transplants, the quality of life for patients in the early years was poor. Although the technology has advanced considerably in recent years, particularly in the field of heart transplants, improving the chances that the patient will live a fairly normal life, there are still tragic cases where the post-operative quality of life for patients and carers is poor. As for the terminally ill, high-technology treatment may perhaps be less humane than the 'low tech' care provided by the hospice movement.

Medical technology has been blamed for increasing the power of the doctor over the patient. The use of technology, it is often argued, confirms the role of the doctor as expert. 'The more decisions are made by experts, the less they can be made by laymen' (Freidson, 1988, p. 336). As knowledge becomes more technical, doctors and other experts can dominate ever more spheres of activity. For example, the medical domination of childbirth was assisted by the emergence of birth technologies introduced by doctors (Oakley, 1980, 1984). However, it is also possible that the reliance on technology might actually work in the opposite direction, effectively de-skilling the medical profession. As the interpersonal and diagnostic skills of doctors are replaced at least in part by new technologies, it is possible that they could become merely intermediaries between the patient and other technical experts (Reiser, 1978).

☐ *Ethical problems*

The final area of concern relates to ethical dilemmas raised by many new technologies. Medical interventions such as organ transplants, genetic engineering, screening and testing for disease raise a variety of ethical issues. For example, under what circumstances should organ donation be permitted? Should genetically manipulated organs from animals be used for transplantation into humans? To what extent should genetic manipulation be allowed to alter the characteristics of unborn children? Should patients be screened for diseases which may lead to them being discriminated against by employers, insurance companies and so on? A further set of ethical questions is raised by the availability of life-saving care and treatment, where previously patients would be allowed to die. How should these scarce and expensive services be allocated? Should treatment be withdrawn from those in severe pain or who are unlikely to regain consciousness?

Such ethical questions are not easily resolved. They often produce a controversial debate, frequently polarised on the basis of firmly-held moral and religious convictions. These issues also increasingly raise complex questions of law, bringing health care more closely into the realm of legal decision-making.

☐ *Managing new technology*

Those who are pessimistic about health care technologies are themselves often attacked for wanting to stop progress. Yet even critics of high technology accept that 'it can confer substantial benefits when appropriately employed' (Jennett, 1986, p. 141). No one would wish to prevent the emergence of potentially effective treatments.

Nevertheless there is unease about the rapid progress of high technology. Clearly, new technologies must be carefully evaluated, and not merely on narrow economic cost–benefit grounds. Evaluation should take into account other important criteria, such as the impact on professional competence and the doctor–patient relationship. It should also take into account the moral and ethical issues raised by the use of new technology.

In the UK, health technology assessment is coordinated by the National Coordinating Centre for Health Technology Assessment in Winchester. This organisation helps to identify and prioritise research projects, provides information on the state of knowledge and disseminates findings of research. The Royal Colleges of medicine also play a role by administering a registration system, issuing guidelines relating to the use of some techniques and make recommendations about training. A more formal system of registering and reviewing new techniques, involving the establishment of a Committee on Safety and Efficacy of Procedures, was in fact recommended in 1993 by the government's own Advisory Committee on Science and Technology. Subsequently the Department of Health established a Standing Committee on Health Technology Assessment to advise on a range of issues including priorities for technology assessment and the need to control the diffusion of new technology.

Finally, not only should new technologies be evaluated, but the implications for the entire system of health care must to be carefully considered and built into plans for future health service provision (Hoare, 1992). As Banta (1993) observes, the take-up of the new generation of technologies will have wide implications for hospital organisation (already over half of the elective surgical cases in the UK are day cases), the workload of primary and community care services, the professions, training, and the costs of service provision.

■ Marxist and other socialist perspectives

Marxists analyse contemporary health care in terms of the class structure of capitalist societies, the search for profits, and the role of the state in ensuring both capitalist domination and capital accumulation (see Navarro, 1978; Doyal, 1979). Other socialist perspectives, examined later in this section, share many of the concerns of the Marxists and sometimes propose similar (though usually less radical) solutions.

To fully understand the Marxist perspective let us begin with the original views of Marx, writing in the nineteenth century. For Marx there was a powerful tendency for capitalists to exploit the workers in an attempt to increase profits and accumulate more capital. He identified three main consequences of this process: inequality, as the material conditions of the workers declined relative to the capitalists; crisis, as the capitalist system found it more difficult to continue exploiting labour in the long term; and conflict between the classes, leading ultimately to socialised control of the means of production.

The implications for health of the unbridled capitalist system were evident during the period in which Marx was writing. Poverty and material deprivation were widespread, and the conditions endured by the working classes were a breeding ground for disease. Although the wealthy were not immune from the infections created by these social and economic conditions, the poor suffered disproportionately (Smith, 1979). There were also wide inequalities in the standards of health care received by the different social classes (Abel-Smith, 1964).

Since the death of Marx, capitalist states have responded to the social problems and economic tensions of capitalism in ways he did not foresee; intervening in the economy to moderate economic crises: replacing capitalist production with public ownership in many areas; and creating welfare states to cushion the impact of capitalism. Neo-Marxists, seeking to apply Marx's philosophy in the modern context, argue that in spite of these changes, the system is essentially the same. The state remains a defender of capitalism, not a guardian of social welfare. It is this general principle which guides their analysis of health care in capitalist states.

☐ *Inequalities, class and capitalism*

In Chapter 1 a number of significant inequalities in health and illness were identified. Marxists attribute these to the material inequalities generated by capitalism. Certainly, specific social conditions are associated with ill-health, such as bad housing and unemployment. Though there are a number of possible explanations for the class gradient, it is undoubtedly true that material conditions are important factors in health (see Chapter 12). Yet it is not clear to what extent health inequalities are directly, exclusively or wholly a product of capitalism. Indeed, health inequalities vary considerably between capitalist countries, while social inequalities persisted in communist countries throughout the post-war period.

Marxists identify inequalities in the provision of health care as a feature of capitalism. They point out that such inequalities are greater in health care systems where private enterprise has a larger role, such as in the USA, but that health care inequalities will also be a feature of state health systems in capitalist societies. There is some evidence to support this. The 'inverse care law' states that areas where health needs are greatest – generally the poorest areas – will be the least likely to receive high-quality care (Tudor-Hart, 1971). This is not just a feature of market-led health systems, though the law is more accentuated by such systems. Studies of the NHS found that poorer areas tended to have poorer health services and that the higher social classes received more health care resources relative to need (Le Grand, 1978). These findings were not universally accepted, however, and the validity of the inverse care law was itself challenged (Powell, 1990). In addition, other studies did not find evidence of significant inequalities in the use of the NHS between the various social classes and income groups (Collins and Klein, 1988; O'Donnell, Propper and Upward, 1991). A further problem, which adds to the problems of measurement, is that equity is a complex concept (see Exhibit 3.6) and can be interpreted in different ways (Pereira, 1993; Whitehead, 1994).

Marxists believe that the health care system is a microcosm of capitalist society. The upper and upper-middle classes are in a position to decide on key questions of resource allocation and the organisation of care. Marxists identify a class bias in the NHS, with upper and middle classes (and increasingly in recent years, business people) dominating health authorities. They further believe that the medical profession, as the most socially exclusive group in health care, is part of the general conspiracy.

As we shall see in Chapter 6, it is true that health authority membership in recent years has been far from representative of society. But to equate socio-economic class with support for capitalism is rather crude. Many health authority members have strenuously opposed moves to commercialise the NHS. Similarly, the fact that doctors are drawn from higher social classes does not necessarily make them allies of business. British doctors have been broadly supportive of the NHS, though they have been opposed to certain models of state ownership. Moreover, one should note that the internal market – the most explicit attempt yet to introduce capitalist values into socialised medicine – was strongly resisted by most doctors and health professionals.

□ Profits and capital accumulation

Marxists accept that state health care has moderated to some extent the health problems generated by the capitalist system, but has been unable to counteract them. They further point out that state health services allow some scope for private enterprise, which has never been totally eradicated even in nationalised health care systems such as the NHS. When the NHS was created, consultants retained the right to treat private patients and GPs secured their status as independent contractors. The profit motive has also survived in many areas vital to health care, such as the supply of medical equipment, pharmaceuticals, hospital building and construction: the so-called medical–industrial complex (McKinlay, 1979).

In recent years private sector involvement in UK health care has increased substantially, with the contracting out of ancillary services and the growth of private health care. Policies such as the Private Finance Initiative and the growing interest in 'managed care' offer further opportunities for private corporations (see Chapter 7) Moreover, the introduction of business-style management processes and market mechanisms into the NHS has placed new emphasis upon commercial motives and judgements. This mirrors developments elsewhere. Even in the US, for example, where the private sector has traditionally had a larger role, observers talk of a corporate transformation in health care involving a so-called invasion by investor-owned 'for-profit' enterprises (Relman, 1980; Salmon, 1995).

Marxists argue that state health services assist capital accumulation in other ways. They make more palatable the problems which arise from capitalist production. Industrial pollution, accidents and injuries, and stress-related illness are seen by Marxists as side-effects of the quest for profits. Health problems associated with consumption of commercially-produced goods such as alcohol, tobacco and junk food can be viewed in a similar way. Marxists believe that the people are fooled into thinking that 'what is politically and collectively caused can be individually and therapeutically cured' (Navarro, 1978). Individuals who suffer ill-health can obtain treatment from state-financed health services in a such a way that public awareness of the root causes of illness is obscured. Protest is thereby neutralised, allowing capitalists to continue making their profits at the expense of public health.

Yet the existence of state health services has not dispersed public protest nor prevented public health campaigns. Governments in capitalist states have been persuaded to take action against pollution, accidents at work, alcohol and tobacco and so on, even where this has offended vested interests. Commercial organisations have formidable lobbying powers to prevent this, but they are not invulnerable.

There are a number of other ways in which health services are seen as assisting profit-making and capital accumulation. Modern capitalism needs high-quality labour in order to thrive. Marxists argue that the productivity of labour can be maintained by protecting the health of key workers (that is, of skilled and technical workers) Moreover, the quantity of labour available to capitalists can be increased when necessary by relieving people of at least some of their caring duties. At the same time, health services become the dumping ground for the 'economically unproductive' (the mentally and physically ill; the elderly) who cannot be used by the capitalist production process. This process appears now to be operating in reverse. A major strand of policy in recent years has been to reduce state responsibilities for health and health care. Informal carers increasingly shoulder the burden of looking after the sick and elderly. The government has also encouraged self-care and more private health care expenditure.

Marxists explain these new trends by arguing that we have entered a new phase of capitalism (O'Connor, 1973; Offe, 1984). This takes the form of an initial crisis, the main features of which are rising tax burdens, high inflation, trade union militancy, and a stifling of capitalist activity. In response, the state adopts policies to curb welfare expenditure and to encourage private enterprise. This leads to a reinvigoration of capitalism, but also produces greater social conflict and inequality.

□ *The contribution of the Marxist approach*

The value of the Marxist perspective, rather like the public health approach discussed in Chapter 2, lies in its focus upon the social and economic roots of ill-health. The Marxist emphasis on inequalities in health care also reminds us that we should never assume that access to health care will always be fair, even in state systems. Marxists help to explain the motives of private health care providers. This is particularly important in view of the expansion of private care and private-sector management practices in the NHS. Finally, Marxism sheds light on why commercial activities harmful to health may be tolerated to some extent by governments.

There are, however, a number of general criticisms. The Marxist critique of the NHS is unfair. The NHS has done much to improve health care in the UK, and is widely judged as being an improvement on the system it replaced. Furthermore, as we have seen, the Marxist approach to class relations in the NHS is flawed, and the evidence of class inequalities in access to health care ambiguous.

Another general criticism is that Marxists are long on analysis but short on specific recommendations for improving health care. Hard-line Marxists point out that health and health care will only improve significantly when the general social and economic organisation of society is changed; that is, when the capitalism itself is superseded. However, as already noted, health and health care inequalities persisted under communism. Communist countries also appear to have a poor record on industrial pollution, alcohol and tobacco-related problems, and other public health problems linked with industry and industrialisation.

□ *Other socialist approaches*

The declining appeal of Marxism, not least within the British Labour Party, does not mean that it is a redundant perspective. To be unpopular is not the same as being inaccurate. Yet one should mention other socialist perspectives, which though they share some of the concerns of the Marxists, are based on other considerations and promote a more pragmatic approach to reform. These perspectives also happen to be shared by many in the 'new' Labour Party and for the foreseeable future will exert far more influence over health policy.

Socialism is a broad church, but one can identify three principles that are particularly important in relation to health and which most socialists would agree with. First, a concern for humanity: that society must protect the weak and vulnerable. Secondly, that capitalism is often (but not always) inefficient, particularly where the provision of collective goods is concerned. Thirdly, that the state, through taxation, public spending and direct service provision, is the key instrument for redressing the inequities and inefficiencies of capitalism.

When applied to health care, these principles have underpinned a range of policies: the creation of state health services, efforts to redress inequities, and policies for vulnerable groups (Carrier and Kendall, 1990; Tudor-Hart, 1994; Widgery, 1988). Perhaps it is a testament to the power of these principles that in spite of nearly two decades of government fired by a very different ideology, they still exert an enormous influence on the parameters of policy debate.

But it would be foolish to argue that nothing has changed. Indeed socialism has itself changed. While retaining their humanitarian concern, many socialists have begun to question whether or not the state can deliver the gains in efficiency and equity in health care and in other fields of provision. Some envisage a greater role for the non-state sector in the provision of care and for individual contributors to the cost of care (see Hutton, 1996; Jones, 1995; Mandelson and Liddell, 1996) and accept the purchaser–provider split introduced by the Conservatives (see Abel-Smith and Glennerster, 1995). There is also a growing interest by socialists in communitarianism (Etzioni, 1993), which combines humanitarian concern with an emphasis on responsibilities. Applying this creed to the health sector provides support for greater self-help and voluntary provision, for individuals taking more responsibility for their health in general, and also for more private funding of health care, such as charges and insurance coverage for those who can afford to cover themselves for health risks.

■ The feminist critique

Contemporary health care can be viewed from a feminist perspective (see Wilkinson and Kitzinger, 1994; Doyal, 1995; Miles, 1991), which has two main strands. First, it is claimed that the delivery of health services is male-dominated. Second, and arising out of this, there is criticism of the way in which the health care system, and in particular the medical profession, view female patients and their health problems.

In traditional societies women were invariably cast in the role of healer. As societies developed, this role became professionalised (Leeson and Gray, 1978). Where women were still allowed to undertake health care roles, they were subservient to the male-dominated medical profession.

Exhibit 3.6   Equity in health care

The concept of equity in health care is complex. In the context of the NHS the following principles of equity have been identified:

1. *A universal health service*. The service should be available to all irrespective of ability to pay. It should not be not means tested. The service should be open to those who make use of private facilities, ensuring that system is not simply 'for the poor'.
2. *Sharing financial costs*. The service should be free at the point of use. Contributions to the cost of the service through taxation should be linked to the size of income.
3. *Comprehensive service*. All aspects of health care should be covered by the service and there should be no exclusions.
4. *Geographical equality*. Services should be of the same quality and accessibility in different parts of the country.
5. Selection on the basis of *clinical need*. People should receive services on the basis of their needs, not their financial situation or because of social position or connections.
6. The encouragement of '*a non-exploitative ethos*'. This involves the maintenance of high ethical standards and the removal or minimisation of economic incentives that might lead to exploitation of patients.

Source: Whitehead (1994, p. 1285) and Cmnd 7615 (1979) *The Report of the Royal Commission on the NHS.*

This domination continued even where female health care roles became professionalised, as illustrated, for example, by the emergence of the 1902 Midwives Act (Donnison, 1988). This Act established state regulation of the midwifery profession and was the product of a protracted battle between doctors and midwives over who should control childbirth. It introduced a number of safeguards to protect the doctors' role and limit that of midwives. During the latter part of the nineteenth century, nurses also successfully pressed for professional recognition, but on terms acceptable to the doctors (Abel-Smith, 1960).

The professionalisation of nursing and midwifery enhanced the social status of these occupations but did not challenge the power of the medical profession, which remained hostile to women. Even today women are still under-represented in the ranks of doctors and find it difficult to penetrate the higher echelons of medicine, as discussed in Chapter 2. They are also under-represented in the managerial ranks: only a tenth of senior NHS managers are female (Maddock, 1995; EOC, 1991). Women have made considerable progress in the professions allied to medicine – physiotherapy, occupational therapy, radiography, dietetics, speech therapy, and so on – but these, like nursing and midwifery, invariably played a supporting role to medicine.

Women tend to perform health care roles which place them in a subservient position relative to men. Medicine is male-dominated: nursing (which is 90 per cent female) and other non-medical health professions are predominantly female. Other health occupations are also mainly female. Seventy per cent of ancillary workers in the NHS are women, as are over four-fifths of clerical workers. In addition, almost two-thirds of those who provide informal care for relatives at home are female (Green, H., 1988). Some writers have focused on the caring roles of women and how the performance of these roles often undermines their health status (Graham, 1984, 1993).

How can subservience and exploitation of women within the health care system be explained? According to Davies (1995) in the context of the nursing professions, this is not simply a result of poor political organisation. The answer lies in the gendering of social institutions – health care delivery is deeply affected by cultural codes of gender in which masculinity is associated with achievement and activity, and femininity with the caring role. Nursing, and other health occupations predominantly undertaken by females, stand for these gendered characteristics. This devalues their role and places them at a distance from real policy debates. Witz (1992, 1994) similarly notes that the 'problem' of nursing is a problem of gender. Nursing is, therefore, seen as 'women's work', which (wrongly) devalues both the task undertaken and the person undertaking it.

It is further argued that male domination of medicine and health care leads to a failure to understand women's health care needs. This is often seen as a historical, and in particular a Victorian, legacy. During the Victorian period the health of women, particularly those in the upper and middle classes who had access to medical care, was defined by male doctors very much in terms of reproduction. Many social and psychological problems experienced by women were therefore attributed to disorders of the sexual organs. Some women were subjected to surgical 'cures' such as the removal of the sexual and reproductive organs (Dally, 1991).

Doyal (1979, 1995) argues that doctors still hold a peculiar view of female health problems, shaped by the belief that men are normal and women abnormal in respect of intellect, emotion and physical functioning. Abnormalities in women are still associated with their reproductive role. Doctors assume that motherhood and the maternal instinct is the main driving force in women's lives, and that a denial of this instinct causes depression and other health problems. They also see women as prone to being neurotic and emotionally unbalanced (Miles, 1991).

Some complain that the medical profession fails to take into account the particular needs of women and actually places them in a position where they can be exploited and even abused (Jenkins, 1985; Roberts, 1992;

Foster, 1995). A commonly cited example is childbirth (Oakley, 1980, 1984). Women feel they have lost control of the birth process, which is treated primarily as an illness. This process, as noted earlier, has been assisted by the use of technology. Most births still take place in controlled conditions in hospital, the seat of medical power and technology. Women have questioned the effectiveness and efficiency of this technology, suspecting its main function to be one of control.

The prevention and treatment of breast cancer is another area where women believe their concerns are not being heeded by doctors (Hann, 1996). For example, radical mastectomy (the removal of the breast) can have a devastating psychological impact on women. There have been criticisms, not only of the inappropriate use of such techniques but of the absence of counselling facilities and the failure to explain beforehand the nature of the operation.

☐ *Feminist solutions*

Feminists blame failures of the health care system on wider social processes of male domination. The overall solution proposed is to change society by strengthening the status of women. Within health care, the position of women could be strengthened through greater participation in medicine and medical decision-making. There has been in recent years a considerable increase in the proportion of women training as doctors, so much so that half of new medical students are now female. However, this alone will not guarantee that women will stay in medicine, or that they will rise to the highest echelons. Flexible career development programmes may help more women to move up the ladder, but other obstacles such as the male-dominated culture of some medical specialities will persist until the proportion of women at senior levels begins to increase significantly.

The situation for women could also be improved by shifting the balance of power in health care away from doctors and towards those professions where women predominate. This could be secured through greater professional autonomy for midwives, nurses, and professions allied to medicine (see Exhibit 3.7). Women are also likely to benefit from moves which give them more choice in health care, and in particular from services which are specially designed to cater for their specific needs such as Well Women Clinics (Foster, 1995) The 'consumer' movement in childbirth is a further aspect of this. Self-help groups offer women a greater opportunity to make decisions about their health (Phillips and Rakusen, 1989). Furthermore, women's health groups represent an important political force with the potential to shape health services (Doyal, 1995; Foster, 1995).

Although attempts to improve the role and status of women in health care must be applauded, it is important to realise that some changes may not provide clear benefits for all women. It is possible that so far the benefits have accrued only to women in the higher social classes, who are more articulate, more vociferous and highly motivated to do something about the problems they experience. This raises the possibility of the emergence of a two-tier system of care, to the disadvantage, perhaps, of working-class women. It must be noted though that the concept of universality of women's experiences has much less attraction for feminists today and as a result the variations in the health experiences of women – relating to ethnic background, social class, disability and so on is increasingly recognised (Doyal, 1995; Graham, 1993).

It is also ironic, as noted in Chapter 1, that many of the illnesses from which women now suffer increasingly have arisen from the adoption of male lifestyles. Many women are also nowadays expected to combine the traditional role as mother/housekeeper with that of worker, which for some is stressful and possibly harmful to their overall health. So the health consequences of a changing role for women are far from straightforward.

■ Iatrogenesis: Illich's thesis

It is one thing to argue that contemporary health care is inefficient, insensitive or misdirected; to argue that the medical establishment is a direct threat to health is far more radical. Yet this is precisely the argument advanced by Illich (1975) in his examination of the nature and extent of iatrogenesis – illness caused by medicine. Illich identifies three dimensions of iatrogenesis: clinical, social and cultural, and each will now be examined in turn.

□ Clinical iatrogenesis

Clinical iatrogenesis occurs when illness is caused by diagnosis or treatment undertaken by medical practitioners. Illich begins by claiming that the successes of modern medicine are overrated. In accordance with those who support the public health approach, he observes that better housing, better nutrition and an improved environment were more effective in reducing mortality and morbidity. He then goes on to argue that a number of aspects of medical treatment are actually useless and ineffective, while others are positively dangerous. He identifies several types of clinical iatrogenesis: diagnostic errors, accidents during the course of treatment, and the side-effects of treatment.

There is much evidence of clinical iatrogenesis. One tends to focus on the high profile cases (such as the misdiagnosis of bone cancers in South Birmingham, uncovered in 1992). Yet errors are not confined to isolated

---

Exhibit 3.7   *Nurses and midwives: challenges to medicine?*

Nursing

The nursing profession has long complained that the skills of nurses are being under-utilised, that nursing is too often subservient to medicine, and that the status of nursing as a profession should be raised. However, in recent years a number of developments have taken place which may affect the future role and status of nursing (see Schober, 1995). The reform of nurse education and training – *Project 2000* – is one of the most significant changes. Apprentice-style training for entrants to nursing has been replaced with an eighteen-month common foundation course, followed by specialisation in a particular area of nursing (adult, mental health, learning disability, children). Trainees are now regarded as supernumeraries rather than an 'extra pair of hands' on the ward. At the same time nursing schools have been integrated with institutions of higher education (HE). Although the implementation of the reforms has been far from smooth – the manpower implications of the shift to supernumerary status and the task of integrating nurse education with HE were particularly problematic – there have been many positive aspects which bode well for the future. In particular the status of nurse education has been raised. It is no longer as subordinate to the day-to-day staffing needs of the service, and nurses themselves have greater opportunities to influence and shape nurse education. Furthermore, the focus on education has moved beyond the preparation of trainees. As with medicine (see Exhibit 2.4) there has been a greater emphasis in recent years upon continuing education – ensuring that qualified nurses update their skills and knowledge.

Another key development was the creation of the UK Central Council for Nursing, Midwifery and Health Visiting (UKCC) in 1983. This body, which replaced a number of separate statutory professional bodies, is responsible for nurse registration and deregistration in cases of misconduct. The UKCC is also responsible for establishing and improving standards of training and conduct. Among other activities, the UKCC (1992a) has drawn up a code of professional practice to act as a guide to nurses. Though widely welcomed as an effort to set principles of professional conduct, the code was criticised for being too general and open to wide interpretation (see Schober, 1995, p. 96). It has since been supplemented with more specific guidelines for professional practice (UKCC, 1996)

Further developments include the transfer to nurses of tasks normally regarded as the responsibility of doctors. This trend has been driven primarily by the need to reduce the workload (particularly of junior doctors) rather than the demands of nurses (Read and Graves, 1994; UKCC, 1992b). Nurses increasingly perform routine tasks normally undertaken by junior doctors.

⟶

Exhibit 3.7 continued

⟶

But they also are taking on more important clinical roles in relation to the assessment and treatment of patients (Kendrick, Weir and Rosser, 1995; Salvage, 1992). Nurse Practitioners, of which there are only a few hundred in England and Wales at present, can examine patients, prescribe drugs, order tests and stitch minor wounds. Clinical Nurse Specialists possess expertise which may relate to specific conditions, such as diabetes for example, or to specific technical procedures. There is also a small but growing number of nurses who perform minor operations under the supervision of doctors.

Other changes are occurring in the role of nurses. For example, the emergence of primary nursing – where nurses are given broad responsibilities for the care of particular patients – and the creation of nursing development units where patient care is directly managed by nurses (see Salvage and Wright, 1995). Furthermore, the promotion of community-based care has implications for nurses working in this setting, leading not only to an increase in their workload, but in the technical complexity of the tasks they must perform (see also Chapters 9 and 10).

Midwifery

The Royal College of Midwives has for many years argued that women should have the right to choose a midwife-led approach to pregnancy, which in contrast to the medical approach emphasises the normality of childbirth. Studies have indicated that midwife-managed care for healthy women is both clinically effective and enhances women's satisfaction with maternity care (Turnbull *et al.*, 1996).This view has recently attracted official support. In 1992, the Social Services Committee (House of Commons, 1992) called for greater choice for women and expressed support for the midwife-led approach. The Department of Health then established its own committee of enquiry. Its report *Changing Childbirth* also endorsed change (DoH, 1993b), proposing that mothers should be actively involved in decisions about care, that good communication and dissemination of accurate information were essential to facilitate choice, and that maternity services should be based on clinical effectiveness. It also stated that there should be greater continuity of care, that there was a need for a lead professional to give a substantial part of the care which for normal pregnancies should be the midwife. The government accepted the findings of *Changing Childbirth* and subsequently promoted a number of initiatives within the NHS with a view to implementing its recommendations. These initiatives have been broadly welcomed though there have been warnings about the pace of change (Allen, Bourke Dowling and Williams, 1997).

cases, and there is a growing body of more systematic evidence which provides considerable support for Illich's argument. Misdiagnosis appears to be a serious problem. In one study, autopsies confirmed clinical diagnoses in only 61 per cent of the cases (Cameron and McCoogan, 1981). Another analysis found that doctors had failed to diagnose treatable diseases in 13 per cent of cases (Mercer and Talbot, 1985). More recently, a study of the diagnosis of PVS (persistent vegetative state) discovered that 43 per cent of patients had been misdiagnosed (Andrews *et al.*, 1996). Another survey found that three-quarters of doctors did not have sufficient knowledge to read an electrocardiogram (ECG), with 59 per cent of consultants failing to interpret findings properly (Montgomery *et al.*, 1994).

Evidence concerning illness directly caused by medical diagnosis and treatment is more difficult to obtain, though there are plenty of case studies of adverse effects in drug therapies – as with Opren and Thalidomide (Collier, 1989). Another approach is to examine cases of medical negligence. According to a study by the Medical Defence Union, a quarter of medical negligence cases won by patients against GPs were directly related to errors in prescribing, monitoring or administering medicine (Mihill, 1996). There is evidence of clinical iatrogenesis in other countries too. The Harvard Medical Practice Study (1990), for example, found that 4 per cent of admissions to hospital in New York experienced adverse events. In a quarter of these cases doctors had actually been negligent. More recently an American study found that almost one in five hospital patients had experienced at least one adverse event leading to longer hospital stays and increased costs (Andrews *et al.*, 1997).

Evidence concerning the extent of clinical iatrogenesis in the UK was revealed by the report of a National Confidential Enquiry into Perioperative Deaths (NCEPOD) (Buck, Devlin and Lunn, 1987). The overall death rate from surgery was low, at 0.7 per cent, and most of these deaths were due to the fact that the patients in question were elderly or suffered from other medical conditions. Nevertheless, the inquiry found that death was avoidable in over a fifth of the cases. Surgical intervention was an associated factor in 30 per cent of the deaths, and was wholly responsible for 7 per cent of deaths. The inquiry found evidence of inappropriate operations, poor pre-operative management, a failure to apply knowledge, and in some cases operations being undertaken by inexperienced and under-qualified doctors. In addition, 2 per cent of deaths were associated with anaesthesia. Subsequent reports by NCEPOD have continued to identify shortcomings in care, though they have also detailed how organisational and external factors can affect both death rates and the quality of care (Camplin, Lunn and Devlin, 1992; Camplin *et al.*, 1995). Meanwhile, more specific enquiries have detected serious problems; a confidential enquiry into deaths in normal babies during birth found that 40 per cent were linked to suboptimal care (DoH, 1995a).

□ *Social and cultural iatrogenesis*

Turning from clinical to social iatrogenesis, Illich argues that health is undermined by the impact of medical organisation on social life. Illness is created as more and more social and individual problems are labelled as medical problems (see also Zola, 1975). Illich argues that this process of medicalisation is harmful because it gives the medical profession enormous power to judge others. As individual conditions and experiences are defined as illnesses, they fall within the judgement and control of the medical profession. Social iatrogenesis is therefore a kind of medical imperialism, with doctors identifying illness in ever more aspects of an individual's life. A further reason why Illich believes medicalisation to be harmful is that it moves the focus away from activities which deal more effectively with the problems faced by society and the individual. It also stifles lay initiatives which otherwise might arise to tackle these problems.

The third type of iatrogenesis identified by Illich is cultural. Medicine seeks to alleviate pain. Most people would agree that this is a noble aim. However, Illich argues that pain is an important part of human experience. To overcome suffering, to cope with pain, to face and accept death, are not necessarily negative experiences. By denying these experiences and turning them into technical matters, medicine therefore undermines the individual's personal capacities. Moreover, because most pain and suffering in industrial society is man-made, there are wider implications. Illich argues that the alleviation of pain and suffering leads to the neutralisation of political forces which might otherwise arise to prevent the underlying causes of illness.

□ *Illich's solutions*

Attempts to assert political control over medicine and therefore redirect health care are doomed to failure, according to Illich. Moves to increase consumer control of health care and to impose a more rational organisation of health care will, in his view, be ineffective in reducing medical power and may actually worsen the situation. He argues against a public health approach, because it implies that individuals are presumed ill until proved otherwise, and because medical influence will spread to other areas of social and economic life, leading to more social iatrogenesis.

Illich does accept that health and health care may be improved by focusing on equity, which in turn raises questions about the social and economic causes of illness. But he goes on to argue that iatrogenesis will not be checked if the concern with equity is confined to matters of health service provision. The only real solution is therefore to limit the scope of professional monopolies and to extend personal responsibility for health. In his own words 'that society which can reduce professional intervention to the minimum will provide the best conditions for health' (Illich, 1975, p. 274).

☐ *Challenges to Illich*

Illich's thesis arises out of a more general critique of industrialisation, institutionalisation and professional power in modern societies. His arguments have not gone unchallenged (see Horrobin, 1977). Doctors argue that much clinical iatrogenesis is an inevitable consequence of the advancement of medical science. According to this view, the frontiers of knowledge can only be moved forward by attempting new treatments, some of which may prove initially to be harmful to the patient. This is the price of long-term success. The failure to try new therapies, doctors argue, would have kept medicine in the Dark Ages.

A further counter-argument is that much clinical iatrogenesis is due to patient ignorance. For example, the failure to follow medical advice properly, particularly in the taking of drugs, is a well-known source of adverse reactions. From this viewpoint, clinical iatrogenesis may be reduced through doctors educating patients and communicating with them more effectively, increasing rather than reducing the scope of professional responsibility.

Another point is that Illich ignores the positive aspects of medicine. Though iatrogenesis has to be recognised and reduced, modern medicine has contributed to the improvements in health, particularly by improving the quality of life for many sufferers. Illich's thesis can therefore be criticised as being polemical and unbalanced in that he does not appear to accept that modern medicine has any redeeming features.

Illich is criticised for being utopian. The processes of industrialisation, institutionalisation and professionalisation, which are the main causes of the problems he identifies, cannot simply be rolled back. It could be argued that professionalism combined with self-regulation and peer review are the most effective safeguards against malpractice in an industrialised society, given the complex division of labour and the diversity of knowledge and expertise. It may be more fruitful to reform the professions rather than undermine or bypass them. The introduction of systems of quality control and medical audit, discussed in later chapters, may be less radical but yet provide a more practical way of reducing clinical iatrogenesis.

■ Conclusion

The various perspectives explored in this chapter, along with the critiques of orthodox medicine discussed previously, highlight a range of problems and issues facing modern health care systems. These include: a lack of accountability in health care; the dominant role of orthodox medicine and the medical profession; the lack of responsiveness to consumer wants and patient needs; thorny questions of priorities and rationing; the need to evaluate the quality and cost-effectiveness of health care in general, and the contribution of new technologies in particular; the problems of health inequalities; and the need to tackle the wider social, economic and environmental causes of ill-health. All health care systems in the developed world are confronting these issues and developing their own particular response to them.

Critical perspectives on health care have provided a wealth of ideas for would-be reformers of the health care system. Some of the ideas and arguments may be regarded as extreme – certainly to defenders of the status quo. Some are flawed and have attracted justified criticism. But this has not stopped them from infiltrating debates about the future of health care, nor has it prevented policy-makers from drawing on these ideas when reforming health care policies and programmes, as we shall see in subsequent chapters.

■ *Chapter 4* ■

The Evolution of the British Health Care System

An understanding of how the British health care system evolved is necessary to place contemporary developments in context. We begin by looking at the system of health care which existed before the emergence of the NHS. This is followed by an examination of how and why the NHS was created. The experience of the NHS in the post-Second World War period up to the Royal Commission's inquiry in the late 1970s is then considered. Finally, there is an analysis of the distinctive approach of Margaret Thatcher's Conservative government which posed a challenge to the ideas which underpinned the postwar health care system in Britain.

■ The health care system before the NHS

Before the creation of the NHS, Britain's health care system was a rather disorganised and complex mixture of private and public services (Webster, 1988; Abel-Smith, 1964). The private sector consisted of voluntary hospitals, private practitioners, and other voluntary and commercial organisations. The public sector comprised municipal hospitals and community health services run by local government. In addition, local government was responsible for sanitary and environmental health services and health-related services such as housing. Let us now look in more detail at these sectors and how they evolved.

□ *The private sector: voluntary hospitals*

The voluntary hospitals were established by philanthropy or by public subscription. Most were created in the eighteenth and nineteenth centuries, although some were older, having been founded in the early Middle Ages. Many voluntary hospitals, however, were of more recent origin: of those existing in 1938 over a third had been founded after 1911 (Webster, 1988, p. 2).

Traditionally, the voluntary hospitals gave their care free of charge, reflecting the charitable motives behind their foundation. When originally founded the prestige of these hospitals was such that doctors often waived their fee for the privilege of being associated with them. The doctors would make a living by treating the rich philanthropists whose contributions supported the hospital. The wealthy were treated at home rather than in hospital. Hospitals catered mainly for the less well-off who could not afford to pay for treatment. Yet admission to these hospitals was quite selective: the very poor and those with infectious diseases were frequently denied access (Abel-Smith, 1964).

By the outbreak of the Second World War in 1939, the voluntary hospitals had changed considerably. Only about a third of their income now came from charitable contributions. They began to charge patients for services to a much greater extent. Patients, in turn, took out health insurance or subscription plans to cover these payments. Voluntary hospitals continued to face financial problems, despite efforts to raise funds. Yet they retained their prestigious status, and continued to make a major contribution to health care. In 1938 one in three patients still received their treatment in a voluntary hospital.

☐ *General practice*

Prior to the creation of the NHS, general practitioners (GPs) were private practitioners who charged a fee for their services. In Victorian times the fear of being unable to pay doctors' fees led to the development of club practice. The more affluent sections of the working class would subscribe to friendly societies, who in turn hired the services of GPs for their members. Club practice covered around a third of the working class by the end of the nineteenth century (Honigsbaum, 1990). However, concern arose that such schemes tended to exclude those not in work, such as the unemployed, married women, children and the elderly. Meanwhile, doctors became increasingly worried about lay interference in medical practice and poor remuneration, evident in some club practices.

In 1911 the Liberal government introduced its own plans for general practice in the form of the National Insurance Act. This led to the provision of sickness benefits, free GP services and free drugs for the employed working class. Employers, workers and the government each contributed to the compulsory scheme. The scheme was administered by local insurance committees, which included the representatives of approved societies (friendly societies and industrial insurance offices and trade unions), local authorities and GPs (Honigsbaum, 1979).

The government's initial plans angered the British Medical Association (BMA). The BMA believed that remuneration for GPs was inadequate. It also feared that GPs would be subject to the same kind of interference experienced under the club practice system. This fear was understandable, given that approved societies had a majority on the insurance committees which administered the scheme. The government did make several compromises, removing the power of insurance committees over doctors' remuneration, and establishing the principle that patients would be free to choose their doctor. These concessions, coupled with the fear of an alternative scenario – a state medical service employing salaried GPs – won the day (Brand, 1965).

By the outbreak of the Second World War, 43 per cent of the population were covered by the National Health Insurance (NHI) scheme, and 90 per cent of GPs participated in it (Webster, 1988, p. 11). This scheme marked a new departure in state intervention in health care. Yet it only applied to the services of GPs, not specialist hospital services (except for the treatment of tuberculosis). Moreover, the scheme excluded the unemployed and dependants, such as married women and children.

☐ *Other voluntary organisations*

The health care system prior to the creation of the NHS involved an array of other voluntary health care organisations. As well as running hospitals, voluntary organisations provided community health services. They increasingly worked in partnership with local authorities in fields such as child welfare, maternity, aftercare, district nursing, and mental and physical handicap.

☐ *The public sector: municipal health services*

Even before the creation of the NHS, the public sector had the largest share of hospital-based care. On the eve of the Second World War, two-thirds of patients were being treated in local authority municipal hospitals. Local government operated a considerable and diverse network of hospitals. These included the isolation hospitals for infectious diseases, hospitals specialising in the treatment of tuberculosis, maternity hospitals and mental hospitals. From 1875 onwards local government had the power to run general hospitals, but few authorities actually did so.

The local authorities also inherited a hospital service which had grown out of the nineteenth century system of relief known as the Poor Law (Hodgkinson, 1967). This notorious system, introduced by the Poor Law Amendment Act (1834), effectively institutionalised poverty. Local Poor Law authorities established workhouses where relief was given on the principle of 'less eligibility' in an attempt to discourage the poor from seeking help. This system, despite its defects and inhumanity, actually exposed a high level of illness among the workhouse inmates. This had two important consequences. First, the development of publicly-funded health services in the form of Poor Law infirmaries, which developed later into separate institutions for the 'sick poor'. In addition, the poor were eligible for free GP services, following a rigorous means test. Second, the recognition of the cost of the 'sick poor' led to a series of inquiries into the environmental (but not the economic) causes of their condition, such as Edwin Chadwick's famous report on the sanitary condition of the labouring population (Chadwick, 1842). These inquiries led in turn to the development of public health legislation, beginning with the Public Health Act of 1848 which gave localities the power to promote a healthier environment.

Although public health legislation was introduced at national level, it was down to local government to implement the statutes, enforce the regulations and develop public health services. Local health committees were set up to administer this process. Local medical officers of health (MOHs) were also appointed to act as guardians of public health. Gradually, local authorities began to provide a wide range of health-related services. These included water supply, sanitation, food and hygiene inspection, and pollution control, and later housing as well as personal and community health services such as school health services, midwifery, community nursing, and child welfare clinics.

The system of public health administration grew up separately from the Poor Law hospital network. The latter fell under the responsibility of the Poor Law Boards until their abolition in 1929. After this date most of the former Poor Law hospitals became municipal hospitals under the control of local public health authorities. However, many chronically ill people continued to reside in institutions under the control of the Public Assistance Committees which took over the remainder of the hospitals.

Suggestions had been made on a number of occasions with regard to integrating health services and local authority hospital, community and environmental health services. In 1909 members of the Royal Commission on the Poor Laws produced a dissenting minority report which argued for a unified state health service run by local authorities (Cd 4499, 1909). The minority report, which was considered too radical, also sought to establish the principle of free health care for the poor as a right, though it fell far short of recommending a comprehensive state health service, available to all and free at point of delivery, an idea widely accepted only three decades later.

☐ The acceptance of a comprehensive state health system

Criticism of the British health care system began to accumulate after the First World War. Health care was fragmented into hospital, community and public health services. There was little coordination of health care to tackle the complex needs of vulnerable groups, such as children and the elderly. Moreover, access to health care was limited for many of these groups. The growth of health insurance and charging for hospital services meant that, for many, health care depended on ability to pay. Furthermore, access to high quality health care varied throughout the country and was apparently unrelated to the level of need (Political and Economic Planning, 1937). According to some, the mismatch between geographical need and availability has been exaggerated (Powell, 1992). Nevertheless, it was widely believed at the time that some form of national planning was required to relate the need for services more closely to availability.

A series of reports in the 1920s and 1930s exposed the problems of the health services and charted future paths for reform. The Dawson report of 1920 argued for the integration of preventive and curative medicine under a single health authority, which would coordinate a network of local hospitals and health centres. The report stated that the provision of the best medical care should be available to all, but did not elaborate on the question of how this would be financed (Cmd 693, 1920).

A further contribution to the debate was made by the Royal Commission on National Health Insurance, which reported in 1926 against a background of concern about access to specialist medical services. It urged the approved societies which operated the NHI scheme to pool their surplus resources to fund such care. It also indicated that the long-term future lay in direct funding of health care by the state (Cmd 2596, 1926).

The failure of the health care system to cater for the needs of those requiring specialist care was also a concern in a report by the BMA in 1929 (BMA, 1929). This report argued that NHI should be expanded to cover specialist services provided by the hospitals. It suggested that the scheme should be extended to the families of insured workers. But the BMA plan was not fully comprehensive: it intended to exclude the wealthier classes from the scheme. The issue of how the higher cost of the extended service would be funded was also side-stepped by this report.

The interwar period, with its high rates of unemployment, created conditions that undermined the operation of the NHI system. In 1932 alone, 200 000 workers lost their right to the benefits of the national health insurance scheme because of unemployment. There was also growing criticism of the insurance companies in relation to the system of health insurance, mainly from trade unions and GPs (Honigsbaum, 1989).

It is often thought that the Second World War, which led to a dramatic expansion in government intervention in health services, was a major reason behind the creation of the NHS. The government created an Emergency Hospital Service (EHS) to coordinate the patchwork quilt of public hospitals and voluntary hospitals. The task of organising the EHS, according to Abel-Smith (1964, p. 440), 'brought home to all concerned the failings of Britain's hospital system'. The experience of the EHS was no doubt useful in showing how the state could coordinate the health care system. But it is generally accepted that the irrationality and inadequacy of the British health care system was evident long before the scheme was created. There was a general consensus about the need for some form of national health service well before hostilities began.

■ The creation of a National Health Service

□ *Towards a comprehensive health system*

In the years before the Second World War, the government actively considered the integration of existing health services. In 1936 the Minister of Health asked his Chief Medical Officer (CMO) to report on the feasibility of a comprehensive health care system. The CMO recommended that local authorities should provide the basis for any comprehensive scheme. From then on the Ministry of Health began to develop policy ideas along these lines. These plans included transferring responsibility for NHI to local authorities and extending coverage of this scheme to dependants.

Such long-term plans were stopped by the need to address short-term emergencies. The first emergency was the financial crisis which hit many voluntary hospitals, including the London teaching hospitals, in 1938. The second was the outbreak of war, which led to the creation of the EHS, discussed above.

During the war, the idea of a comprehensive health service became bound up with the broader aim of reconstructing Britain. A major landmark was the ministerial announcement of October 1941, which set out the government's intention to create a comprehensive hospital service after the war. It was not clear at this stage that the service would be free. Moreover, there was no question of voluntary hospitals being taken into public ownership, though it was expected that they would cooperate closely with local authorities to produce a more coherent pattern of hospital provision.

Meanwhile, the medical profession was busy formulating its own plans for a new health service. In 1940 the BMA established a Medical Planning Commission to consider the future development of medical services. The Commission produced an interim report two years later which set out many features which were eventually incorporated in the NHS (BMA, 1942). These included the regionalisation of hospital administration; a prohibition of full-time salaried service for GPs; and the remuneration of GPs, mainly by a capitation fee (a fixed payment for every patient registered with them). The Commission supported an extension of NHI to pay for hospital and community health services, but did not come to any clear conclusions about the coverage of the new scheme. Later the BMA came out in favour of a scheme which provided for the whole community rather than just sections of it (Grey-Turner and Sutherland, 1982, p. 38).

Then came the Beveridge report (Cmd 6404, 1942). In setting out a broad framework for the postwar welfare state, Beveridge supported the idea of a comprehensive health service, available to all. Yet the final version of the Beveridge report left open the precise financial and organisational details of the service. In the event, it was these detailed matters which produced the most controversy.

☐ *The shape of the new health system*

In contrast with the broad agreement on the need for a comprehensive health service, there were widely differing opinions surrounding the organisational and financial principles of such a service. The Ministry of Health favoured a municipally-controlled health service, as set out in a confidential memorandum of 1943 named (after the Minister of Health) the Brown Plan. This plan gave local government the responsibility of organising services and sought to bring general practitioners and the voluntary hospitals under the wing of local government. The GPs were not happy with this arrangement. Their discontent was shared by a number of local authorities depressed by the prospect of running such an expensive new service. The voluntary hospitals were also unhappy, fearing the loss of independence implied by the prospect of central government funding being channelled through the local authorities. In short, the Brown Plan pleased no one.

The government offered a compromise. A White Paper containing revised proposals was eventually published in 1944 (Cmd 6502, 1944). Under this scheme, health services would be comprehensive and free at the point of delivery, and GPs would come under the control of a Central Medical Board. They would not be directly under the influence of local government except where they worked in health centres run by local authorities. GPs working in such health centres would be salaried, as would new entrants to the profession, and other GPs could be salaried if they wished. Private practice was permissible and the right to buy and sell practices was retained, though some restrictions would be imposed on these activities. Finally, the hospital service was to be operated by joint local authority boards responsible for controlling municipal hospitals and coordinating the activities of the hospital network in the area.

The doctors, fearing a loss of autonomy, rejected the White Paper. Their lobbying was effective in that all the major proposals were dropped, including the establishment of the Central Medical Board. The government agreed that the responsibility for GP services would remain with local committees on which the GPs would have a majority. The local authorities' control over doctors working in health centres was eroded to the point that their function was to be little more than that of landlord. The provision that doctors working in health centres would be salaried was also dropped.

The local authorities also obtained concessions. The joint boards that would have taken control of municipal hospitals were subsequently confined to a local planning role, leaving control in the hands of individual local authorities. This made it politically possible to allow medical representation on these boards, a move which had been resisted strongly by local authorities as long as the boards had control over municipal hospitals. In addition, expert regional planning bodies were proposed. This was mainly to satisfy the demands of the voluntary hospitals, in particular the more prestigious teaching hospitals, which had lobbied for a regional tier to advise on planning and developing specialised medical services.

A further White Paper embodying the revised proposals was planned, but meanwhile Labour had left the war coalition government. This second White Paper was suppressed before the 1945 election and, as a result of the Conservative Party's defeat at the polls, was never published. Even so, some of its proposals reappeared in the Labour government's plans, namely the regional structure and the separate local administration of GP and hospital services, discussed below.

☐ Bevan's plan

The 1945 General Election produced a clear victory for the Labour Party. Clement Attlee, the new Prime Minister, appointed Aneurin Bevan as Minister for Health, giving him the task of rescuing the plans for a new health service. Despite the support within his own party for a comprehensive health service based on local authority control, Bevan opted for nationalisation of the entire hospital sector within a tripartite system of provision.

This option was chosen not on ideological but on practical grounds. As Honigsbaum (1989, p. 95) correctly notes, 'far from being a dogmatic socialist, Bevan proved to be a pragmatic reformer'. Yet there was considerable opposition to his plan. Bevan was challenged by his Cabinet colleague Herbert Morrison, a staunch defender of local government interests, who argued against the nationalisation of the municipal hospitals. Bevan won this battle, but local authorities continued to have a significant role in health care through their provision of community services, personal social services and public health functions.

The other main source of opposition to Bevan's plan came from the medical profession, particularly the GPs, whose views were forcefully put by the BMA. Many GPs were alarmed not only about the principle of nationalisation, but also about proposals to ban the sale of practices and to control the geographical distribution of new entrants to general practice. Their biggest fear, however, was the prospect of a salaried medical service. In an attempt to attract their support Bevan permitted GPs to remain as independent contractors. They would be allowed to provide services to NHS patients on the basis of a contract negotiated between the Ministry of Health and the profession's representatives, and would be paid mainly by capitation payments. A part-time salary element for all GPs was included in Bevan's original plan, though this was later restricted to new GPs for a limited period only. As a further concession, which was instrumental in securing the cooperation of the profession, Bevan agreed to a ban on full-time salaried medical services.

The interests of the GPs as independent contractors were also protected by the creation of a separate administrative branch. It was agreed that GP contracts, and those of dentists, pharmacists and opticians, would be administered by executive councils. These bodies would consist of part-time appointees nominated by the Minister of Health, the local authorities, and by the independent contractor professions themselves, with the last of these groups providing half the members.

The local authorities and the executive councils formed two parts of the tripartite structure (see Figure 4.1). The third was the hospital service which, with the exception of the teaching hospitals (see below), had a two-tier structure. The top tier consisted of Regional Hospital Boards (RHBs) responsible for the overall planning, coordination and supervision of hospital services within a large area. The RHBs were appointed by the Minister of Health after consultation with local authorities and the medical profession. The second tier, responsible for the actual running of the local hospital service, consisted of Hospital Management Committees (HMCs). The HMC members were appointed by the RHB, following consultation with local authorities, the medical profession, and voluntary associations.

The prestigious teaching hospitals were administered by a separate board of governors appointed by and accountable to the Minister of Health. Though the hospitals themselves did not regard their position as being privileged, the treatment given to the élite hospitals was seen by the rest of the hospital sector as favourable. This appears to have been part of a strategy by Bevan to buy off the medical élite – the top consultants – who worked in these hospitals. The consultants were also courted with generous salaries, merit awards, the retention of pay beds within NHS hospitals, and the option of combining private practice with NHS work.

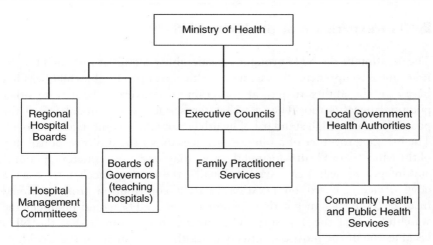

Figure 4.1   *The original National Health Service structure (England and Wales), 1948–74*

The strategy was apparently successful in promoting the support of the consultants. Hence the famous comment attributed to Bevan that he 'stuffed their mouths with gold'.

Aside from these concessions, the consultants tended to take a more favourable view of the NHS than their colleagues in general practice. Many consultants believed that a comprehensive state health system would lead to a more efficient and more technically advanced service. The GPs, on the other hand, were more concerned about the threat to their independence. These differences were reflected in the divisions between the BMA, a stout defender of GPs' interests (and which was strongly opposed to Bevan's initial plan), and the Royal Colleges, representing the consultants' views, which were more supportive. Indeed, the BMA only agreed to advise its members to join the NHS at the 'eleventh hour', following a series of concessions from Bevan and several ballots of its membership. Senior members of the Royal Colleges – such as Lord Moran, the president of the Royal College of Physicians – were active behind the scenes in building support for the NHS and in promoting a compromise between Bevan and the GPs (Webster, 1988, p. 116).

Aneurin Bevan is popularly remembered as the father of the NHS. Yet as Honigsbaum (1989, p. 217) has observed 'Bevan had the good fortune to spearhead a movement that already had force'. Yet one should not belittle Bevan's contribution. His vision, skill and strategy made possible the political settlement that allowed the NHS to emerge. Moreover, this political settlement forged an organisational structure, which, though flawed in many respects, was to last almost thirty years.

■ The experience of the NHS: 1948–79

The creation of the NHS brought considerable benefits. It provided for the first time a comprehensive system of health care, open to all, which was not based on the ability to pay at the point of delivery. There were other potential benefits too. The fact that the service was national raised the possibility that a high standard of health care could become available to all. The bringing together of a range of services under the direct responsibility of the Ministry of Health created the potential for a more coherent, planned and integrated health care system. Finally, the funding mechanism for the new service – based on taxation (with a contribution from National Insurance funds) – meant that spending on the NHS would be under the watchful eye of the Treasury. This arrangement ensured that the NHS became one of the most cost-effective health care systems in the world.

The NHS became a popular institution. For the generation that lived under the previous system, it represented a major achievement. It was similarly popular with the generation that grew up with the welfare state. However, despite its popularity, the NHS has faced a number of problems during its lifetime and has not always tackled these successfully (Webster, 1988; 1996). By the late 1970s the situation became so serious that even the considerable achievements of the NHS appeared to be under threat. The NHS came to be widely perceived as in a constant state of crisis (Haywood and Alaszewski, 1980). This impression continued throughout the 1980s and into the 1990s.

Some of the difficulties facing the NHS plagued it from its earliest days, arising from its original structure. Others were new, a reflection that the challenges facing the NHS, and indeed the expectations of the service, had changed since its creation. Another set of problems was caused, at least in part, by botched attempts to reform and reorganise the service, while others were caused by changes in the wider political and economic environment.

☐ *Problems with the structure of the NHS*

As noted earlier, the original structure of the NHS was tripartite, comprising the family practitioner services (GPs, dentists, pharmacists and opticians) administered by executive councils; local authority community health services (such as community nursing and midwifery), personal social services and public health; and the nationalised hospital service.

It soon became evident that the original NHS structure was flawed. The major problems were overlap, duplication and lack of coordination between the three parts of the structure (Ministry of Health, 1959; 1963; BMA, 1962). During the 1960s the structure came under increasing pressure, leading ultimately to government proposals to reorganise the service (Ministry of Health, 1968; DHSS, 1970). After some deliberation, and two changes of government, new proposals were brought forward (DHSS, 1971; Cmnd 5055, 1972) and a reorganisation eventually implemented in 1974.

The new structure embodied three tiers of health service management below the Department of Health and Social Security (DHSS) (which had succeeded the Ministry of Health in 1968): at regional, area and district level. New health authorities, responsible for planning and development of services were established at regional and area level. Like the RHBs and HMCs which preceded them, these bodies were accountable to, and appointed by, ministerial authority.

The reorganisation did not solve the structural problems of the service. The family practitioner services supplied by GPs, dentists, pharmacists and opticians were not fully integrated. They remained separate, under new family practitioner committees (FPCs) which replaced the former executive councils. The NHS became responsible for community health services, transferred from local government. But the latter retained responsibility for environmental health services and social care. So there remained three separate agencies involved in the provision of state health care. Tripartism proved remarkably resilient.

The new NHS structure was criticised for having surplus tiers of management and requiring too many administrators. New systems of planning and management which accompanied these organisational changes were similarly criticised. These were held responsible for slow decision-making and a lack of accountability. Yet the search for an 'organisational fix' (Klein, 1983, p. 90) continued. Despite the problems associated with the reorganisation, policy-makers still placed their faith in structural reform (McLachlan, 1990) giving rise to a further reorganisation in 1982.

☐ *Accountability, control and planning*

The problems of the NHS went beyond the original structure. It became clear that there was a fundamental contradiction at the heart of the NHS with respect to the powers and responsibilities of Health Ministers. Health Ministers had full responsibility for health policy, but had little direct control over the activities of the NHS. It was well known that power over service developments was concentrated at local level, in the hands of doctors, who were not accountable to ministers for their actions or for the resources they used. At the end of the day the medical profession had an effective veto power over the implementation of policies. But health authorities, responsible to and appointed by ministerial authority (yet drawn in part from local government and the health professions) could not be relied upon to impose policies designed by central government. (Haywood and Alaszewski, 1980; Elcock and Haywood, 1980).

Ministers nevertheless attempted to influence service developments through the health authorities. Instead of clarifying the goals of the service, ministers preferred to emphasise the importance of specific service developments. They began with the Hospital Plan of 1962 (Cmnd 1604, 1962). This was essentially a plan for capital expenditure in the hospital sector, though it did set out norms for the provision of beds for various medical specialities. In the following year a similar plan was introduced for the community health services (Cmnd 1973, 1963).

A more elaborate planning process for the NHS was introduced in 1976. Ministers explicitly set out their priorities, emphasising the so-called 'Cinderella services' (the services for the elderly, the mentally ill, and the mentally and physically handicapped), primary care, and preventive medicine (DHSS, 1976a, 1977). This guidance was filtered down to the lowest tiers of the NHS, which formulated their own plans within this framework. These plans were then passed back up the structure to enable the DHSS to monitor the consistency of the local and national plans and the overall development of services.

The planning process was persuasive rather than directive. Health authorities (and the medical profession at local level) were thus able to resist a dramatic shift in priorities. The planning process was also criticised as being too cumbersome, and involving too many advisory and planning bodies. This prolonged the planning process, confused the setting of objectives, and inhibited the achievement of new priorities.

☐ Funding, efficiency and resource allocation

Since its creation, the resourcing of the NHS has been a constant issue of debate. The NHS had hardly begun its life before it was faced by a financial crisis (Webster, 1988). In the 1950s the Conservative government, worried about the resources consumed by the service, established the Guillebaud inquiry into the NHS. The report of this inquiry (Cmd 9663, 1956) was unexpectedly favourable, concluding that spending on the NHS was not as extravagant as some had suggested, and that in many respects it provided good value for money. The Guillebaud report also pointed out that there were deficiencies in some services and that this required more spending rather than less.

The Guillebaud report strengthened the case of those who argued for greater NHS expenditure. Health expenditure began to grow both in real terms and as a proportion of national expenditure. This continued until the late 1970s, when the government attempted to exert a much tighter control over public expenditure in view of the deepening economic crisis. The NHS, like many other public services, faced financial restraint. This in turn focused attention on the need for greater efficiency in order to maximise the use of existing resources.

At the same time it also became evident that something had to be done about the distribution of resources. Ministers were concerned to redirect resources to 'neglected' groups, such as the elderly, in line with their priorities. Also there was an increasing emphasis on geographical inequalities in health service funding. In the 1970s the highest-spending NHS regions spent around two-thirds more per head than the lowest-spending regions (Griffiths, 1971). In an attempt to iron out these inequalities, and to ensure that health authorities received a budget more appropriate to the health needs they faced, the Labour government introduced the RAWP (Resource Allocation Working Party) formula in 1977 (Mays and Bevan, 1987).

RAWP sought to allocate resources on the basis of a formula reflecting each region's relative health care needs. First, an assessment of relative need was established based on indicators of illness, such as regional population size and structure, standardised mortality ratios for specific conditions and so on. Second, a target level of funding for each region was calculated by dividing the resources available by the estimate of relative need. Third, in view of the likely disruption caused by changing the funding system immediately, budgets were allocated in such a way as to move the regions towards their target funding levels. Hence, over a number of years, those regions below their target received a greater increase in their resources than those regions over target.

Scotland, Northern Ireland and Wales had their own equivalents of RAWP which similarly sought to relate budgets to indicators of need. Yet while the case for a more rational allocation system was widely accepted, there was much concern about the operation of these schemes in practice (Goldacre and Harris, 1980; Radical Statistics Health Group, 1977). This centred mainly on the accuracy of the indicators of need within the redistributive formula. There was particular criticism of the use of standardised mortality ratios. Many observers regarded morbidity data as being a better indicator of the need for health services, while others argued that indicators of deprivation provided a better measure given the relationship between poverty and ill-health.

The formula was also attacked for failing to account for the different costs facing each region (and each district therein). Some modifications were made to the formula to reflect the higher costs of delivering services in London, teaching hospitals, supra-regional specialties (provided for the benefit of populations in more than one region), and cross-boundary flows (the treatment of patients from another region). Despite these changes,

RAWP was still regarded by many as a rather blunt instrument which in times of financial stringency could have serious effects on services in those districts which lost out in the redistributive process.

Finally, there was the related question of health inequalities and the access to health services. The NHS had been created as a free service. Yet despite the removal of financial barriers to care, social class differences in health status persisted. It was also alleged that the provision of health services favoured the middle classes, and that the working classes faced problems of access to services. The Labour government of the 1970s responded to increasing concern by setting up a working party under Sir Douglas Black, to examine health inequalities (see Chapter 12).

□ Industrial action, professional power and the consumer

The 1970s saw a marked deterioration in industrial relations in the health service, reflecting general trends in British society. The government became embroiled in pay disputes with all classes of NHS staff: nurses, doctors and ancillary workers. In addition, the government faced the threat of industrial action from hospital doctors (and some of the unions representing ancillary workers) over the issue of pay beds in the NHS.

Industrial action in the NHS was not new. In 1965 GPs had threatened to resign from the NHS in a dispute over pay and conditions. The differences between the 1970s and previous disputes were in terms of scale, regularity and intensity. The 1970s not only saw more days lost (298 000 working days were lost to the NHS through industrial action in 1973 compared with only 500 in 1966), but the ferocity of the disputes was of a different order.

Industrial action, based mainly on the protection of the interests of workers and professionals, disrupted services for patients. Yet, surprisingly, this, along with other problems such as the length of waiting lists and the occasional scandals of malpractice or ill-treatment, never seriously damaged the public's support for the NHS and it remained a popular institution. There was, however, no room for complacency. The growth of the private sector in the late 1970s illustrated that some people were beginning to vote with their feet. There was also a feeling that once support for the NHS began to subside, the whole edifice might cave in.

Certainly, there were signs that patients were not quite as passive as they once had been. Wider concerns about the quality of health services and their responsiveness to consumer pressures grew in the 1960s and 1970s. This was enhanced by a number of developments. The 1974 reorganisation introduced Community Health Councils to represent patients' views. In 1973 Parliament created the Health Service Commissioner to investigate maladministration in the NHS. Also there were moves to improve

complaints procedures at around the same time, though these efforts did
not come to fruition immediately (see Chapter 11).

☐ The Royal Commission on the NHS

The accumulation of these various problems by the mid-1970s contributed
to a growing sense of crisis in the NHS. The Labour government
responded in May 1976 by establishing a Royal Commission to consider
'the best use and management of financial and manpower resources of the
NHS' (Cmnd 7615, 1979, p. 1). The Royal Commission was not intended
as a tool of radical change, indeed its membership was carefully selected to
avoid such an outcome. Yet, ironically, when it reported three years later it
did so to a radical Conservative government headed by Margaret
Thatcher.

The Royal Commission noted the absence of clear objectives in the NHS
and sought to remedy this by setting out seven key objectives. These were:
to encourage and assist individuals to remain healthy; to provide equality
of entitlement to health services; to provide a broad range of services to a
high standard; to provide equality of access to these services; to provide a
service free at the time of use; to satisfy the reasonable expectations of its
users; and to remain a national service responsive to local needs.

The Royal Commission's assessment of the situation facing the NHS
was less gloomy than most. It identified social and geographical
inequalities as being a particular problem, but added that this could not
be tackled by the NHS alone. It also urged greater efforts to prevent illness.
Nevertheless, the Commission believed that the performance of the NHS
could be improved in many areas, and that much of this improvement
could be achieved through greater efficiency.

Many of the Commission's 117 recommendations fell on stony ground.
For example, it unsuccessfully urged the abolition of charges and direct
accountability of the regional health authorities to Parliament. The
Commission's argument for the abolition of a tier of management below
the regional level, however, was enthusiastically pursued, as was the
recommendation for a limited list of prescribed medicines. The passage of
time also saw the Commission's recommendations for medical audit, the
extension of screening programmes and the merger of health authorities
and family practitioner authorities taken up by government.

The acceptance of some of the Royal Commission's conclusions and
recommendations by the incoming Conservative government exemplifies
certain continuities in health policy-making. Nevertheless, change was the
theme of the 1980s in health care as in many other areas of public policy.
These changes arose from the general approach of the Thatcher
government, explored in the next section.

■ Thatcherism and health care

□ *The Thatcher government*

The election of a Conservative government in May 1979 was a watershed. The style and approach of this government, and particularly of its leader Margaret Thatcher, represented a considerable break with the past (see Jenkins, 1987; Riddell, 1991; Young, 1991). During her time in office, Thatcher presided over a government which attempted to transform many aspects of the welfare state established after the Second World War. The NHS, as a cornerstone of the welfare state, employing over a million people and accounting for more than a tenth of public-sector expenditure, could never be insulated from these wider changes in British politics.

□ *The New Right*

The Thatcher government's direction was strongly influenced by the political philosophy of the New Right. Though, as Gamble (1994) has noted, this was neither a unified movement nor a coherent doctrine, one can identify within it a number of common themes. Generally, the New Right favoured more freedom for business, more choice for individuals in the market, the removal of 'impediments' in the market (such as trade unions or regulations restricting trade), a greater role for markets generally and a smaller role for the state in economic affairs. This was combined with a belief in the authority of the state in social matters, where morality, social order and individual responsibility have to be preserved. The New Right philosophy was therefore in essence a fusion of conservative and liberal thought, favouring a limited but authoritarian state and a free market economy (see also King, 1987; Green, 1987).

The Thatcher government's appetite for this brand of political philosophy predisposed it towards certain social and economic policies: the privatisation of the financing and provision of public services; public expenditure control and cuts in direct taxation; the encouragement of self-help and voluntary services; and restrictions on trade unions. For similar reasons it was also predisposed against other policies, such as restrictions and regulations on business activity and policies aimed at reducing social inequalities and deprivation. As we shall see in later chapters, this had important implications for the adoption of certain health policies.

This government also pursued a distinctive approach to the management of public services which was to have equally wide-ranging effects. This has become known as 'new public management' (see Farnham and Horton, 1993; Pollitt, 1993a). Its main features are: politically-driven management reform initiated by central government; the introduction of management techniques drawn from the private sector; a focus on efficiency, financial accountability and cost control; and marketisation – ranging from the use of market-style institutional arrangements in the allocation of resources within the public sector to the transfer of specific functions out of the public sector altogether. The new public management has not been confined to services of a commercial or industrial nature, such as the public utilities. Welfare services, including the NHS, have increasingly been subjected to its influence (Cutler and Waine, 1994; James, 1994; Laughlin and Broadbent, 1994).

Superficially, and in retrospect, the Thatcher government's programme was a well-planned assault on British postwar society, and in particular on 'socialist' institutions: the trade unions, the welfare state and the nationalised industries. But 'Thatcherism', as Gamble (1994, p. 222) notes, did lack symmetry, coherence and purpose. The Thatcher government, like all governments, tended to react pragmatically to events rather than responding according to some master plan. Young observes that Thatcher herself was not an ideologist nor a long-term thinker, but 'a pragmatist and a problem solver' (Young, 1991, p. 603). Her government was prepared to tread more carefully, particularly as general elections drew near. Indeed, as Kavanagh (1990, p. 97) pointed out, some of the more hard-line adherents of the New Right philosophy believed that the Thatcher government was not radical enough. Furthermore, in practice there was often a gap between the radical intention of the government and the outcome of the policies once implemented (Marsh and Rhodes, 1992).

Nevertheless, the Thatcher government was unusual in the degree to which it did adhere to a particular vision of the world while in office. The postwar history of Britain is filled with government 'U-turns' and party political rhetoric operating within a broad consensus. The Thatcher government was, by contrast, a conviction government, not afraid of offending established interests. It also had the benefit of an environment conducive to the pursuit of these convictions, namely a long period in office, a passive (and when it mattered, a supportive) electorate, and a feeble political opposition. This enabled it not only to promote radical change in many areas of public policy, but also to change the political agenda and the terms of debate. Although Margaret Thatcher was ousted as leader, the Conservatives continued in office for a further seven years. Moreover, her legacy was to change the landscape of British politics and policy-making in ways which would persist well into the future.

☐ *Thatcherism and the health care system*

The Thatcher government's approach to health and health care was typical of its overall approach to public policy: a vision in harmony with the New

Right ideology, consistent with the tenets of the new public management, yet tempered with short-term expediency and pragmatism. Thatcher (1993, p. 606) herself has denied that she intended to reform the NHS in a fundamental way. Yet her government inherited a health care system faced with a number of internal problems and external challenges, and in attempting to deal with these issues often fell back on its ideological predispositions. But it also drew on existing ideas, and developed policies in the light of experience. There were continuities, as well as significant changes.

In the remainder of this book these continuities and changes will be explored in an attempt to assess the extent to which the Thatcher government – and its successor under John Major – attempted to deal with the fundamental challenges facing the British health care system. The chapters in the second half of this book analyse key areas of health policy touched by the reforms of the 1980s and 1990s: structural and management reforms; privatisation and public expenditure constraint; the introduction of market mechanisms into the NHS; primary care; community care; reforms relating to patients and users; and, finally, public health. There is also a deliberate attempt to look forward, in the light of the Labour Party's victory at the 1997 General Election, to examine the likely pace and direction of future health care reform.

■ *Chapter 5* ■

The British Health Care System Today

The main purpose of this chapter is to outline the major features of the British health care system today. Before doing so, however, it is important to place it in a broader context, by looking at the variety of health care systems found in advanced industrial societies.

■ Health care systems

Field (1989, p. 10) uses the general term 'health system' to identify 'the totality of formal efforts, commitments, personnel, institutions, economic resources, research efforts (both basic and applied) that a nation state or a society earmarks or devotes to illness, premature mortality, incapacitation, prevention, rehabilitation and other health-related problems'. This definition is very broad and, as Field himself recognises, boundaries have to be set for analytical purposes. One way forward is to focus on a more narrowly defined set of health care services.

Alternatively, Moran (1991, p. 3) has defined the 'health care state' as 'that part of any state concerned with regulating access to, financing, and organising the delivery of, health care to the population'. This is helpful because it focuses upon a key feature of modern health care systems – the nature of state intervention – though this should not divert our attention away from the significant role undertaken by voluntary and commercial organisations in health care.

Most classifications of health care systems are based on characteristics related to state involvement and the scope for independent provision. Field's (1989) typology of health care systems shown in Figure 5.1 is one such example. Field's classification is mainly based upon allocative mechanisms. Health care systems allocate resources primarily through the market (for example, emergent and pluralistic systems), or through the state (state insurance, national health service and socialised systems). State involvement ranges from direct ownership of health care facilities and the employment of health care workers (as in the NHS), through to the provision of funding schemes to reimburse the population's health care

Type 1:   EMERGENT
Health care viewed as item of personal consumption
Physician operates as solo entrepreneur
Professional associations powerful
Private ownership of facilities
Direct payment to physicians
Minimal role in health care for the state

Type 2:   PLURALISTIC
Health care viewed mainly as consumer good
Physician operates as solo entrepreneur and in
    organised groups
Professional organisations very powerful
Private and public ownership of facilities
Payments for services direct and indirect
State's role in health care minimal and indirect
Example: USA

Type 3:   INSURANCE/SOCIAL SECURITY
Health care as an insured/guaranteed consumer good
    or service
Physicians operate as solo entrepreneurs and members
    of medical organisations
Professional organisations strong
Private and public ownership of facilities
Payments for services mostly indirect
State's role in health care central but indirect
Example: France

Type 4:   NATIONAL HEALTH SERVICE
Health care as a state-supported service
Physicians solo entrepreneurs and members of medical
    organisations
Professional organisations fairly strong
Facilities mainly publicly owned
Payments for services indirect
State's role in health care central and direct
Example: UK

Type 5:   SOCIALISED
Health care a state provided public service
Physicians are state employees
Professional organisations weak or non-existent
Facilities wholly publicly owned
Payments for services entirely indirect
State's role in health care is total
Example: Former Soviet Union

Source: M. G. Field (ed.) *Success and Crisis in National Health Systems* (London: Routledge, 1989) p. 7.

Figure 5.1   *Health care systems*

expenses. The relationship between state and market is increasingly complex, as countries adapt their systems both in the light of common problems and in view of other countries' experiences.

□ *Different systems: common problems*

Increasingly, different health care systems are facing similar problems. Countries such as the USA, France, Holland and Italy, like the UK, face growing dissatisfaction with their health systems. The majority of OECD (Organisation for Economic Co-operation and Development) member countries have undertaken significant reforms in their health care systems in recent years. The UK is far from alone in considering radical reform (OECD, 1990, 1994a, 1996; Ham, 1997).

Health systems in industrialised countries face similar demands. They must respond to lifestyle and environmental factors associated with ill-health, tackle new patterns of disease, and deal with rising expectations about the quality of service. At the same time they must respond to the demands of ageing populations and manage the introduction of new technologies. These countries also experience similar problems in terms of organisation and funding of health care, such as the need to control costs, improve accountability and efficiency, monitor the effectiveness of care, establish priorities, and ensure health care is accessible. In view of these common problems, it is not surprising that similar solutions are being sought.

Policy imitation is a recognised feature of health planning where countries borrow ideas from each other (Leichter, 1979). Some identify convergence, with health care systems becoming increasingly similar to each other (Jönsson, 1990; Moran, 1994). Even so, considerable differences persist. While there may be a long-term trend towards convergence in some aspects of health care finance and organisation, considerable differences are likely to remain as systems retain their own particular identities (Taylor-Gooby, 1996).

■ The British health care system

□ *Organisation*

Let us now look at the British health care system. Essentially, it has four main aspects: central government; the NHS; local government; and the independent sector. The picture is complicated by the fact that each part of

---

Exhibit 5.1   The health care systems of France and the USA

France

Finance   Around three-quarters of health care costs are funded by the state social security fund, raised by levies on employers and employees. For certain illnesses (for example, cancer) the state funds 100 per cent of the cost. In other cases individuals pay the balance of care costs, usually financed by subscriptions to non-profit-making insurance societies. The scale of medical fees is negotiated between the profession and the health ministry.

Ownership of facilities/employment   About two-thirds of hospital beds are in publicly-owned hospitals under the responsibility of the health ministry, the remainder are in private hospitals. Private hospitals tend to be smaller and outnumber public hospitals by about 2:1. Most hospital physicians are salaried, but family doctors are independent. In all, over half the doctors in France are private practitioners.

Reform   In recent years the health care system has been in a state of financial crisis (due as much to the impact of unemployment and low economic growth on insurance contributions as to rising health costs). The French government has made various efforts to balance the books (see Wilsford, 1991; Bach, 1994), introducing new taxes on income and expenditure to raise revenue. There has been tighter regulation of medical fees, nationwide computerisation to reduce administrative costs, and encouragement of generic prescribing to reduce drug costs. A new system of hospital management has been introduced, strengthening the role of hospital directors and requiring strategic business plans in the context of tighter budgetary controls. In France patients are not assigned to a GP's list as in the UK, but can consult any doctor. The government has sought to limit this by encouraging referral networks (ie: referral to specialists only through a general practitioner), clinical guidelines and a new system of record-keeping where all doctors must enter details of each consultation. These and other reforms have provoked a hostile response from health professions, and more than once in recent years they have taken to the streets in protest at the government's plans.

United States of America

Finance   The state operates two main schemes: Medicaid for the poor, and Medicare for the elderly and disabled, which reimburse the medical fees of these groups (state schemes also exist for those who have served in the armed services). These schemes are far from comprehensive. Medicare patients often have to make top-up payments for care, and long-term care is not covered by the scheme. Medicaid does not cover single people, the childless, or the

→

Exhibit 5.1 continued

→

low-paid, but it does cover long-term nursing care for low-income elderly and disabled people. A further two-thirds of the population is insured privately, the majority as part of their employment package. A growing proportion of the privately insured (amounting to a quarter of the total population) are enrolled with Health Maintenance Organisations (HMOs – see Chapter 8). This leaves around 16 per cent of the population – approximately 40 million people (Hellander *et al.*, 1995) – without health insurance. Limited free care is provided by the public hospitals and some private hospitals cross-subsidise patients who cannot pay.

Ownership of facilities/employment   Three-quarters of hospitals are privately owned, of which a minority are operated for profit. However, the involvement of 'for-profit' corporations in the financing and provision of US health care has increased in recent years and is expected to grow further (Salmon, 1995). The remaining hospitals are run by local or state authorities. Traditionally, the majority of the medical profession has taken the form of independent private practitioners charging a fee for services provided. But increasing numbers are employed directly by hospitals and by third-party organisations such as HMOs.

Reform   Following his successful election campaign in 1992, during which health care was a key issue, President Clinton announced plans to create a managed market in health care, while guaranteeing health insurance to all citizens. Regional alliances would be established to manage enrolment on insurance plans (except for large businesses), negotiate fees and premiums, monitor the quality of health plans, and means test low income subscribers. Yet in spite of the initial support from the general public, big business, large insurers and from parts of the medical profession, the proposals were defeated. Explanations have been advanced for this (see Navarro, 1994; Peters, 1996; Ranade, 1995a). Certainly, the institutional sclerosis of the American system of government played a part. The plan was also criticised for its growing complexity, which promoted confusion and suspicion among the public. Moreover, the opponents of reform – particularly small business interests and parts of the insurance industry – mounted an effective campaign against the legislation.

The collapse of the plan has not discouraged individual states from experimenting with a wide range of reforms (see, for example, Exhibit 3.4). Moreover, it appears that the health insurance market is already moving in the direction set by the Clinton plan. Increasingly, hospital doctors and doctors are forming provider networks to negotiate fees with purchasing pools formed by employers (see Roberts, 1994) the UK has its own separate structure. In this section the focus is mainly upon the health care system in England, though important differences with Wales, Scotland and Northern Ireland will be highlighted.

☐ *Central government*

In England, the Department of Health is responsible for overseeing health services. The specific functions of the department are to determine policy and priorities, circulate advice to NHS authorities, review their performance, and allocate resources to them. It also advises, inspects and provides some resources for personal social services operated by the local authorities.

Political responsibility for health and personal social services lies with the Secretary of State for Health, the senior minister and constitutional head of the department. The minister is formally accountable and responsible to Parliament for a range of matters. This involves explaining and justifying the department's policies to individual MPs and Parliamentary committees. The Secretary of State is accountable for the financial resources spent by the department and the NHS and has a general responsibility to promote the health of the people.

The Secretary of State for Health is responsible to Parliament for the detailed operation of NHS services, though not strictly speaking for local authority personal social services. However, the Secretary of State is responsible for the statutory framework within which personal social services are provided and has specific responsibilities for issuing guidelines to local authorities with regard to the care of the elderly, child welfare, mentally and physically handicapped persons, and those suffering from mental illness. The minister has acquired a range of powers for inspecting and approving arrangements and services provided by local authorities for these groups. The rising profile of issues such as child protection and community care, and criticism of arrangements in these areas, have led health ministers to take a much closer interest both in policy development and in the details of personal social services in recent years.

Furthermore, as the Secretary of State is responsible for health and social care generally a whole range of other issues fall within his or her brief. These include matters relating to the voluntary and private sector, professional standards, the education of health professionals, research and development, public health, the safety of medicines and ethical issues such as euthanasia and organ transplants.

The extent of ministerial responsibility was captured in Aneurin Bevan's phrase: 'when a bedpan is dropped on a hospital floor its noise should resound in the Palace of Westminster' (quoted in Nairne, 1984). Given the enormity of the task, detailed responsibility for health services is, as the Royal Commission on the NHS noted, largely a constitutional fiction. Yet the Department of Health has been a political hot-seat for a number of years. Ministers are fully aware of the extent to which they can be held personally and publicly responsible for unpopular policies and short-comings in services (Castle, 1990; Crossman, 1977; Fowler, 1991).

The Secretary of State for Health is assisted by a number of junior ministers, currently four. All have specifically defined responsibilities for aspects of health policy and operate with the delegated authority of the Secretary of State. One is drawn from the House of Lords and acts as the department's spokesperson there.

The Department of Health employs 3700 civil servants, who advise ministers and who are responsible for implementing policy decisions. Civil servants can have considerable influence over policy in view of their permanence (the civil service is a career but ministerial tenure is short, lasting on average only thirty months), knowledge of departmental activities, and experience of the procedures of policy-making (Hennessy, 1988). Civil service influence is at its greatest where ministers are not committed to a particular policy. In general, decisions on technically-complex issues, matters currently attracting little attention from the public or from major pressure groups, and issues of low party-political significance tend to be determined largely by civil servants in view of the relatively low levels of ministerial interest in these matters.

There are two types of civil servant within the Department of Health: the generalists, who have a general administrative background; and the specialists, who have specific professional backgrounds in health or social care. The department employs civil servants drawn from medicine, nursing, social work and a range of other caring professions, who contribute to policy-making and implementation with regard to their specialist training and knowledge.

The structure of the Department of Health reflects the need to combine generalist administrative skills and specialist advice. Although the department is headed by a generalist permanent secretary, professional advice is incorporated at every level. At the top there is the Chief Medical Officer (CMO) who has direct access to ministers and is also the chief medical adviser to the government as a whole. Although the CMO is in effect the professional head of the department, the other professional groups have their own chief officers (such as the Chief Nursing Officer, for example) to whom they are professionally accountable.

Specific advice on policy is given by professional officers within the various groups and divisions in the department. Their expertise is supplemented by outside advice from a range of sources. The department often establishes expert groups to advise on policy development (recent examples include maternity services, variations in health, research and development). Some advisory committees are permanent – such as the Standing Medical Advisory Committee and the Clinical Standards Advisory Group. The department also consults a range of interest groups, representing professionals, patients, health authorities, and commercial and voluntary organisations. In addition it may consult single issue cause groups on issues such as smoking, drug abuse and abortion.

Given the complexity of health policy and its increasingly controversial nature, there have been moves in recent years to reduce the burden on health ministers through reorganisation of the department's functions. From 1968 to 1988 the responsibility for health and social security was combined within the Department of Health and Social Security (DHSS). The departments were de-merged in 1988, partly because it had become apparent that the DHSS was unable to formulate and coordinate such a wide range of politically controversial policies in an effective manner.

Attempts have been made to devolve the responsibility for the day-to-day running of health services to the NHS, in an effort to limit ministerial responsibility and to distance politicians from some of the more detailed matters relating to the service. Following the Griffiths report of 1983, separate policy and management boards were established for the NHS. For reasons discussed in Chapter 6 this arrangement was not initially successful. The attempt to divide policy and management was revived again in a slightly different form in 1989 with the creation of a new Policy Board and the NHS Management Executive (subsequently renamed the NHS Executive).

The Policy Board, which is responsible for the overall policy and strategy of the NHS, is chaired by the Secretary of State for Health, and consists of ministers, senior civil servants from the Department of Health, the Chief Executive of the NHS, special advisers, and others appointed for their knowledge of large business organisations and public-sector management. In addition eight non-executive directors, each drawn from one of the areas covered by the NHS regional offices (see the section on regional organisation below) are members of the Policy Board.

The NHS Executive (NHSE) has two functions: it advises ministers on NHS policy and is responsible for day-to-day management of the NHS. It is led by a Chief Executive, who is directly accountable to the Secretary of State for Health. The NHSE consists of senior managers, each of whom takes responsibility for a particular directorate, such as finance, human resources and so on. The heads of each directorate, along with the directors of the eight NHS regional offices, sit on the NHSE management board chaired by the Chief Executive. The management board is the focus for implementing the policies and strategies formulated by the NHS Policy Board.

☐ *Further developments*

The NHSE is not a separate agency but remains part of the Department of Health. It is however physically separated from the wider department. In 1992 the NHSE headquarters was moved from London to Leeds. Further upheaval followed with the establishment of an internal inquiry (the Banks Inquiry) into the organisation of the Department of Health, the findings of which became known in 1994. Its report made a number of recommendations (DoH, 1994b). First, that the department should be organised into groups, each focusing on one of the three main business areas – public health, social care and health care – plus a separate support services group. Second, each group should be responsible for policy, implementation, monitoring and accountability within their areas of responsibility. Hence the NHSE would be responsible for policy as well as implementation in the field of health care (entailing the transfer of functions from other parts of the department). Third, that civil servants with a health professional background should be integrated into a single management structure within each group. Fourth, the report argued for a continuing need to focus on client groups (such as the elderly, for example) that would be enhanced by clearer lead responsibilities. It proposed that the lead responsibility for the elderly, disabled people and those with learning difficulties should lie with the social care group. The NHSE would have lead responsibility for mentally-ill people. Finally, the report recommended a more proactive style of management. To this end it was proposed that the Departmental Management Board (consisting of ministers and senior civil servants) should have a more strategic role, supported by a small high level Policy Management unit (PMU).

These recommendations were accepted by ministers and the Department of Health was subsequently restructured along these lines. Figure 5.2 shows the current structure of the Department of Health including the NHSE.

☐ *Other departments and agencies*

Other government departments and agencies have responsibility for health services and policies. The Secretaries of State for Scotland, Wales and Northern Ireland are responsible for health policy and services in these parts of the UK. The Ministry of Defence is responsible for health care issues in the armed services, while health care in prisons falls within the brief of the Home Office. The Department for Education and Employ-

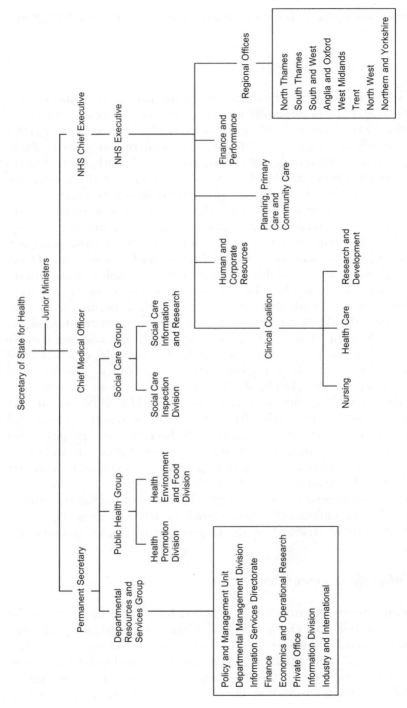

Figure 5.2 *The Department of Health and the NHS Executive*

ment's involvement in health care is related mainly to the education of health professionals, and health-related research in higher education, but it also has other interests including health education in schools. The Department of the Environment, Transport and the Regions has general responsibility for local government funding and services, and for specific policy areas which have an important bearing on health, such as housing, water, transport, road safety and environmental pollution. The Department of Social Security's functions include the financial support of low-income and vulnerable groups, including disabled and chronically-ill people, elderly people, children, all of whom have significant health needs.

The Ministry of Agriculture is responsible for food and drink policy (though some of its functions may be transferred to a new food standards agency – see Chapter 12). Many of the health issues of the 1980s and 1990s – nutrition, food labelling, food-borne infections, and alcohol abuse – have involved this department. The Department of Trade and Industry has also been involved in health issues through its sponsorship of health-damaging industries, such as chemicals and tobacco.

In theory, the policies of government departments are coordinated by the Cabinet and its various committees and secretariats. Health policy is considered by the Cabinet, but as this body meets infrequently (usually only once a week) and is large (over twenty members) most work is undertaken by smaller subcommittees of cabinet or by interdepartmental committees of civil servants. Examples include the Interdepartmental Group on Disability and the Interdepartmental Group on Public Health. In practice, coordination between the departments is often weak and sometimes involves considerable conflict. It is therefore by no means unusual for different departments to pursue conflicting policies, as revealed by, for example, the salmonella and eggs crisis during the 1980s (Doig, 1990).

Finally, a number of government agencies have been established to handle particular areas of health policy and administration. An example is the Health and Safety Executive, responsible for promoting health and safety in the workplace, and whose work relates to a number of government departments, including the Department of Health. The special health authorities, on the other hand, are directly focused on health matters and are directly accountable to the Secretary of State for Health. These include the Health Education Authority, which implements the government's health promotion programme; and the Special Hospital Authorities responsible for high-security mental hospitals. Other agencies include the Medicines Control Agency, which regulates medicines, and non-departmental public bodies such as the Human Fertilisation and Embryology Authority, whose task it is to license those involved in scientific and medical activity in this field.

☐ The National Health Service

The structure of the NHS at December 1997 is shown in Figure 5.3. It should be noted that this will change following the Labour government's White Paper on the NHS (Cm 3807, 1997). The proposed changes are noted in Figure 5.3 and in the following sections.

☐ Regional organisation

In 1996 the Regional Health Authorities (RHA) in England were abolished and replaced by regional offices of the NHSE. The former RHAs, which replaced the old regional hospital boards in the 1974 reorganisation, were initially created as strategic management bodies. They acted as a buffer between the Department of Health and district health authorities (DHAs), planning services within their boundaries, allocating resources to lower-tier authorities, holding them to account and arbitrating in disputes between them. The RHAs had important responsibilities with regard to education, training and public health. They also provided services above

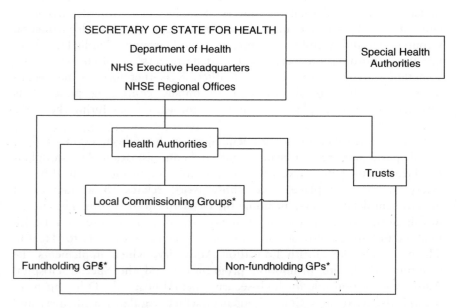

*Note: It is envisaged that fundholding and non-fundholding GPs will be absorbed into local commissioning groups (to be known as Primary Care Groups) by 1999.

Figure 5.3   *The structure of the National Health Service, 1997*

district level, such as blood transfusion services and, in some areas, ambulance services. However, in the years prior to their demise the RHAs had mostly divested themselves of such functions in order to concentrate on a strategic management role.

Following its review of the NHS structure in the early 1990s, the Department of Health announced that the RHAs would be 'slimmed down', reduced in number, and eventually replaced by regional offices of the NHSE (DoH, 1994c). The new regional offices also superseded NHSE regional outposts established in the early 1990s to monitor the growing number of NHS self-governing trusts.

The NHSE regional offices are headed by a regional director, accountable to the Chief Executive of the NHS. The regional directors are represented on the NHSE management board. In addition, a non-executive director is drawn from each region to sit on the NHS Policy Board, preserving in a much-reduced form the tradition of lay participation at regional level. Regional non-executive directors in consultation with regional directors are also responsible for recommending health authority appointments to the Secretary of State.

The key role of the regional office is to supervise the performance of NHS commissioning bodies and service providers and to arbitrate in disputes between them. It was intended that regional offices should act as a conduit through which central initiatives flow, such as the development of clinical audit or the promotion of primary care. Regional offices must ensure that medical education and research is appropriately supported by the NHS. Regional Postgraduate Deans commission postgraduate medical education and provide input on decisions affecting medical education and training issues at regional level. Research and development directors have also been appointed at regional level to develop strategies in this field. The regional offices also play a role in resource allocation, advising NHSE headquarters on revenue allocations and major capital programmes. In addition they hold small funding allocations for pump-priming schemes and have delegated powers to approve smaller capital schemes.

Finally, the regional offices retain the principal public health role of the former RHAs and each region must appoint a Director of Public Health. However, certain public health functions – such as responsibility for screening programmes and the surveillance of communicable disease have been devolved to health authorities.

☐ Health Authorities

Health authorities have a statutory responsibility to evaluate and promote the health needs of their resident populations in the context of national policies and regional strategies. They are the agents of the Secretary of State for Health and are accountable to ministers through the regional offices of the NHSE, which set objectives (in the form of a corporate contract) and monitor performance. The health authorities commission health care for those needs not covered by other commissioning arrangements. In this capacity they reach agreement with providers for a particular level and standard of services. The precise nature of this process is discussed in Chapter 8.

The health authorities are expected to work alongside other commissioning bodies and service providers in the field of health and social care (such as GP fundholders, local commissioning groups, local authority social services departments and trusts) in an effort to promote a coordinated and efficient service. They are expected to plan for the health needs of their populations and produce strategic plans setting out local priorities and how these can be achieved.

Health authorities in England and Wales consist of a chairperson and other non-executive members, appointed by the Secretary of State for Health. The remaining members include five executive members (including the health authority's general manager, finance director and director of public health). Where the health authority area contains a teaching hospital, one of the non-executive members must be drawn from the medical school.

Following the creation of the internal market in 1991, the old DHAs (of which there were 190 in England) sought to combine their purchasing power by merging with each other, their number being virtually halved by 1995. In many areas the DHAs also joined forces with the FHSAs (Family Health Service Authorities), which were responsible for managing family practitioner services. These informal arrangements (called health commissions) were given a statutory basis in 1995 with the passage of the Health Authorities Act, which created 100 integrated health authorities in England. The number of health authorities is likely to fall further following the 1997 NHS White Paper (Cm 3807, 1997). This document set out proposals to strengthen the health authority planning role and devolve commissioning functions to local primary care groups (see Chapters 6 and 8).

☐ *GP fundholders and other commissioning bodies*

From 1990 onwards the Department of Health invited applications on an annual basis to join the GP fundholder scheme (see Chapter 8). By 1996 over half the population of England and Wales was covered by the scheme. However, in 1997, following the election of a Labour government, further applications to join the scheme were halted. The government also introduced new rules on budget-setting and referrals. Then in the White Paper of 1997 it was announced that fundholding would end by 1999. It was envisaged that all GPs would join new Primary Care Groups responsible for commissioning services. These new arrangements build on a range of schemes developed since 1991, described below.

Under the standard fundholding scheme each practice receives a budget which covers the cost of running the practice, buying drugs, and a range of elective (that is, non-emergency) hospital services and community health services. When first introduced in England and Wales the scheme was confined to larger practices with over 9000 patients and later extended to those with practice lists of 7000 and over (in Scotland the eligibility threshold was 6000 patients subsequently reduced to 4000 from April 1996). In 1995 a three-tier system was introduced in England and Wales: community fundholding for practices with over 3000 patients covering the costs of staff, drugs, tests and community health services but not hospital services; a revised system of standard fundholding for practices with over 5000 patients, covering most elective and outpatient services; and total purchasing, confined to a number of pilot schemes, where the budget covers all services including accident and emergency and maternity care.

In addition there are 'multifunds' (20 schemes in operation by 1996), where GPs pool management budgets to pay for a common administrative structure to support their commissioning activity. There are also other forms of GP involvement in commissioning at local level (see Exhibit 8.3). These arrangements provide a range of models for the development of the new Primary Care Groups.

Fundholding practices and other local commissioning bodies agree levels of service provision with a range of NHS trusts and independent provider units caring for their patients. But they are expected to plan services in accordance with national and local priorities. Indeed the White Paper of 1997 envisaged a strengthening of the requirement to participate in efforts to achieve locally agreed objectives. The operation of these schemes and recent changes made since 1997 are discussed further in Chapter 8.

□ *Self-governing trusts and directly managed units*

The internal market involved the creation of two types of organisation providing NHS hospital and community health services: trusts and directly managed units (DMUs). The DMUs were directly managed by the local health authority, most being prepared for trust status. As with fundholders, trusts were created in a series of annual 'waves'. By 1997 virtually all providers on mainland Britain and in Northern Ireland had achieved trust status.

Trusts are directly accountable to the Secretary of State for Health, formerly through the NHSE outposts and now through the regional offices. They are expected to operate within guidelines set by the NHSE and are normally required to break-even within each financial year while making a return of 6 per cent on their capital. They generate income by providing services to fundholders, other NHS commissioning bodies, the independent sector and private patients.

Trusts have a number of freedoms. They can determine their own management arrangements within the guidelines set by the Department of Health. Recently, health ministers have stressed that non-executive members must be draw from the communities they serve. In addition there have been changes to the procedures for selecting non-executive members. Trusts have considerable discretion in principle over the employment terms and conditions of service of their staff, though in practice most have been unwilling or unable to move away from national terms and conditions. Finally, they have some flexibility in handling investments, borrowings and assets, though again the Department of Health has sought to restrict these freedoms though guidance.

It has been stressed that trusts must continue to provide essential health services at local level and that their services must remain free to NHS patients. Trusts have also been urged by government to respond to national and local policies. The White Paper of 1997 sought to strengthen trusts' commitment to locally agreed health plans. It also envisaged new responsibilities for trusts to guarantee high quality services as well as meeting financial targets.

☐ *Community Health Councils*

Community Health Councils (CHCs) were established in England and Wales in 1974 to give patients a voice within the NHS. Normally there is one CHC for each local health authority. Similar bodies are found in Scotland and Northern Ireland. CHCs are statutory bodies established by the Secretary of State for Health and are resourced from a central NHS budget. The regional offices of the NHSE are responsible for overall budget management and agree levels of support services. The regional offices require CHCs to develop annual plans reflecting priorities and monitor their performance in relation to these plans. Local health authorities hold the employment contracts of their staff

CHC members are nominated by voluntary organisations and local authorities. One-half are nominated by local authorities, one-third by voluntary organisations and a sixth of the membership are appointed by the regional office. Although they lack specific powers, they have a number of rights to enable them to perform their function of representing patients' views. These include rights to information, to be consulted about substantial variations in service and to observe certain proceedings at health authority meetings. In addition CHCs are increasingly asked for their views on priority setting, the commissioning of health care services, and the development of quality standards. They also have a greater level of contact now with social services departments on issues such as hospital discharge arrangements, complaints procedures and community care planning. Some have also forged better links with general practitioners in their area.

Deprived of formal powers and financially-constrained (English CHCs have a budget of around £120 000 and two full-time staff), the CHCs nevertheless play a useful role in informing patients, assisting them with complaints and representing the views of the community. In the 1990s they have faced a number of problems, including exclusion from health authority meetings. There has been concern about their independence, particularly following the abolition of the RHAs which were formerly responsible for establishing and resourcing them. These issues are discussed more fully in Chapter 11.

☐ The NHS in other parts of the UK

There are important differences in the structure of the NHS in Wales, Scotland and Northern Ireland. Further changes may be expected in the light of the Blair government's devolution plans, which provide for a range of independent powers over NHS services in Wales and Scotland, and its plans to replace the NHS internal market.

The Secretary of State for Wales has overall responsibility for the NHS in the principality. He or she is supported by the Welsh Office Health Department, which has its own Chief Medical Officer, Chief Nursing Officer and other professional heads. The Director of NHS in Wales, appointed by the Secretary of State, along with the chief officers and the heads of the administrative divisions of the Welsh Office are members of an executive committee responsible for the management of the NHS. There is also a Policy Board which sets objectives for the NHS in Wales.

There are no regional offices in Wales. The Welsh Health Common Services Authority (formerly known as the Welsh Health Technical Services Organisation) is charged with providing support services for health authorities and trusts in Wales which in England were formerly undertaken by RHAs, including estates, information technology and supplies. In the 1990s, however, this body was subject to a more commercial regime. As a result, non-clinical functions were subjected to market-testing with a view to privatisation.

As in England, the creation of an internal market involved the establishment of GP fundholders and trusts in Wales. Health authorities were reorganised in 1996, DHAs and FHSAs being amalgamated into five health authorities. The Welsh authorities undertake planning and commissioning like their English counterparts. Their composition is similar: a combination of executives and five non-executive directors plus a chairperson. Chairpersons and non-executives are appointed by the Secretary of State for Wales.

In Scotland, the NHS falls under the responsibility of the Secretary of State for Scotland, assisted by civil servants in the Health Department of the Scottish Office – which in 1995 became a free-standing department. As in England, the Scottish Health Department contains a Management Executive for the NHS. In contrast to England, the chief executive of the NHS in Scotland also serves as the chief executive of the Health Department as a whole. Policy objectives are set by a policy advisory board within the Scottish Office which contains health professionals and lay people alongside civil servants.

The Scottish NHS, as in Wales, has a Common Services Agency which provides support services to the central administration, health authorities and trusts. It too has been subjected to market-testing and privatisation, its building division being privatised in 1995.

The planning and commissioning function in Scotland is undertaken by fifteen local health boards. Since 1972 Scottish health boards have been responsible for family practitioner services as well as hospital and community health services. Scotland has therefore had considerable experience of integrated health authorities. Members of Scottish health boards are appointed by the Secretary of State for Scotland. In Scotland there are usually six non-executive members on each board, in addition to the chairperson.

NHS trusts and GP fundholders operate along similar lines as in England and Wales, though there are slightly different eligibility rules for fundholding as well as some differences in the budgetary regulations. A final point is that the NHS internal market reforms were a little slower to take off in Scotland, so the number of trusts and the percentage of the population covered by fundholders has tended to lag behind the rest of Great Britain. Nevertheless, by 1996 all providers of health care on the mainland had become trusts (health care providers on the Scottish isles remain directly managed by health authorities). In the same year GP fundholders covered 43 per cent of the Scottish population.

The NHS in Northern Ireland differs considerably from the rest of the UK. In particular the responsibility for health and social services is combined, both at departmental level and at health authority level. Overall responsibility for these services in the province lies with the Secretary of State for Northern Ireland, assisted by the Department of Health and Social Services within the Northern Ireland Office. Departmental policy is developed by a Health and Personal Social Services (HPSS) Group, while the HPSS Management Executive is responsible for the day-to-day management of services. The Management Executive is led by a Chief Executive accountable to the Secretary of the State.

As in Scotland and Wales, a central agency provides support functions, though its role is different. The Central Services Agency in Northern Ireland undertakes some functions which elsewhere are the responsibility of health authorities (such as the payment of GPs). In addition, some functions, such as information technology services, which in the rest of the UK are the responsibility of health authorities or central service agencies are directly provided by the NHS Executive in Northern Ireland.

The Health and Social Services Boards are responsible for planning social services as well as hospital, community and family health services. The boards consist of a chairperson and six non-executive members who are appointed by the Secretary of State for Northern Ireland. As in the rest of the UK, the remaining members are executive directors, and include the general manager.

Reform of administrative and management arrangements in Northern Ireland has proceeded at a much slower pace than the rest of the UK. General management (see Chapter 6) was introduced over a much longer period. Similarly, the internal market reforms were slow to develop in Northern Ireland. Even so, by the mid-1990s, change was well underway. By 1996 GP fundholders covered over half the population of Ulster and all the providers had converted to trusts.

☐ Local authorities

As shown in the previous chapter, local government has been heavily involved in health service provision in the past. Although most of these responsibilities have since been removed, local authorities still have an important role in relation to personal social services and public health.

Personal social services cover a range of caring, protective and support services for children, the family, the elderly, mentally-ill people, and those who are mentally and physically handicapped. Local authorities are responsible for residential and community-based care and support services. In some cases these services are jointly provided in collaboration with the NHS or the independent sector.

Local authorities have a particularly important role as lead agencies in the field of community care with responsibility for assessing people's needs and arranging an appropriate package of services (see Chapter 10). Local authorities also provide a variety of environmental health services aimed at the protection of public health, ranging from pest control and noise pollution to the inspection and registration of food premises. Other local authority services such as housing, education, cleansing, waste disposal, and the provision of sport and leisure facilities also have the potential to make a major contribution to a healthy environment and a healthy society.

Some have argued that the health role of local authorities should be expanded, even to the extent of taking over some of the functions of the NHS (see Hunter and Webster, 1992; Regan and Stewart, 1982; Association of Metropolitan Authorities, 1994). Indeed some local authorities, such as Wandsworth for example, have shown an interest in acquiring the planning and commissioning roles of health authorities. Proponents argue that this approach has a number of benefits. First, it would help address some of the concerns about the lack of accountability of local NHS authorities (see Chapter 6), bringing them under democratic control. Secondly, given the potential which local authorities have for influencing health of the population through their other functions and responsibilities, it makes sense to bring the organisation of health services within their ambit. Thirdly, by bringing health services under local authority control, the prospects for coordinating the planning of health, social and environmental services could be improved.

However, it is unlikely that the transfer of responsibility for health services to local authority control would improve democratic account-ability. Democratic participation in local government is at a low level, turnout at elections rarely exceeding 40 per cent. Furthermore, as numerous scandals in the social services (notably with regard to child abuse in local authority homes) have illustrated, local authority responsibility does not guarantee public accountability. A further point is that despite being 'under one roof', there are many examples of poor coordination between existing local authority services such as housing, education and social services. Finally, there are political problems. Local authority control of health services was not supported by the Thatcher or Major governments and has not been endorsed by the Blair government. There is also much resistance to local authority control from many of those working in the NHS (see Hunt, 1995).

☐ The independent sector

The independent sector consists of the commercial provision of health care (the commercial sector), that provided by charitable and voluntary organisations (the voluntary sector), and the care provided by friends, neighbours and families (the informal sector). At the margins, however, a clear-cut distinction between these categories is not easy to maintain. The main distinction between commercial providers and the rest of the independent sector is that the former expects to make a profit from its involvement, though charitable organisations often make a surplus which could be seen as the equivalent of profit in a commercial organisation.

The independent sector often interacts with the public sector. For instance, the NHS sells its services to the private sector. This takes the form of hiring out equipment to private hospitals or treating private patients. Likewise the independent sector provides services to the NHS. As we shall see in the next section, a considerable amount of funding for commercial, voluntary and informal care is provided by national and local government and the NHS.

The independent sector provides a considerable proportion of Britain's health care and its contribution of has grown substantially in the 1980s and 1990s. In 1984, private and voluntary hospitals and nursing homes supplied only 7.5 per cent of UK hospital based treatment and care. By the mid-1990s this had grown to 20 per cent (Laing, 1996).

☐ *The commercial sector*

Commercial providers are involved in many aspects of health care: including acute hospitals, nursing and residential care homes, and the provision of health insurance. With the advent of competitive tendering for NHS ancillary services, commercial firms have secured a substantial role in the provision of NHS cleaning, catering and laundry services. More recently they have shown interest in delivering a wider range of other services on behalf of the NHS including health care.

Commercial health care is more common in some sectors than others. This is because some treatments and forms of care are more profitable than others, while some are not profitable at all. The involvement of the commercial sector has been highest in routine, non-emergency surgery, and abortions. In recent years the commercial sector has also increasingly been involved in long-term care, particularly the care of the elderly, and in primary care, for example the provision of health screening facilities. Furthermore, it should be remembered that the provision of medical equipment, medicines and appliances is in the hands of commercial suppliers.

All forms of independent provision of health care were actively encouraged by the Conservative government in the 1980s and 1990s, but within the independent sector it is the commercial providers that have shown the most significant growth (Laing, 1996). For example, 'for profit' organisations now control over 60 per cent of beds in independent acute hospitals and a similar proportion of places in private residential care homes.

□   *The voluntary and informal sectors*

The voluntary and informal sectors have been actively encouraged by the government over the past decade or so. The term 'voluntary sector' covers a diverse range of activities. These activities can range from the rather small-scale activities of local volunteer groups to large national charities and non-profit-making bodies.

The voluntary sector has long been involved with the provision of health services. In the past hospitals were created and financed by voluntary action. Today, voluntary organisations supplement NHS provision in both the hospital and the community health sectors. An example is the Womens' Royal Voluntary Service (WRVS) which assists with patient services in hospital, meals on wheels, old peoples' clubs and so on. The scale of this effort is reflected in the following statistics: WRVS provides 15 million meals every year; it has 125 000 members working 500 000 hours a week. Other examples of voluntary organisations at work in the health field include the London Lighthouse which provides advice and support for those suffering from HIV and AIDS, and the National Childbirth Trust (NCT) which provides help and advice for parents-to-be.

Although voluntary bodies are increasingly large-scale and professional in their organisation, they continue to depend on unpaid volunteers to raise funds and to deliver services. Over a quarter of women and over a fifth of men participate in various forms of voluntary activity in the health field and elsewhere, such as fund-raising and voluntary work (Central Statistical Office, 1996).

Voluntary work is a relatively cheap (though not costless) and flexible way of delivering services. Yet there are worries about an over-reliance on voluntary services. Voluntary organisations could be led into performing roles for which they are unsuitable, and replacing rather than complementing services currently provided directly by the NHS and local authorities (see Chapter 10).

Informal care refers to the care undertaken by friends, relatives and neighbours. If adequate support from statutory and other services is provided, such care may well be far more humane and effective than institutional care. However, it is argued, with some foundation, that the informal sector is used as a dumping ground for long-term patients in order to save public money, and that support for carers is patchy and in some cases non-existent.

There has been a movement in recent decades towards self-help and greater personal responsibility regarding health. Given the growing importance of lifestyle factors in producing ill-health, it is important that individuals take some responsibility for their own well-being. However, government also has a role to play, both in the prevention of ill-health and in the provision of an adequate level of caring services when individuals and families are unable to help themselves.

■ Funding the health care system

The organisational structure of health services is, of course, an important aspect of the health care system. But equally important is the way in which services are funded, and how these resources are spent.

□ Private funding

Services provided by the independent sector are not necessarily privately funded. Private health care may be purchased out of public funds; for example, a health authority may try to reduce its waiting lists by buying services from a private hospital. Conversely, health care can be provided by the public sector and funded by the private sector; for example, a private clinic may hire equipment from the NHS. These various partnerships are explored in more detail in Chapter 7.

In 1995, 16 per cent of the cost of health care in the UK was privately funded. This is low when compared with other industrialised countries (see Figure 5.4). But, as with the provision of services, there are wide differences in the levels of private funding for various types of care. Private funding is higher than the UK average, in the long-term care of the elderly, abortions, non-emergency surgery, medicines and ophthalmics (see Table 7.1).

Private financing takes two forms. People can subscribe to an insurance scheme, which then pays for health care when the subscriber requires treatment. Or they can pay directly for health care as they receive it. The second method is obviously more popular for low-cost health care items such as medicines. The first method is used mainly for medical care, where costs are high and cannot be spread over time. It has also been identified as a means of funding long-term care where, even though costs are divisible, payments are high relative to income (see Chapter 10).

□ The public sector: income

The majority of health care in Britain is publicly funded. But how is this money raised? Since the NHS began in 1948, the vast majority of funding has been in the form of general taxation (around 80 per cent during the

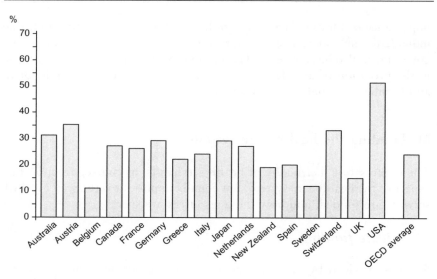

Source of data: Office of Health Economics, *Compendium of Health Statistics* (1995).

Figure 5.4   *Proportion of health care privately funded (selected OECD countries), 1995 (private expenditure as a percentage of total health care spending)*

1990s). This is supplemented by a contribution from the National Insurance Fund (about an eighth of the cost of the NHS). Most of the remaining funds are raised from patient charges for dental treatment, prescriptions, equipment, and other receipts such as the sale of assets.

Local authority spending on health and social services is funded in several ways: through central government grants, the council tax, business rates, and charges for specific services. A significant amount (about a tenth of the total expenditure on personal social services) is raised in fees and charges. The majority of the funds (around two-thirds of the total) take the form of central government grants.

☐ *Public expenditure*

Having explored the sources of public finance for health care, it is now possible to look briefly at the broad categories of expenditure. The majority of public expenditure on health care has in the past been allocated to the hospital sector, and within this category, in-patient care. Figure 5.5 illustrates that the UK appears to spend a large proportion of health expenditure on in-patient care. Yet, taking into account the difficulties of international comparison of such expenditures, the UK is not significantly

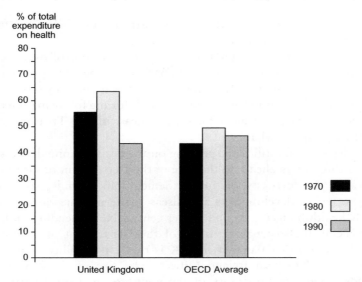

Source of data: OECD, *Health Systems: Facts and Trends 1960–1991* (Paris, OECD), p. 100.

Figure 5.5 *Spending on inpatient care as a percentage of total health care spending, 1970–90*

out of step with others in terms of the balance between hospital and community health care spending.

However, the picture is definitely changing and there are signs that the dominance of the hospital sector has been challenged. Figure 5.5 illustrates that there is a general trend among industrialised countries away from expenditure on hospital-based care. These issues are explored more fully in Chapter 9.

☐ *The public expenditure process*

The NHS (and central government financial support for local authority personal social services) must compete for resources at a national level with other priorities such as defence, education, housing, social security and so on. The budgets for these services are determined through the annual public expenditure exercise.

The method of determining public expenditure was altered in 1993. Under the previous system departments bid for funds, then bargained with the Treasury within an overall target of expenditure set by the Cabinet. The bargaining process was regarded as being rather irrational since it did not explicitly identify expenditure priorities. In addition, it proved difficult to control overall spending when the departments lobbied successfully for higher budgets on politically sensitive issues.

The new system was intended to exert tighter control over aggregate spending as well as facilitating a comparison of spending priorities. The government, in the light of economic circumstances, initially sets an overall level of expenditure (the New Control Total) for the following three years. Each government department then negotiates with the Treasury over the size of its particular share.

The departments still plan spending on the basis of annual assessments, looking three years ahead. In the case of the Department of Health, plans are based on forecasts of future demographic trends, technological changes, service developments and disease patterns. The vast majority of the UK health budget – around 80 per cent of NHS spending, in fact – is contained in the expenditure plans of the Department of Health. NHS expenditure in other parts of the UK is the responsibility of the Welsh, Scottish and Northern Ireland Offices. The size of the health budget depends largely on the ability of the ministers in these departments to bargain and negotiate effectively within the government. The outcome of the public spending process is examined in Chapter 7 along with the debate about the appropriate level of funding for health care.

Once the overall size of the health allocation is determined it is then distributed within the NHS. In the past this was done largely on an historical basis, with service providers receiving similar shares of the budget as in previous years. This changed with the introduction of RAWP in the 1970s (see Chapter 4). Following the advent of internal markets, a new system of allocation was introduced. Budgets were given to commissioning authorities (such as health authorities and GP fundholders), to agree levels of service with provider units (hospitals and community health service units), in allocate resources accordingly.

☐ The British health care system in transition

The British system of health care is still predominantly state-dominated. The vast majority of non-informal care is given by public-sector organisations. The public sector of health care is, in turn, dominated by the NHS, though local authorities play an important role through their responsibilities for environmental health, community care and other services which affect public health. The overwhelming majority of health expenditure is public expenditure, raised mainly through general taxation.

The expansion in the independent sector, discussed in more detail in later chapters, is a significant development. However, as this sector is still small in comparison with the public sector, the British system of health care remains a 'national health service' in Field's typology outlined earlier. Nevertheless, there have been significant changes over the past two decades. These require further analysis. Each of the remaining chapters explores an area of health policy and service development, identifies the key reforms, explains their origins, assesses their impact, and draws out the implications for the future of health care in Britain.

■ *Chapter 6* ■

The Management of Health Care

Inadequate management arrangements have often been identified as the root cause of the problems of the NHS. During the 1970s, as shown in Chapter 4, governments sought to address these issues mainly through structural reorganisation, accompanied by management reform and the development of new planning procedures and coordination mechanisms. In the following decade, the emphasis was increasingly upon business-style managerialism, with government drawing heavily on ideas imported from the private sector. The 1990s brought further initiatives: some extended the managerialist ethos, others sought to reconcile the new regime with traditional public service values. This chapter examines the reforms of the last two decades and their impact on various aspects of health service management.

■ The 1982 reorganisation

In 1982 the structure of the NHS was streamlined by abolishing the middle tier of the NHS structure – the Area Health Authorities (AHAs) – and establishing new health authorities at district level (DHSS, 1979). Planning and professional advisory systems were also simplified (Hambleton, 1983). In addition, central government replaced the previous practice of giving detailed guidelines to NHS authorities with rather more general statements about priorities (DHSS, 1981a).

During the early 1980s, health ministers emphasised that management responsibility should be delegated downwards to localities. Some saw this as an attempt to evade responsibility for the shortcomings of the service (Chaplin, 1982). In the event, this move was relatively short-lived. Ministers faced increasing pressure from Parliament to improve the accountability of the NHS, and were urged to monitor its performance more closely. A new planning process addressed some of these concerns by introducing annual performance reviews. This in principle enabled central government – in the form of the DHSS – to monitor the performance of health authorities more closely, and in particular their progress towards central objectives and targets (DHSS, 1982).

■ The Griffiths Inquiry: towards a new model of management

Norman Fowler, who became Secretary of State for Social Services in 1981, became convinced that the real problem of the NHS lay in its management processes (Fowler, 1991). He established a small inquiry team with business experience to examine NHS management arrangements in England, chaired by Roy Griffiths (then Deputy Chairman and Managing Director of Sainsbury's, the supermarket chain). Although its original remit did not cover Scotland, Wales or Northern Ireland, its recommendations were later applied to these parts of the UK as well.

□ *The Griffiths report*

The Griffiths Inquiry (DHSS, 1983) focused on the absence of a clear line of management responsibility in the NHS, summed up in its observation that 'if Florence Nightingale were carrying her lamp through the corridors of the NHS today, she would almost certainly be searching for the people in charge'. Much of the blame was laid at the door of 'consensus management', the existing method of decision-making introduced following the 1974 reorganisation. Under this system, management teams were drawn from a variety of backgrounds including administration, finance, nursing and medicine. In principle, no member of the management team had superior status and each had the power to veto decisions. Although this form of decision-making had advantages, in that the management team was forced to consider a wide range of perspectives before arriving at a decision, it was held responsible for delays in decision-making, avoidance of tough decisions, and blurring of responsibility.

The inquiry also identified a confusion of responsibilities between the DHSS and the NHS. Echoing an earlier inquiry (DHSS, 1976b), it found that the DHSS continued to intervene directly in the detailed affairs of health authorities, contrary to the declared policy of decentralisation and delegation, and that intervention was undertaken in a haphazard and inconsistent way. Furthermore, the inquiry was highly critical of failure to address the needs of the consumer and to achieve national policy objectives. It identified an absence of clear objectives for the NHS, and too little performance monitoring, though it acknowledged that the newly-adopted regional and district annual performance reviews were a step in the right direction.

☐ *The Griffiths Inquiry recommendations*

The Griffiths Inquiry recommended the creation of two new boards within the DHSS. A Health Services Supervisory Board (HSSB), chaired by the Secretary of State, responsible for NHS strategy, reviewing performance and allocating overall resources. Meanwhile, the NHS Management Board, was accountable to the HSSB for the management of the NHS. The aim was to separate and distinguish policy (and, by implication, politics) from management. This arrangement initially failed, for reasons discussed later.

Second, Griffiths recommended that existing management arrangements be replaced by general management, defined as 'the responsibility drawn together in one person, at different levels of the organisation, for planning, implementation and control of performance'. It was intended that general managers would take overall responsibility for service performance and management at regional, district and unit level. The rationale for general management was rooted in the belief that it would clarify responsibility within the NHS and promote greater accountability. It was seen as crucial to the attainment of greater cost-efficiency. Griffiths himself argued that general management would also provide better leadership, producing an improvement in the motivation of staff working in the NHS.

Third, the Griffiths Inquiry argued that accountability would be strengthened further by including units within the annual review process currently used to monitor the performance of regions and districts. Districts would be responsible for reviewing the performance of units, thus creating a line of accountability from service providers up to the Management Board.

Fourth, Griffiths identified a special role for health authority chairpersons at regional and district level. These people would drive forward the implementation of general management, taking a leading role in the identification and appointment of the general manager, and reviewing his or her performance. They would be expected to take on an important leadership role in the organisation of health authority business as well as having a specific brief to promote efficiency.

The Griffiths report made other specific recommendations concerning efficiency, such as the introduction of cost improvement programmes (discussed in the next chapter). A further recommendation was the development of management budgeting as a means of relating clinical workload directly to resources. Griffiths also urged that doctors should become more closely involved in processes of management and budgeting.

Finally, the report concentrated on the quality of service by recommending that managers took steps to evaluate performance, particularly from the patient's perspective. It urged that this perspective be incorporated in the planning and management of services, along with improved information about the effectiveness and efficiency of services.

□ *Implementing Griffiths*

Health ministers were keen that a substantial proportion of candidates be appointed from outside the NHS, in particular from business. But the attractions of NHS management were limited. Salaries were lower than in the business sector and fringe benefits virtually non-existent. Moreover, general managers were appointed on three- to five-year contracts and therefore had limited security of tenure. Despite central intervention, the majority of general managers – around two-thirds – were former NHS administrators. Only a fifth of regional and district general managers, and less than one in ten unit general managers, came from outside the NHS. The remainder were drawn from a nursing or medical background.

□ *The impact of Griffiths and other management initiatives*

The Griffiths report laid the foundations of future management reform. Following the implementation of its recommendations other changes were introduced in an effort to encourage a more entrepreneurial and dynamic management culture. These included new financial incentives for managers, such as performance-related pay and more generous remuneration packages. Later, NHS management structures were reformed so that they more closely resembled structures of decision-making found in the business sector. Furthermore, an array of management techniques used widely in commercial organisations were imported into the health service. Finally, the advent of the NHS internal market represented an attempt to create a decision-making environment similar in some respects to that faced by commercial organisations.

The remainder of this chapter explores the impact of the management reforms of the 1980s and 1990s, in relation to three key aspects of NHS management: health authorities and trusts; the relationship between managers and professionals; and the relationships between central government and local health authorities.

■ The management of health authorities and trusts

□ *Management structures*

Griffiths argued for a more streamlined and efficient management system. Central to this philosophy was that once objectives were set, managers should be given the freedom to achieve them. This implied not only the abandonment of consensus management within health authorities, but the weakening of the traditional role of the health authority member.

Following the implementation of Griffiths, general managers (along with chairpersons) took the opportunity to re-fashion their management structures. New posts appeared on the reconstituted management boards (such as director of personnel, director of research, director of information and so on). Because such changes were not uniformly imposed, it became increasingly difficult to generalise about management arrangements. Management structures below board level also began to alter and diversify, with the introduction of clinical directorates – discussed later in this chapter. Diversity was further encouraged by the creation of NHS trusts, which were given a certain amount of freedom in determining their internal arrangements.

In spite of the changes there were also important continuities. Consensus management, although formally abandoned, persisted to some extent in an informal way (Strong and Robinson, 1990, pp. 143–4). In some health authorities efforts were made to retain its advantages by emphasising teamwork at board level. Others realised that a 'macho' management style often backfired and that a more persuasive approach, working constructively with the professions and other staff, was more effective. Elsewhere, however, new management styles and structures served only to create further conflict between managers and staff.

Another important aspect of the new management arrangements was the key role played by health authority (and trust) chairpersons. Evidence concerning the role of health authority members since the implementation of Griffiths indicates that the balance of power within health authorities tends to reside with the chairperson and the general manager (Strong and Robinson, 1990; Ferlie, Ashburner and FitzGerald, 1993). The chairperson has a key role, not only in the organisation of health authority business but in the appointment of the general manager and in the assessment of his or her performance.

The powerful combination of chairperson and general manager further undermined the position of the ordinary health authority member. But in this respect the Griffiths reforms accentuated a trend that was already in motion (Ham, 1986; Day and Klein, 1987). It was acknowledged that the 1974 reorganisation of the NHS had strengthened the manager's position with respect to health authority members. Subsequently, in the early 1980s, the roles of the chairperson and senior management had been further enhanced by the annual review process, discussed earlier.

☐ The new health authorities

A further development was the reconstitution of health authorities.

Previously, all health authority members served in a part-time capacity and were drawn from a range of backgrounds. Some were nominated by local councils, providing a link with the local community, while others were drawn from the ranks of NHS staff. In 1990 the general obligation for health authorities to include people from the health professions or representatives of local communities was removed. Half the members – renamed 'non-executive directors' – were in future to be appointed for their relevant knowledge and expertise (with management knowledge and expertise being emphasised). However, district health authorities with a teaching hospital within their boundaries were required to include a member holding a post in a medical or dental school. Meanwhile, trust boards also had to include a medical school member where appropriate, as well as at least two people drawn from the local community.

Non-executive directors, like the chairperson, are part-time appointees acting on behalf of the Secretary of State for Health. They receive an honorarium as a recognition of their input (chairpersons have received part-time remuneration since 1974). They were joined on the new health authorities by executive directors, appointed in view of their management responsibilities. This was a new departure as previously senior NHS managers were not members of the health authority itself. District health authorities were required initially to include the general manager and the finance director (and subsequently, the director of public health), while trust boards had to include the medical director and a senior nurse.

The non-executive members and the chairperson clearly have a key role, not least with regard to the accountability of the NHS. But who are these people? To what extent do they differ from their predecessors on the old-style health authorities? Research has shed some light on these questions (Pettigrew *et al.*, 1991; Ferlie, FitzGerald and Ashburner, 1996; Ashburner and Cairncross, 1993)

First, there was a surprising degree of continuity between the membership of the old and the new health authorities. Almost three-quarters of non-executive members and chairpersons of the new authorities were found to be continuing previous service. However, there were also important differences. The new authorities contained a lower proportion of women than their predecessors. Less than a third of non-executive members were female, though by 1995 this proportion had risen to 39 per cent (*Health Care Parliamentary Monitor*, 1995). Ethnic minorities were also under-represented, with 2.5 per cent of non-executive members being non-white according to earlier studies (Pettigrew *et al.*, 1991), though a subsequent study found this had increased to just under 5 per cent by 1995 (Aanchawan, 1996).

The new authorities had more members with a business or self-employed background. Indeed, the majority of non-executives and

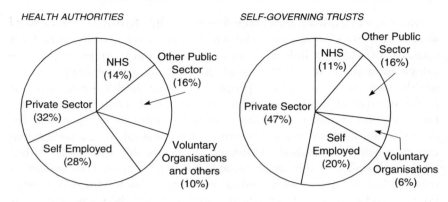

Source of data: A. Pettigrew *et al.* (1991) p. 18.

Figure 6.1   *Backgrounds of health authority and trust members, chairpersons and non-executives (England)*

chairpersons were either employed by the private sector or were self-employed (see Figure 6.1). Nevertheless, health authorities retained some members with experience of the public sector and voluntary organisations. Despite the removal of the obligation to include local councillors, 15 per cent of non-executive members of new health authorities had served in this capacity.

Compared with the new health authorities, a higher proportion of the non-executive directors on 'first wave' trusts established in 1991 were new to the NHS (Ashburner and Cairncross, 1992). Only a third had previous experience of the NHS. Figure 6.1 shows that trusts had a higher proportion of non-executive directors drawn from the business sector. Ethnic minorities and women were similarly under-represented on trusts boards as on health authorities.

A Labour Party survey of trusts showed that 56 per cent of the chairpersons had a business background, and only half had previous experience of the NHS. This survey reported an even greater business presence among trust non-executives, with five out of six being drawn from the private sector (Labour Party, 1992a).

☐ *Criticism of the new health authorities*

The new health authorities attracted much criticism. First, it was alleged that appointments to health authorities were becoming increasingly politicised. Secondly, there was concern about the lack of public accountability in the new arrangements.

An analysis by the Labour Party (1992a) of NHS trust chairs discovered that 67 per cent of those revealing their political background were Conservatives. A further study by the Labour Research Department (1994) provided a more accurate picture. It found that 14 per cent of trusts were chaired by someone linked to the Conservative Party (including individuals connected with companies which had made political donations), while less than 1 per cent were connected with Labour. A quarter of trusts contained non-executive directors who had links to the Conservative Party or who were prominent figures in a donor company. 149 trust chairpersons and non-executive directors were found to have strong Conservative connections, outnumbering those linked to other parties by six to one. Even so, in the context of the total number of chairpersons and non-executives appointed (2629), the number with overt Conservative connections was relatively small.

A survey by the NHS Trust Federation (1995) similarly found relatively low levels of partisanship among trust non-executives. But again, of those who had connections with a political party, the Conservatives were in a large majority. On the basis of each trust chairperson's assessment, only 10 per cent of non-executives were identified as Conservatives, 3 per cent Labour, and 1 per cent Liberal Democrat.

It appears therefore that health authority and trust members are not highly partisan. This conclusion is consistent with other research which indicates that less than one in five are members of political parties (see Pettigrew *et al.*, 1991). Certainly in the 1990s, there has been genuine concern about those connected with the Conservative Party outnumbering those linked with other parties. However, this may have been partly explained by other factors, including Labour Party rules which restricted activists' involvement in trusts until 1995. It remains to be seen whether or not a change in government in 1997 will give health authorities a different political bias, redress the political balance, or lead to a decline in partisan appointments. On the one hand, the new government stressed its commitment to appointment on merit irrespective of partisan allegiance. Yet the suspicion that political interference would continue was reinforced by the swift resignation of half of the regional chairpersons shortly after Labour took office.

Concern about political bias in NHS appointments is linked to a wider debate about the accountability of public and corporate bodies and the quality of the people who serve on them. This debate was influenced by two high profile reports, by *The Committee on the Financial Aspects of Corporate Governance* (Cadbury, 1992) – the Cadbury Report; and *Committee on Standards in Public Life* (Cm 2850, 1995) – the Nolan Report.

The Cadbury Report focused on the operation and accountability of corporate boards, and called for a strengthening of the role of non-executive directors, particularly in relation to audit and the remuneration of executive directors. In addition, it recommended a formal selection process for non-executives and that they should serve for specified terms. It also called for the separation of the roles of chairman and chief executive (as in fact was already the case on NHS boards). Another key recommendation was for the full disclosure of directors' remuneration.

The Nolan Report was concerned with wider issues of public accountability and standards of conduct in public life. Part of its report dealt specifically with public bodies, recommending codes of conduct for members and greater openness in the declaration of political connections and activities. It also called for appointments to be based on merit and on the basis of advice from panels with an independent element, and recommended a Commissioner for Public Appointments to monitor, regulate and approve appointments procedures.

Although dealing with broader issues, the Cadbury and Nolan Reports were extremely relevant to the NHS and had considerable impact. Following the Cadbury Report the Department of Health established a task force to examine its recommendations within the context of the NHS. The Nolan inquiry ensured that these issues stayed on the agenda. Both inquiries struck a particular chord within the NHS, where there was increasing anxiety about the accountability of health authorities and trusts.

There were three related issues. First, probity. In the years following the introduction of the new health authorities a number of financial scandals came to light (see Exhibit 7.2). This added to pressure for explicit standards of conduct not only with regard to fraud, but where any possible conflict of interest might arise. A second concern related to the ability of non-executive directors to promote and secure accountability. As noted earlier, the weakness of ordinary health authority members was not new. But mounting evidence suggested that non-executives faced an increasingly difficult task. Non-executives claimed to be overworked, to be lacking knowledge about the NHS, to be uncertain about their role, and in some cases they reported serious tensions between themselves and executive directors (Ashburner, Ferlie and FitzGerald, 1994; Audit Commission, 1995b; Peck, 1995). Subsequent research indicated that these were continuing problems (NAHAT, 1996; Stern, Martin and Cray, 1995), though some case studies gave grounds for more optimism (Ferlie, FitzGerald and Ashburner, 1996).

The third main criticism related to the lack of openness in the NHS. It was argued that new management arrangements, coupled with the move to trust status, created incentives to conceal information and to prevent those working within the NHS from speaking out on issues of concern. There was some evidence to support this. Many trusts were reluctant to meet in public beyond the statutory minimum of once a year. According to one survey, trust managers believed the NHS had become more secretive (Crail, 1995). Concern was also expressed at the introduction of so-called 'gagging clauses' aimed at preventing clinicians from speaking out, highlighted by the *British Medical Journal* (1994) in a series of articles entitled 'The Rise of Stalinism in the NHS'. After Labour took office in 1997, health ministers declared their intention to outlaw such clauses.

Public concern about secrecy, in the context of pressures for greater accountability, led to a Code on Openness in 1995. An earlier draft was modified following criticism that it was too vague, restrictive and likely to lead to prohibitive charges being imposed on those seeking information. The final version, introduced the following year (NHSE, 1995a), emphasised the need to respond positively to requests for information. It was less restrictive about the criteria for withholding information and recommended that charges should be exceptional. It accordingly received a much warmer reception, although some concerns – relating in particular to charges – remained.

The Major government also responded to criticisms about the lack of accountability in the NHS. Following the task force inquiry into corporate governance, it introduced Codes of Conduct and Accountability for NHS staff, including non-executives (NHSE, 1994a). These Codes, which came into effect in 1994, stressed public service values and required boards to keep registers of members' interests open to inspection by the public. They also defined with greater clarity the role and function of boards and their members. Echoing the recommendations of the Cadbury Report, health authorities and trusts were required to establish audit and remuneration committees. Chairpersons were charged with enabling all members of the board to make a full contribution and to ensure that the board worked as a team. The Codes also placed an emphasis on the proper organisation of business – boards now had to set out clearly their procedures for making decisions. Furthermore, additional requirements were introduced for boards to report on performance and to declare details of board members' remuneration to the public.

A new system of appointing NHS non-executive directors was established in February 1995, pre-empting the Nolan Report recommendations. The NHS was required to advertise for suitable candidates for non-executive directorships, who now had to declare if they have been active in a political party. A selection process by interview was introduced, with successful candidates joining a regional list from which vacancies could be filled. Appointments are scrutinised by assessment panels, one-third of whose members must be independent of the Department of Health, while in Scotland there is an advisory committee on appointments which includes non-NHS members.

Further changes to the appointment system followed the election of a Labour government in 1997. With 900 non-executive posts becoming vacant in autumn 1997, local authorities were invited to nominate candidates. The Secretary of State for Health also asked MPs for nominations. In addition, anyone applying for a non-executive post was required to live locally and demonstrate a commitment to the NHS. It is too early to assess the effect of these changes on health authority composition. The new government also issued fresh regulations on openness in the NHS, requiring NHS boards and trusts to meet more often in public.

■ Management and the professions

The health care professions were suspicious of the Conservatives' management reforms. In particular, they feared the exclusion of professional advice, a reluctance to respect professional views and interests, and domination by lay managers. In this section there is an attempt to assess the actual impact of the management changes upon nurses (the largest professional group) and doctors (traditionally the most powerful professional group).

□ Nurses

Nurses gained much from the structural and managerial reforms of the 1970s. They benefited considerably from the NHS reorganisation of 1974, gaining a place on the new consensus management teams. The retention of consensus management in the 1982 reorganisation consolidated their position. The Griffiths Report, however, threatened to diminish the role of nurses at senior levels in the management structure.

Nurses' fears were to some extent justified. Few were appointed as general managers (less than 10 per cent of general managers had a nursing background). Moreover, as mentioned earlier, the new general managers had considerable freedom to determine their own management structures. These structures often changed in ways unfavourable to nursing, especially at district level where nursing officers began to disappear from the management boards.

Following a campaign by nurses the DHSS vetoed management structures in a number of districts where nursing advisers had been excluded, though it did not guarantee them a place on the management boards. The career prospects of senior nurse managers declined further with the abolition of the RHAs, though the regional offices subsequently created nurse director or nursing advisor posts. At district level, according to a Royal College of Nursing survey, only about half of health authority boards included nurses in an executive capacity (Hancock, 1995). Meanwhile, the merging of district health authorities and FHSAs further reduced opportunities for nurses at this level.

The initial impact of Griffiths' reforms, particularly upon senior nursing staff, was viewed in extremely negative terms (Walby and Greenwell, 1994) and, as Robinson (1992) notes, 1985 was seen very much as the low point. Others believed that nurses' loss of influence would be temporary, noting the opportunities for nurses under the new regime, for example through the development of a quality assurance role (Harrison, 1988). Others argued that nurses were well-placed to compete for general management posts in future and saw the Griffiths management reforms as having a symbolic effect rather than altering actual power relations (Owens and Glennerster, 1990).

Post-Griffiths, the problems facing nursing have been much the same as before. The voice of nursing continues to be disregarded at senior levels (Robinson, 1992; Davies, 1995). And it is widely recognised that nursing still suffers from a lack of strategic management, so that its contribution to improving service quality is not fully realised (Audit Commission, 1991a). Nevertheless some positive signs for the future did begin to emerge post-Griffiths.

The creation of trust status led to structural changes which in some respects increased the opportunities for some nurses to contribute to management. It will be recalled that although trusts have considerable discretion in establishing their management structures, trust boards must include a senior nurse. In addition, the development of clinical management teams, stimulated by the development of trust status and the commissioner–provider split, seems to have facilitated the representation of the nursing perspective below board level – though much seems to depend on local personalities and conditions (Jones, 1994; British Association of Medical Managers *et al.*, 1993). As new forms of management develop, it is possible that the influence of nursing may be extended rather than undermined (Walby and Greenwell, 1994, p. 151). Although clinical management teams are mainly headed by doctors, nurses have been appointed to this role. Indeed, nurses' leaders have argued that in future more nurses should serve in this capacity (Hancock, 1993). Clinical management arrangements are discussed in further detail later in this chapter.

The devolution of certain management responsibilities following Griffiths and other management reforms, while adding to the workload and stress levels of nurses, can be seen in a more positive light (Owens and

Glennerster, 1990). In particular the devolution of budgets to ward level is believed to have increased the financial and management role of nurses (Alaszewski, 1995). Ward managers increasingly have a role in the establishment and maintenance of quality standards. However, they are subject to the overall constraints set by senior managers.

Further opportunities to develop the nursing role may be presented in the future. Some relate to the changes in the nursing process and in nurse education and training discussed in Exhibit 3.7. In addition, as some observers such as Witz (1994, p. 24) and Davies (1995, p. 184) have argued, new managerial structures have opened up a number of possibilities. In particular, the contract culture and the focus on quality of care and value for money have the potential to produce a more explicit recognition of nurses' contribution, on the basis of alliances with managers and other professional groups.

But at the same time management changes contain a number of dangers. Nurses remain, in comparison with doctors, the weaker profession. Changes in skill-mix and task allocation, prompted by management arrangements, may serve to merely extend their traditional 'handmaiden' role as they take on routine functions discarded by doctors. Efforts to change the allocation of tasks may disadvantage nurses in other respects. Replacing nurses with clerical workers and nursing assistants may enhance the status of fully-qualified nurses but is also likely to reduce their numbers. Furthermore, there is the spectre of multi-skilling, with the prospect of replacing professional nurses and therapists with health workers trained in a range of specific tasks (Health Services Management Unit, 1996a). According to this scenario, nurses may find themselves increasingly subject to measures which erode rather than advance their professional status.

☐ *The medical profession*

Much of the impact of management reform on the medical profession has been analysed in terms of conflict between doctors and managers. This is hardly surprising given the perception that general management was a means of undermining medical autonomy. In this respect, at least, doctors need not have worried. The Griffiths reforms did not significantly alter the balance of power between doctors and managers. Doctors successfully resisted efforts to limit their autonomy and externally monitor their performance (Strong and Robinson, 1990). As Harrison and Pollitt (1994, p. 50) observed, most managers steered well clear of issues where the medical profession was likely to raise strong objections. As a result the relationship between the two remained to be renegotiated (Harrison *et al.*, 1992).

In some localities, however, new recruits drawn from outside the NHS (usually from business or the armed services) did overtly challenge the local medical establishment. In the vast majority of cases these managers backed down, many leaving the NHS never to return. Following these early skirmishes tensions occasionally erupted into open conflict usually leading to the resignation of senior management, and in some cases chairpersons and non-executive directors. But although tensions remained and relations between doctors and managers have been in some cases poor (Blackhurst, 1995), overt conflict has not been the norm. A survey by the Hospital Consultants' and Specialists' Association found that only one in eight senior doctors believed that their trust management style was 'very or extremely confrontational' (*Health Service Journal*, 1995). However, two-thirds said their trust was occasionally or moderately confrontational, while only one-fifth of respondents said the trust management was not confrontational at all.

Tensions between managers and doctors might be seen as an indication that the medical profession is being challenged. According to some the continuing process of management reform since the Griffiths Report has strengthened the position of managers. Flynn (1992, p. 183), writes of 'an unprecedented battery of measures and techniques for audit evaluation, monitoring and surveillance' circumscribing the autonomy of doctors. Compounding this was the decision to separate commissioning from provision, which as Harrison *et al.* (1992) note, has placed 'several additional levers of power and persuasion into managers' hands'. Certainly, the need to secure contracts and generate income, added weight to managers' arguments for changes in service organisation and delivery, improved monitoring of service quality, and the matching of workload to resources.

Finally, managers acquired new roles in relation to managing doctors and rewarding their performance. Trusts hold doctors' contracts and can vary the terms and conditions of new appointments. Managers are responsible for agreeing job plans with consultants. They, along with non-executive directors, sit on consultant appointment committees, though doctors still form the majority. Finally, lower level merit awards for doctors are awarded by committees at trust level, and contribution to management is now one of the criteria for awarding merit pay.

Yet, as noted in Chapter 2, the medical profession remains powerful. Doctors do not have to remove an offending manager to secure their objectives. As the Audit Commission (1995c, 1996a) indicated, many of the new powers of managers have not been fully exercised. For example, in spite of the formal requirements for job plans, some hospitals had not implemented this. It seems that lasting change is only possible with the commitment and cooperation of doctors (see Hadley and Forster, 1993). A great deal seems to depend not only on the approach taken by managers, but on the need to overcome the traditional reluctance of doctors to become involved in management.

☐ Doctors in management: resource management

The resource management initiative (RMI) was launched in 1986 on an experimental basis. Resource management has two main features. First, the development of an information base about the cost and quality of services. Second, a management structure which explicitly incorporates clinicians into the decision-making process and gives them responsibility for budgets.

The RMI was an amalgam of ideas, none of which were particularly new (Perrin, 1988). A number of 'management budgeting' projects had taken place in the 1970s to provide clinicians with information about the resource implications of their decisions. However, there were significant differences between 'management budgets' and the RMI. Management budgeting was essentially a 'top-down' exercise, the main aim of which was to provide clinicians with information about costs in an attempt to get them to accept some responsibility for their budgets. Resource management was seen as more of a 'bottom-up' exercise. The focus was upon generating information about resources and activity which could be used by clinicians and managers to identify potential improvements in cost-effectiveness, thereby informing future resource allocation.

Confidence in the RMI was shaken following the report of an evaluation study by researchers at Brunel University (Packwood, Keen and Buxton, 1991). In the six pilot sites chosen for RMI, not one had a fully-operating resource management system up and running within three years of the initiative's launch. Obstacles were encountered in setting up accurate data collection procedures, analysing the data, and in bringing the data into the decision-making process. No conclusive evidence of improved patient care was found by the researchers. But the cost of implementing the resource management system was twice as high as originally expected. In spite of this the scheme was expanded in 1989, before the evaluation of the RMI 'experiment' was complete. Resource management went on to become the cornerstone of the internal market, providing information on the costs of clinical activity, which could then be incorporated in contracts.

Since this time, efforts have been made to devise systems which can produce more accurate and relevant information for resource management. One of the main difficulties has been to devise an appropriate case-mix system which classifies treatments (and patients with particular diseases) in a way which reflects the information needs of all participants. In 1996, a report into the impact of resource management found that less than 30 per cent of sites had fully operational case-mix systems, and that even where systems were up and running clinicians and managers in many cases did not see the originally anticipated benefits. The study also found little evidence that resource management had improved clinical practice, despite the fact that this was one of the primary objectives of the programme. However, on a more positive note it did appear that resource management had influenced clinical participation in management in a positive way (Health Services Management Unit, 1996b).

The development of information systems with regard to resource management particularly reflects a broader problem within the NHS, which continues today. As Spurgeon (1993, p. 96) has observed, much more has been said about the information revolution in the NHS than has actually happened. It is true that much-heralded initiatives in this field have frequently foundered. For example, there have been delays and difficulties associated with the introduction of integrated hospital information support systems (HISS) (National Audit Office, 1996a; Thomas, 1994), and problems associated with the introduction of computer coding systems (Cross, 1996). Meanwhile, the shortage of adequately trained information technology staff has caused additional difficulties (Brittain, 1992).

☐ Clinical management

Resource management, trust status and the purchaser–provider split prompted the formation of new management structures below unit level, known as clinical management teams (CMTs). Although there are a variety of models, the most common is the clinical directorate which itself takes a number of forms (see White, 1993; British Association of Medical Managers *et al.*, 1993).

Clinical directorates are focused on the main areas of a provider's activity. In hospital units they are organised according to the main specialties such as medicine, surgery, specialist surgery, obstetrics and gynaecology, and other clinical services (for example pathology, radiology and anaesthetics). In practice, groupings vary considerably and may be subdivided further into associate directorates based on departments. Some directorates, particularly in non-acute units, are focused around client groups, such as the elderly.

Although clinical directorates are usually headed by a consultant, some clinical directors (particularly of community health services and non-medical therapies) have a non-medical background. The clinical director is usually part-time, maintaining some professional practice. Working with the clinical director and responsible to him are a nurse manager and a business manager. In some directorates these roles are combined into a single post. There are other models, including the specialty directorate model, where a full-time specialty manager, usually from a non-medical background, holds the budget. He or she agrees activity levels with clinicians and with trust management. In this model, clinicians are less directly involved in the management process.

The clinical director has a number of responsibilities which he or she undertakes with the assistance of the other members of the clinical management team (CMT). These include management of the budget, staff, workload and, increasingly, overall quality of service. Clinical directorates produce a 'business plan' and monitor performance against this. Finally, clinical directors represent the directorate within the trust, for example by participating on management boards and committees. Medical clinical directors can also channel views through the medical director, who sits on the trust board and has overall responsibility for monitoring medical performance.

Despite the difficulties inherent in getting doctors to participate in management activities, the experience of the new clinical management systems has apparently been good. One survey found 'a high level of positive attitudes to clinical management' (British Association of Medical Managers, *et al.* 1993), while Marnoch (1996, p. 25), for example, notes that they have attracted a 'certain degree of justifiable optimism'. Potentially, the new clinical management systems can improve teamworking, develop greater flexibility in the provision of services, help to integrate clinical and resource management, and achieve improvements in the quality of care (Capewell, 1992).

There are, however, a number of obstacles. At best clinical management teams work in a consensual way, with all participants sharing views and perspectives. But team-building is undermined in some cases by a refusal to share decision-making (Walby and Greenwell, 1994). Meanwhile, flexibility can be frustrated in practice by the failure to devolve budgetary responsibilities to clinicians (British Association of Medical Managers, 1996). Another problem is that clinical directors have limited influence over their colleagues and cannot be held responsible for their performance (Orchard, 1993). Doctors are particularly suspicious of anything resembling line management, and may ultimately refuse to cooperate with the plans agreed by the clinical director at unit level. As a result most clinical directorates remain a device for managing budgets and balancing the books (Audit Commission, 1995c; Marnoch, 1996).

The lack of managerial authority of the clinical director also threatens potential improvements in service quality. As Marnoch (1996, p. 61) states, 'it will be a rare case where a clinical director is using an audit system to identify underperforming colleagues and subsequently act upon this evidence.' As a result standards are often set, but not effectively monitored

(British Association of Medical Managers *et al.*, 1993). There have been a number of recent cases where doctors have taken early retirement following allegedly poor performance exposed by the audit process. But such cases remain comparatively rare.

☐ *Medical audit and quality assurance*

Although it is still difficult to influence the behaviour of individual doctors, it is nevertheless the case that the medical profession and other health professions have been subjected to greater pressures to set, monitor and improve standards of care. These pressures are associated with the introduction of medical audit (and clinical audit for other professions) and other quality assurance initiatives.

Medical audit is defined by Marinker (1990) as 'the attempt to improve the quality of medical care by measuring the performance of those providing that care, by considering performance in relation to desired standards and by improving on this in performance'. Doctors themselves accept the need for medical audit, but only under certain conditions: that the process remains under their control, that it is highly confidential, that participation is voluntary, and that there is no compulsion to alter practice in the light of the results. An example of this approach is the confidential inquiry, supported by the main professional bodies. As noted in Chapter 3, the National Confidential Enquiry into Perioperative Deaths (NCEPOD) has revealed serious shortcomings in the quality of care and standards of practice.

Such inquiries play a valuable role, not only in highlighting deficiencies in medical practice, but problems with support services, hospital organisation and resources. Indeed, NCEPOD reports have attributed a significant proportion of deaths in hospital to factors outside doctors' control. They have identified the lack of critical care facilities and the inadequacies of medical records as particular problems. In the 1992 NCEPOD report, personnel and resource shortages were associated with 5 and 4 per cent of deaths respectively (Camplin, Lunn and Devlin, 1992).

In 1989 there was an attempt to promote a more systematic approach to medical audit. The Department of Health sought to institutionalise medical audit procedures by establishing advisory committees at district and regional level. Similar arrangements were established for doctors working in primary care. Although managers were given a role in the establishment and broad direction of these committees, the Department of Health agreed that the process should be managed by the doctors themselves.

As a result, medical audit has not directly challenged the clinical autonomy of the profession. Indeed, as Pollitt (1993b) has argued, the scheme was established in such a way that it would not offend medical interests. The objectives and processes of audit fitted in with doctors' own concept of quality, rather than managers' and patient's perspectives. This view is supported by Packwood, Kerrison and Buxton (1994), who note that audit has remained focused on technical processes and has not resulted in stronger external management of doctor's work. In connection with this, Black and Thompson (1993) identified considerable obstacles to medical audit, many of which could only be overcome by a substantial change in doctors' beliefs, knowledge and attitudes. Further criticisms were made by the Public Accounts Committee which noted that a sizeable minority of doctors still did not participate in audit (House of Commons, 1996b). The Committee also observed that in spite of incurring costs of £279m on developing such schemes since 1989, there had been a failure to monitor the benefits accruing to patients.

But perhaps medical audit, in conjunction with other initiatives, may have a longer-term impact. There has been an attempt to shift the focus away from narrow professional considerations to a more multidisciplinary approach to audit, focused on overall quality of service. The move towards comprehensive *clinical audit* aims to integrate the audit processes of all the professions involved (that is, medical audit, nursing audit, and the audit of professions allied to medicine). This has been encouraged by the funding of initiatives through a National Centre for Clinical Audit. Meanwhile clinical audit has become an increasingly important part of negotiations and agreements between commissioners and providers of health care. In 1996 health authorities were given the responsibility for developing clinical audit. As they (and other commissioners of care) specify in greater detail the quality of service they expect from providers, clinical audit will take on a much larger role in ensuring that what was agreed has actually been delivered. Furthermore, commissioning bodies are being encouraged by the NHSE to use audit to identify good practice which can then influence the development of future contracts and agreements.

Efforts to extend clinical audit must be seen in the context of other quality assurance initiatives. A range of initiatives have been introduced, often based upon ideas drawn from the private sector. One approach is accreditation, where health service organisations such as hospitals or general practices seek public endorsement of their service quality from an external body, such as the British Standards Institute (in this case the relevant standard is BS 5750). Another example is the Charter Mark scheme under the auspices of the *Citizen's Charter* introduced by the Major government in the early 1990s.

Other approaches are connected with the idea of 'total quality management' (TQM) defined by Joss and Kogan (1995, p. 37) as 'an integrated, corporately-led programme of organisational change designed to engender and sustain a culture of continuous improvement based on customer-oriented definitions of quality'. It is rooted in four principles: that organisational success depends on meeting customer needs; that quality (defined by the customer) is achieved by the production process; that most employees are motivated to work hard and perform well; and that simple statistical methods can reveal faults in the production process, leading to continuous improvements in quality (Berwick, Enthoven and Bunker, 1992).

Despite growing interest in this approach, which originated in the management and production processes of successful Japanese companies, it has nevertheless been criticised on several grounds (Freemantle, 1992). First, it is argued that health care is a complex personal service not suitable for 'production line' quality evaluation techniques developed for manufacturing industries. Second, it is maintained that the measurement of performance under TQM relates more to superficial consumer reaction rather than to improved quality of service.

In practice there have been difficulties in implementing TQM systems. As Joss and Kogan (1995) observed, there is still a large gap between the rhetoric of quality and the reality of implementing schemes based on TQM principles. They also note that the success of such schemes crucially depends upon the participation of the clinicians at an early stage, a point reiterated by others (Marnoch, 1996, p. 82).

One particular approach that has attracted some attention in the latter part of the 1990s is hospital process re-engineering. This too is based on concepts and techniques imported from the business world. Its aims are to initiate and develop radical thinking about process and organisation in an effort to secure improvements in efficiency and patient satisfaction. In 1994, the Leicester Royal Infirmary was chosen as a pilot site for this approach. This involved teams of staff pooling their knowledge about vital processes – such as the passage of patients through the hospital. This led to recommendations for changing these processes and redesigning hospital organisation, for example with regard to outpatient visits (Millar, 1995). Hospital re-engineering has its critics, many of who dismiss it as the latest 'management fad'. However, in conjunction with other efforts to improve the quality of service it may prove to be a useful component of a strategy to re-think and re-design organisations and methods of working (see Buchanan, 1996).

Finally, the Labour Government's White Paper of 1997 proposed a range of initiatives to improve health service quality. Two new bodies were envisaged. A National Institute for Clinical Excellence, to issue guidance on cost-effectiveness, clinical effectiveness, and on clinical audit. A second body – the Commission for Health Improvement – is intended to promote changes in service quality. This body will check that effective systems to monitor and improve clinical services are in place at local level. The government has suggested that the Commission will be able to investigate persistent problems of service quality and recommend necessary action. In addition trusts will be expected to monitor service quality more closely in future and will be held accountable for any shortcomings identified.

■ Central–local relations

The management initiatives introduced by the Conservative governments of Thatcher and Major were often viewed as centralist: increasing the influence of central government over local health services (Ferlie, FitzGerald and Ashburner, 1996; Paton, 1993). In particular, management reforms were acknowledged as producing a stronger system of line management, or a professionalised management hierarchy (Loveridge and Starkey, 1992) facilitating 'top-down' policy initiatives.

□ *Politics and management*

One of the central themes of the Griffiths Report was the devolution of management responsibility. In theory, ministers and their senior advisers would set policy objectives, and NHS managers would be responsible for efficient and effective implementation. The inquiry team believed that 'the requirement for central isolated initiatives should disappear once a coherent management process is established' (DHSS, 1983, p. 16).

Following the Griffiths Report, as shown earlier, the division between policy and management was institutionalised. It was also intended that the Department of Health's role would be drastically pruned. However, the officials fought a successful rearguard action. They played on the fears of ministers who, given the sensitivity of health issues, insisted that health authorities should be carefully monitored (Klein 1990b; Stowe, 1989). The tension created by the attempt to divide policy and management was clearly illustrated by the resignation of the first chairperson of the NHS management board, the industrialist, Victor Paige. He resigned after only sixteen months following alleged disagreements with ministers, later claiming that 'Ministers took all the important decisions: political, strategic and managerial' (House of Commons, 1988a, p. 94).

A fresh attempt to establish the division between policy and management was made in 1989, with the creation of the NHS Management Executive, subsequently renamed the NHS Executive (NHSE). Notably, its first Chief Executive was a career NHS manager, Duncan Nichol. The NHSE was later relocated to new headquarters in Leeds, establishing a physical separation from the politicians and civil servants in Whitehall. Yet policy and management in the NHS remained closely entwined. The reorganisation of the Department of Health and of the NHS, following the introduction of the internal market, blurred the division even further. The NHSE (which remained part of the Department of Health) was subsequently given responsibilities for health care policy as well as management (DoH, 1994b).

Meanwhile, following a review of the NHS structure in 1993, ministers decided to replace the regional health authorities with regional offices of the NHSE (DoH, 1994c). This was widely seen as a centralist move, as the regional tier of the NHS would in future be run by civil servants within the Department of Health rather than by NHS employees accountable to health authorities that had at least some external representation (see Hunter, 1993). The government rejected this, arguing that the regions would not intervene excessively, but would instead maintain a 'light touch'. Ministers also claimed that management responsibility was in fact being delegated further down the NHS structure, as functions formerly undertaken by the regional tier were devolved to district level.

☐ *Accountability*

Efforts to devolve management responsibility, a major theme in the reforms of the 1980s and 1990s, have added to the problems of NHS accountability. The main problem is that while ministers have attempted to strengthen central control of the NHS, they have at the same time sought to devolve the responsibility for services to local managers. The intention was that when things went wrong, managers rather than ministers and civil servants would get the blame. This was widely seen as unfair and inappropriate. For instance, as the former head of the Audit Commission, Sir John Banham, noted, health authorities cannot influence the level of resources nor the demand for services (Limb, 1995). However, in practice central government continued to attract most the flak for the problems of the NHS.

For the Conservative governments of Thatcher and Major, management accountability appeared to take priority over broader notions of public accountability (see Wall, 1996; Bruce and McConnell, 1995). This was reflected in complaints by MPs who found difficulties in obtaining information and holding ministers to account (House of Commons, 1996c). For example, the percentage of Parliamentary Questions relating to health answered 'no' or 'not collected centrally' rose from 3.4 per cent to 8.5 per cent between 1989–90 and 1991–2. It later fell to 4.5 per cent (*Health Care Parliamentary Monitor*, 1995b).

In other respects, however, there was a tightening of Parliamentary accountability. In 1995 chief executives of health authorities and trusts became designated as accountable officers, becoming directly accountable to MPs for the money spent by their organisations. In addition Parliamentary scrutiny of the NHS improved considerably with the extension of the role of the Audit Commission, the greater interest taken in health management matters by the National Audit Office, and the detailed inquiries of the Health Select Committee (see Chapter 7 for further discussion of these bodies). Moreover, despite efforts to shift responsibility from the centre to the periphery, it was clear that health ministers continued to face enormous pressure on specific issues, particularly where there was significant Parliamentary and media interest.

□ *Planning, monitoring and review*

As mentioned in Chapter 4, from the 1960s onwards central government sought to improve health service planning. These initiatives, and further plans introduced in the 1970s and early 1980s, were largely 'indicative' and did not seek direct control over service developments. However, from 1982 a more centralised approach began to emerge. The new planning system introduced that year emphasised the importance of strategic planning. The establishment of regional manpower targets the following year reinforced a more centralised approach, while the introduction of an annual review process reflected a growing concern with service provision at the periphery. This process was strengthened further with the creation of the NHS Management Board (and subsequently the Management Executive and later the NHSE) which took a greater interest in management performance review.

Some believed that the new review processes were overrated. Former health minister Ray Whitney (1988) claimed that the reviews of the mid-1980s were an exercise in cajolery rather than management. Moreover, in some important specific areas of policy including preventive medicine, the management of doctors, and the introduction of market testing, the evidence points to a clear failure to promote the desired response from health authorities in line with stated priorities (Audit Commission, 1995c; Butler, 1995b; National Audit Office, 1996c). A further problem with the central planning approach was that priorities tended to multiply. For example, during the late 1980s it was not uncommon for the RHAs to have between forty and fifty priorities (Flanagan, 1989). As ministers themselves admitted, such a large number of priorities meant in reality no priorities at all (Whitney, 1988).

Subsequently, the focus shifted away from specific targets towards broader initiatives aimed at improving sectors of service provision – maternity care, for example – and overall standards of service, such as waiting times. The Department of Health began to focus on a smaller number of medium-term priority areas alongside a larger number of baseline requirements and objectives (NHSE, 1995b; Department of Health, 1996a) that related to particular initiatives and standards of service.

Another important departure during the 1990s was a much greater emphasis on locally-specific objectives and targets. Objectives are agreed between NHSE and regional offices and in turn between regional offices and health authorities (see Figure 6.2). Further changes in the planning system were generated by problems exposed and in some respects exacerbated by the internal market (see Chapter 8). These changes included a greater emphasis on the role of commissioning plans, drawn up by health authorities, which set out key objectives and priorities locally and how services might develop in such a way to meet these aims. The commissioning plan was intended to be the framework within which service contracts and agreements should be negotiated. Commissioners and providers were expected to cooperate in the formulation of these plans and share relevant information. However, as we shall see in Chapter 8, there were considerable obstacles to this in practice.

In 1997 the Blair government signalled its intention to develop a more cooperative planning regime. Health authorities, trusts, GPs, other commissioning groups, local authorities and other relevant interests would in future have to establish Health Improvement Programmes in an effort to improve health and health care locally. Meanwhile, the broad priorities for the NHS remained much the same: to develop a leading role for primary care, to improve mental health services, improve clinical and cost-effectiveness of services generally, give greater voice to users and carers, provide better services for the elderly and other vulnerable people, and develop the NHS as a good employer. However, there was now more emphasis on tackling inequalities in health and ensuring fairness in access to health services than under the previous government.

☐ *Performance indicators*

It is widely believed that central intervention has been enhanced by the availability of more information about the performance of health authorities. Performance indicators were introduced in September 1983, the first set being grouped under the headings of clinical activity, finance, manpower, support services, and estate management. They were seen by

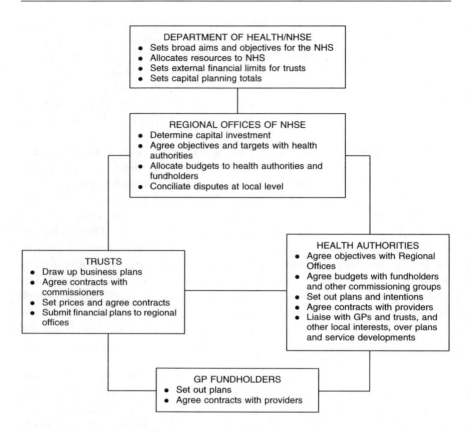

Figure 6.2   *The NHS planning process (1998–9)*

some as essentially a 'centre-run exercise focused on a narrow, finance dominated notion of performance' (Pollitt, 1985, p. 9).

Yet the immediate impact of performance indicators was slight. Neither health authorities nor professionals took much notice of them, though planning and finance staff took them more seriously. Since then indicators have become more refined and extensive. New sets of performance indicators were introduced in subsequent years. These were influenced by the need to improve the use and collection of information in the NHS, in the light of the Körner reports (Windsor, 1986) and the national strategy for health services information (DHSS, 1986a).

An added pressure behind their development was the need for ministers to demonstrate to the public that all was well in the NHS. So official statistics were able to show that the NHS was able to deliver, year-on-year, more care with greater efficiency. The efficiency index, a measure of health service output per unit of resource, was introduced in the 1990s as a means of deflecting such criticism. However, given the narrow measurement of output it adopted the index itself attracted much criticism (Clarke *et al.*, 1993). The particular measure of output, the Finished Consultant Episode (FCE), was attacked for inflating estimates of hospital workload (Benster, 1994; Radical Statistics Health Group, 1995). The Department of Health undertook a review of the index, but this was overtaken by a change of government in 1997. A new performance framework has since been proposed. It has six dimensions: fair access; efficiency; health improvement; effective delivery of appropriate healthcare; health outcomes; and patient/carer experience.

In the 1990s the development of performance indicators was influenced by other initiatives such as resource management, clinical audit, the purchaser–provider split, the national health strategy, *The Patient's Charter*, and the drive to promote evidence-based medicine. There was also a greater emphasis on the need for information about health outcomes, rather than simply inputs or outputs. In recent years there has been a greater effort to produce evidence on clinical outcomes. North of the border, clinical outcome statistics have been published since 1995, making it possible to identify differences in post-operative survival rates between health board areas and readmission rates between different hospitals. Though it is often stressed that no conclusions should be drawn from the data regarding the comparative quality or efficacy of treatment, the information is beginning to have an impact on the commissioning process (Scottish Office, 1995; 1996a). England and Wales are set to follow this path. In 1997 the Department of Health proposed 15 new clinical indicators for the NHS, including deaths in hospital following surgery and emergency readmissions.

Performance indicators are generally viewed as a centralist tool. In theory, health authorities that underperform can be identified and their managers held to account. The use of such indicators dovetails neatly with the processes of accountability review and general management. However, there is concern about their inappropriate use, with 'league tables' coming in for particular criticism. Those who are 'bottom of the league' may have very good reasons for being there – their workload and the population they serve may differ considerably from providers at the top of the table. It has been noted that outputs are often influenced by more factors outside the control of institutions than those for which they are held accountable (Goldstein and Spiegelhalter, 1996). The authors of this study warn that caution should be applied when making comparisons and that results should be regarded as 'suggestive rather than definitive'.

Moreover, continuing inaccuracies in the collection and processing of data undermine confidence in performance appraisal (Skinner, Riley and

Thomas, 1988). One clinical director tells a revealing story about how his department was criticised for detaining patients too long in hospital. It was later discovered that in two cases the patient's date of birth had been erroneously recorded as the date of admission. Hence two octogenarians had been recorded as spending 80 years in hospital, thus grossly inflating the average length of stay statistic (Phillips, 1996). Conspiracy as well as cock-up can distort the figures. As we shall see in Chapter 11, some hospitals have found ways of meeting performance targets without necessarily achieving better quality care.

Even if the quality of the data improves there is no guarantee that the information will be properly used, or that performance will actually improve (Birch and Maynard, 1988). Furthermore, performance indicators may turn out to be less effective in controlling and monitoring clinicians' performance than was initially believed. Indeed, doctors have been urged to use indicators in view of their potential to demonstrate the contribution of clinical activity (Lowry, 1988). According to this perspective, rather than simply providing information to support the review process, performance indicators become an important factor in the battle for additional resources.

■ Conclusion

The reforms introduced during the 1980s and 1990s represented a departure from earlier attempts to alter health service management. The main aim was not merely to promote organisational change in order to produce a more coherent health service, but cultural change to make the NHS more 'businesslike' and efficient. It also involved the creation of a professionalised management hierarchy to fulfil the aims and objectives set by the centre.

It was widely acknowledged that new 'managerialist' values would have to infiltrate the mind-set of clinicians before they could dominate the culture of the NHS. So far there is no hard evidence that such a cultural change has taken place (see Walby and Greenwell, 1994; Laughlin and Broadbent, 1994; Harrison and Pollitt, 1994). Nor has the development of a professionalised management hierarchy significantly undermined professional power. We have seen that initially nurses were adversely affected by some of the changes. But even here new opportunities have been presented. Moreover, the 'corporate rationalisers' (Alford, 1975) still have much to do to tame the medical 'professional monopoly' of the doctors. Although some of the foundations might well be in place (Harrison et al., 1992), management reform has not as yet produced an unambiguous shift in the balance of power between doctors and managers.

During the Thatcher/Major era, central government acquired more tools with which to monitor the NHS and to promote particular policies and initiatives. There was also a clear attempt to politicise appointments and infuse the NHS with people from a business background. But, ironically, many of the government's own reforms promoted a greater delegation of responsibility to the local and unit level, where the medical profession remains powerful. Moreover, as we have seen, doctors have so far been able to tame the 'new managerialism' by using performance indicators, clinical management and medical audit to their own ends.

The distinction between policy and management in the NHS still remains cloudy. Time and again central government has interfered in detailed aspects of NHS management and has been unable or unwilling to confine itself to a strategic or coordinating role. This has fuelled complaints about a lack of accountability in the service, particularly the accountability of services to the local community. There are real fears that the NHS has become something of a black hole in terms of accountability, with delegation producing a system where it is possible for all to escape blame when things go awry.

And yet the politicians who head the service have not escaped overall responsibility for NHS policy and funding, despite efforts to delegate managerial responsibility. Responsibility for the NHS is rather like throwing away a boomerang. When things go seriously wrong ministers have great difficulty in distancing themselves from the problems of the service. As long as the NHS continues to be perceived by the public as a national service, remains centrally funded out of taxation, and as long as health care remains high on the political agenda, ultimate responsibility for the service will continue to be focused at the centre.

■ *Chapter 7* ■

Resourcing Health Care

In the postwar period the public sector has dominated health care funding and provision to a greater extent in Britain than in most other comparable countries. Since the late 1970s, four major developments have influenced this model of resource allocation. These are: the growth of the private sector; pressure to restrict public spending; the focus on greater efficiency and selectivity; and the introduction of a 'purchaser–provider' split into the NHS. The first three are discussed in this chapter, the fourth in Chapter 8.

■ Privatisation

The arguments against the allocation of health care by the market are formidable (Normand, 1991). Markets are poor at allocating resources to those most in need of health care, and in a private health care market sick people are less able to afford the costs of treatment. This is partly because illness is linked to socio-economic status and poverty (see Chapters 1 and 12), and partly because health insurers have an incentive to exclude those with a record of previous illness or who are prone to develop serious illness.

Individual transactions in a private market cannot reflect the wider importance of health and health care for the whole community. Providers of health care tend to locate where the population is generally prosperous, and poorer areas will be under-provided for. Furthermore, if individuals cannot for financial reasons obtain the health care they need, this is a social as well as an individual problem. Inability to obtain treatment imposes further costs on the community in the long run in the form of outbreaks of infectious disease, premature mortality and chronic illness. Taking a broader public health perspective, health care can be seen as a special good which should be allocated on the basis of need rather than by ability to pay.

Choice in a private market is limited by a number of factors. In particular, consumers lack information and expertise in health care matters: health care providers have a monopoly of knowledge and skills. In an unregulated market there is great potential for exploitation of consumers and oversupply of services. Furthermore, market-led health care systems create obstacles to effective planning and coordination. It is difficult to coordinate the activities of different buyers and sellers in the marketplace, particularly when they are free to respond to individual demand rather than community needs. In addition, the commercial secrecy required by private markets inhibits the sharing of information which is essential to effective planning.

Finally, private health care markets do not seem to promote efficiency. Bed occupancy rates are generally lower in private hospitals compared to the NHS (Laing, 1996). Administrative costs also tend to be higher in health care systems dominated by the private sector. Around a quarter of the cost of the US health care system is allocated to administration (Woolhandler and Himmelstein, 1991), while in the NHS prior to the introduction of the internal market, administrative costs accounted for just under 7 per cent of total spending (Office of Health Economics, 1984).

The experience of the USA is often identified as the main example of how private markets can adversely effect health care (Ginzberg, 1990). The USA spends a seventh of its national income on health care, twice as much the UK. Yet infant mortality is higher, and male life expectancy lower than in Britain. There is also evidence of a higher level of unnecessary surgery and over-doctoring in the USA (see Chapter 3) while, paradoxically, 16 per cent of Americans are uninsured and cannot obtain the treatment they need.

□ *Privatising the NHS?*

The warnings about the failure of private health care markets has not prevented efforts, at home and abroad, to alter the public/private mix in health care (Newbrander and Parker, 1992). In Britain the private sector began to grow during the 1970s at a time of industrial unrest within the NHS. This trend was later boosted by the Thatcher government which believed that the private sector was more efficient, better managed, and more responsive to the consumer than the public sector. However, the main obstacle to a greater role for the private sector in health care was the popularity of the NHS, which remained high even after the industrial strife of the 1970s.

The constraint imposed by public opinion was clearly illustrated in 1982, when the government 'think tank', the Central Policy Review Staff (CPRS) suggested partial privatisation of NHS services. The report, which was leaked to the press, argued that if the government were serious about their stated aim of reducing public spending, radical measures would have to be considered including a move away from a tax-financed health service towards a private insurance system, and for increased charges for health services. In the face of public and media hostility, ministers disowned the report (Fowler, 1991). The affair culminated in the now famous statement by Margaret Thatcher at the Conservative Party Conference in October 1982, that the NHS was 'safe with us' in which she restated the principle that 'adequate health care should be provided to all, regardless of the ability to pay' (Thatcher, 1982).

While the Thatcher government was not prepared to pursue outright privatisation of the NHS, it did initiate a programme of what might be called 'creeping privatisation'. This included the introduction of business-style decision-making heralded by the Griffiths Management Report, the selling-off of assets owned by the NHS, the introduction of market testing for certain NHS ancillary services, and finally, the expansion of private health care.

☐ Selling-off NHS assets

From the early 1980s, health authorities were encouraged to sell property in order to raise funds. The revenue raised increased sharply during the property boom of the late 1980s, but then fell with the ensuing slump. In addition, RHAs were pressured to reduce directly-managed services by privatising certain functions, such as building design and computer centres, through management buy-outs or by selling-off functions to private companies. The abolition of the RHAs in 1996 hastened and extended this process of divestment.

☐ Competitive tendering and market testing

The Thatcher and Major governments saw competitive tendering as a means of reducing the power of trade unions, improving the efficiency of the public sector, and increasing opportunities for private enterprise. Competitive tendering involves allowing the private sector to bid for work currently undertaken by public sector. In theory, the bid that offers the best value for money will be invited to provide the service for a given period. At the end of this period a further competitive tender may be held, with others perhaps taking part.

Competitive tendering, whether compulsory or not, does not necessarily lead to privatisation. There is no guarantee that private firms will inevitably replace the 'in-house' workforce which also usually puts in a bid for the work. Furthermore, even if a private bid is successful services may continue to be publicly funded. However, it is wrong to assert that competitive tendering makes no difference. Irrespective of who wins, the process can produce changes in the delivery of services and can have potentially far-reaching consequences for the workforce and for patients.

In 1979 the private provision of ancillary services was at a low level. Private firms provided around 2 per cent of NHS domestic cleaning services, 14 per cent of laundry services and a negligible proportion of catering services. The government sought to increase this in 1983 by introducing compulsory competitive tendering into the NHS in England and Wales. This was strongly resisted by trade unions and by some health authorities. In this hostile environment, private firms secured only a small number of contracts. Believing they had been unfairly treated, they lobbied for a change in the tendering rules. This pressure paid off as the DHSS and the RHAs began to lean heavily on health authorities that awarded contracts to in-house bids, in some cases over-ruling their decisions. In spite of this, in-house bids continued to win the majority of contracts.

In 1991 the Major government issued a White Paper, *Competing for Quality* which attempted to extend competitive tendering through systematic 'market testing' of public service provision (Cm 1370, 1991). Units were required to report annually to the NHSE on their plans. It was envisaged that the competitive tendering would be extended to other services, including clinical support services such as pathology and pharmacy, and acute services such as ophthalmology and abortions. This was welcomed by some NHS managers who saw market testing not only as a way of reducing costs but as a means of improving quality, enhancing flexibility and improving performance (Decker, 1995).

This extension of policy proved difficult to implement. In 1995, the NHSE revealed that around 30 per cent of units had failed to test catering and laundry services, while a fifth had not subjected domestic services to competitive tender. The private sector continued to win a minority of contracts by value (40 per cent in 1995). Market testing of clinical and clinical support services was undertaken on a very small scale (NAHAT, 1995), with only a tiny minority (less than 3 per cent of contracts by value in 1995) being subjected to this process.

There are many reasons why market testing did not expand at the rate ministers envisaged. First, the situation was complicated by legal action undertaken by trade unions and other groups to protect workers' rights. In a series of judgements in the 1990s, British and European courts agreed that certain conditions and rights for staff should be guaranteed when contracting work out to another organisation (Kerr and Radford, 1994). This, in combination with other legal judgements relating to part-time workers' rights, reduced the incentive to undertake market testing. Notably, the cost reductions achieved by market testing arise mainly from redundancies, reduced pay and conditions and the replacement of full-time with part-time employees (Kerr and Radford, 1994; Milne, 1987).

Secondly, many NHS managers learned that market testing was not the best way of improving efficiency, and was in some respects counterproductive (see Decker, 1995; Dix 1996). The main problems perceived by managers were lack of competence of outside suppliers, the cost of market testing services and monitoring performance. Managers began to show interest in other less costly methods of assessing efficiency. For example, benchmarking, which involves comparison of performance between service providers, without necessarily exposing them to direct competition. Market testing was also seen by managers as a threat to good industrial relations and as a challenge to the traditional values of the NHS (Decker 1996).

Third, experience of competitive tendering of ancillary services revealed examples of contract failure. The Joint NHS Privatisation Unit (1990), an organisation supported by the health service unions, found 103 instances where standards were judged to have fallen following the introduction of a private contractor, representing at the time one failure for every four contracts. However, as yet there has been no comparative study of contract performance between public and private sectors in this field. It is clear that the problems associated with competitive tendering are not confined exclusively to the private sector. In one study, Pollock and Whitty (1990) identified inadequate staffing levels and poor supervision of catering staff as major factors in an outbreak of food poisoning in a psychiatric hospital. These shortcomings were attributed to a combination of factors: limited supply of labour, poor wages and conditions, and insufficient recognition of the problem of recruitment by managers, all of which were believed to have been exacerbated by the tendering process.

Finally, even basic cost savings may fail to emerge from market testing. NHS ancillary contracts are concentrated among a small number of private companies. As a result contract prices may rise in future in the absence of competition. This is particularly the case with larger contracts where only the major players have the resources to get involved.

The future of compulsory market testing in the NHS is currently in doubt. In 1997 the Blair government initiated a review of market testing, which examined, among other things, alternative methods of appraising efficiency such as benchmarking, mentioned above. In view of this, it is likely that a more flexible approach to market testing will be pursued in future, with health authorities no longer being pressured to contract functions out to the private sector.

☐ *The growth of private health care*

There are two ways of looking at the contribution of the private health care sector: the extent to which services are privately funded, and the extent to which they are provided by independent organisations. Yet no matter how one looks at this sector, its expansion in the 1980s and 1990s has been significant.

Private health care grew for a number of reasons, but perhaps the key factor was political support. Those wishing to see an expansion of the private sector had a powerful ally in Margaret Thatcher who was both a supporter and a consumer of private medicine. Notwithstanding her statement that the NHS was a 'fixed point' in her policies (Thatcher, 1993, p. 606), there is no doubt that her government wished to encourage a massive expansion in private medicine. It was constrained only by the strong level of public support for collective provision. Subsequently, the Major government re-emphasised its commitment to the NHS, but nevertheless encouraged the private sector through promoting joint working arrangements and through a continuing squeeze on public spending.

☐ *Private funding*

According to official figures, by the mid-1990s almost 16 per cent of health care spending in the UK was private expenditure (OECD, 1996). This compares with 9 per cent in 1975. A number of factors lie behind this trend.

In 1979, approximately 4 per cent of the UK population were covered by private health insurance. Ten years later this had risen to 13 per cent. Subsequently this proportion fell in the recession years, recovering to almost 11 per cent in 1995 (Laing, 1996). This growth of private health insurance was a deliberate policy during the 1980s (Higgins, 1988). In the 1981 budget, employers and employees were given tax incentives to encourage health insurance as a fringe benefit. Later, in 1989, tax relief on private health insurance was extended to those over sixty years of age. This was subsequently abolished by the Labour government in 1997.

Other factors contributed to the growth in private health insurance during the 1980s (Besley *et al.*, 1996) A series of industrial disputes in the early 1980s led to an acceleration in the number of subscribers. Growing dissatisfaction with lengthening waiting lists and, more importantly perhaps, with the perceived quality of NHS services were important factors (Calnan, Cant and Gabe, 1993). Yet it is important to note that the principles of the NHS continued to attract wide public support. Furthermore, patients were often deceived about the comparative quality of service between the NHS and the private sector (Wiles and Higgins, 1992; Consumers' Association, 1992). Indeed, there is little to suggest that those with private insurance behave like the 'rational consumers'. Few shop around for the best price and quality of services on offer, and choice is restricted by doctors and insurers (Calnan, Cant and Gabe, 1993). In addition, patients have little understanding of health insurance policies and are often ignorant about the extent of their cover (Office of Fair Trading, 1996).

The fact that individuals are enrolled in private schemes tells us little about the true extent of private-sector involvement in the funding and delivery of health care. There is no guarantee that the insured will make a claim on their policies. Nor is it certain that they will opt for treatment in the private sector when they become ill. Those with insurance are not barred from using NHS facilities if they so desire. To complicate matters further, the NHS itself has the largest share of private beds in the UK, and consultants have considerable freedom to practise private medicine. Indeed, for reasons explored later, the NHS began to compete more aggressively for private patients during the 1990s.

In addition many individuals pay directly for private health care without the benefit of insurance schemes. In 1986 just over a fifth of private patients (excluding those having abortions) were self-financing (Nicholl, Beeby and Williams, 1989b). However, this proportion had almost halved by 1993 (Williams and Nicholl, 1994). Added to this, patients pay directly for a range of low cost treatments such as over-the-counter medicines (where a prescription is not required) and a wide range of appliances and therapies supplied by the private sector.

Many people contribute towards the costs of the NHS through specific charges. Patient charges for spectacles and dentures were introduced by the Labour government in 1951, which also paved the way for prescription charges introduced by its Conservative successor. However, in the 1980s charges rose sharply. By 1991 they represented 4.5 per cent of the NHS budget twice the level of the 1970s. By the mid-1990s the contributions of charges had fallen to 3 per cent. In 1979 individual payments for NHS dental treatment represented 20 per cent of the total cost of the service. These contributions rose steadily to around 40 per cent by the late 1980s. The proportion of NHS dental care privately funded has since fallen back to just under 30 per cent in 1995, though for reasons discussed in Chapter 9 private dentistry has grown in the intervening period. Prescription charges rose twenty-fold between 1979 and 1996, though a larger proportion of prescriptions (currently over 80 per cent) are now exempt from charges than was the case in 1979 (65 per cent). The net effect was a rise in patients' contribution towards NHS prescription costs, from 4 per cent in 1979 to around 10 per cent by the early 1990s, falling to 8 per cent by the middle of the decade. Moreover, in 1985 a range of medicines was removed from the NHS list, and must now be paid for in full as with other over-the-counter medicines. Finally, in 1989 charges were extended to eye tests and dental checks. The impact of increased charges here is discussed further in the context of primary care in Chapter 9.

Another aspect of private funding is the financial contribution of charities and voluntary bodies to health care. Such organisations have a long history of funding health services. Since the creation of the NHS, charitable funds have been mainly devoted to medical research and the provision of supplementary services for patients. Charitable funding has grown considerably in the 1980s and 1990s (Chamberlain, 1993). Some believe that charities are not merely providing optional extras but funds for core services, including capital and running costs. (Fitzherbert and Giles, 1990; Fitzherbert, 1992).

The Conservative governments of Thatcher and Major emphasised the importance of charitable contributions, and encouraged donations through the tax system (for example, by giving tax concessions to charities and by payroll contributions schemes). They also encouraged independent fund-raising by the NHS. The rules on hospital fund-raising were simplified in 1980. This was followed in 1988 by measures extending the powers of health authorities to develop commercial activities, such as the marketing of clinical services, video advertising in hospitals, and leasing space for shops, in an effort to generate income. Many did so, though the overall contribution to funding has remained fairly small (National Audit Office, 1993).

Table 7.1 shows that private funding is higher in certain areas of care and treatment than in others. Private expenditure is relatively high in pharmaceuticals, ophthalmics and dentistry, abortion and long-term care of the elderly. It also represents a significant proportion of spending on elective surgery.

☐ *The relative contribution of the private sector: provision*

Another way of looking at the growth in the contribution of the private sector is to consider the amount of money spent on private provision relative to NHS services. Laing (1996) estimated that the private-sector share of UK hospital-based health care increased from 7.5 per cent in 1984 to 20 per cent in 1995. More specifically, there was a 58 per cent increase in the number of in-patients treated by private hospitals between 1981 and 1993 and a 440 per cent increase in day cases (Nicholl, Beeby and Williams, 1989a, 1989b; Williams and Nicholl, 1994). In comparison, acute and general NHS in-patient cases rose by over a quarter and day-cases by almost 160 per cent over the same period

Private-sector provision is extensive in the long-term care of the elderly, in pharmaceuticals, ophthalmics and abortion, which, as noted above, are heavily financed by private means. In addition, private provision, largely funded by the public sector, is significant in other areas of long-term care

Table 7.1   *Public and private sectors in health care*

| Care supplied by: | | Care funded by | | | |
| | | % public sector | | % private sector | |
		Public sector	Private sector	Public sector	Private sector
Elective surgery	1992/3	86	*	2	12
Long-term care elderly	1995	28	33	3	37
Acute psychiatric treatment	1995	93	2	*	5
Long-term mentally ill	1995	39	61	*	*
Long-term mental handicap	1995	45	55	*	*
Maternity	1994	99	*	*	1
Abortion	1995	48	16	*	36
General practice	1983	99	0	0	1
Pharmaceuticals	1995	61	0	5	35
Ophthalmics	1989	24	9	0	67
Dentistry	1988	62	0	27	10

Notes:
Figures have been rounded to avoid decimal amounts.
* indicates small percentage (less than 1 per cent).
Bases for comparison: surgery, abortions (cases); care of elderly, pharmaceuticals, dentistry, ophthalmics (cash); maternity (births); acute psychiatric treatment, care of mentally ill and mentally handicapped (beds); general practice (consultations).

Source: Table compiled by Laing, 1996, p. A62 (reproduced with permission).

(for example, care of mentally-ill and mentally-handicapped people). Commercial and voluntary homes together now supply over three-quarters of the residential and nursing home places available in the UK, compared with a third in 1979. During the 1980s the number of places available in local authority homes increased slightly and the number provided by charities fell, while those provided by the commercial sector more than quadrupled. The implications of this particular trend for these client groups is discussed more fully in Chapter 10.

A range of specific surgical interventions are performed increasingly in the private sector. For example, 28 per cent of hip replacements and 16 per cent of varicose vein operations were performed in the private sector during the mid-1980s (Nicholl *et al.*, 1989b) and though no recent figures are available it is widely believed that these percentages increased in the 1990s (Yates, 1995).

There are significant regional variations in the level of private hospital provision, reflecting the uneven distribution of facilities. The usage rates of private hospitals vary fivefold (Williams and Nicholls, 1994), being highest in London and lowest in the north of England. Most private beds are also concentrated in London and the South East.

Private provision was encouraged by recent Conservative governments through a number of technical changes. Consultants' contracts were modified in the early 1980s enabling them to take on more private work. The Health Services Board, a body charged with phasing out NHS pay beds and controlling the building or extension of private sector facilities, was abolished in 1980. The restrictions imposed on pay beds had prompted a decline in the NHS share of private health care from 40 per cent in the late 1970s to 11 per cent by the mid-1980s (National Economic Research Associates, 1995). This trend was reversed in the late 1980s for several reasons. First, in 1988 hospitals and health authorities were given powers to raise extra income from private patients. Second, the restriction on the number of private beds which an NHS hospital could provide was abolished in 1990 (prior to this no more than 10 per cent of beds in an NHS hospital could be allocated to private patients). Third, the advent of trust status from 1991 onwards stimulated income generation plans, and as a result services for private patients were marketed more aggressively. NHS hospitals began to improve their private facilities, making them more attractive to private patients. They began to create new dedicated private sector units – sometimes in partnership with private operators – with high quality hotel facilities to compete more effectively for business. By 1995 there were around 72 such units in England providing 1370 beds (National Economic Research Associates, 1995).

Gradually the NHS began to claw back a greater share of the private health care market. By the mid-1990s it had a 16 per cent market share and this was expected to rise even further before the turn of the century (Health Care Information Services, 1995). Private hospitals, worried at the prospect of losing even further ground, accused the NHS of unfair competition. In particular, they argued that the NHS was engaged in a price war by failing to base prices on the full cost of treatment. A report by the National Economic Research Associates (1995) did find some evidence of this, though even in the most pessimistic scenario only 5 per cent of costs were shown to be excluded. Even if NHS hospitals had taken these costs into account, they would still have set competitive prices and made a considerable surplus from their private work.

The competition for private patients intensified further in the mid-1990s. The situation was complicated by the movement of general insurance companies into the health insurance market. Some introduced low-cost schemes allowing access to NHS paybeds only. Meanwhile, some traditional health insurers responded by offering incentives to patients not to use NHS private facilities. Some also restricted their policies, in

---

Exhibit 7.1   *Private finance and the* NHS

The Private Finance Initiative (PFI) was introduced in 1992 in an effort to increase private involvement in the financing and operation of public sector projects and services. Under PFI, the private sector may take on the responsibility for the running of public services as well as supplying capital. A variety of possible joint arrangements can be established, involving various degrees of private and public sector participation.

The Major government saw the NHS as a key area for the extension of PFI. In 1993 the NHS was given greater freedom to develop smaller-scale projects without Treasury approval, and trusts were urged to 'rigorously explore' private finance for larger projects. It was made clear that public funding for capital investment would not be given unless it could be demonstrated that private finance had been actively sought. To reinforce this point the NHS capital budget was cut sharply.

Health authorities and trusts began to explore private finance options. Some plans were very ambitious involving the building of entirely new hospitals. However, as it became clear that many projects involved the private sector in the management of services as well as infrastructure, fears that the NHS was being effectively privatised began to mount. In England, ministers sought to reassure the public and the medical profession by ruling out private provision of medical care in PFI schemes. However in Scotland the scope of such projects was wider, though no project actually went ahead on this basis.

In the event, the PFI scheme in the NHS did not expand as quickly as the government hoped. In the 1995/6 and 1996/7 financial years only £130m was raised through the PFI, well short of expectations. By November 1996 only one major PFI contract had been signed – that relating to the building of a new district hospital in Norwich at a cost of £140m. The process proved highly complex, and the cost of bidding for contracts was often prohibitively high from the point of view of the private sector. A number of deals were scuppered by the withdrawal of potential partners. The private sector was increasingly worried about the risk involved in such ventures. As a result the law was amended in 1996 (and again by the Blair government in 1997),

⟶

---

particular with respect to intensive care, to limit their liability when private patients are treated in the NHS.

☐ *Collaboration between the public and private sector*

The Conservative governments of Thatcher and Major encouraged collaborative ventures between the public and private sector. By the end of the 1980s, Leadbeater (1990) found that about half of all health authorities had used the private acute sector to care for NHS patients. A fifth had been involved in a joint purchasing or leasing arrangement for medical equipment and a similar proportion had used private-sector screening services.

Exhibit 7.1 continued

⟶

making it clear that the NHS would honour its liabilities should a project fail once established. Political factors also discouraged the expansion of PFI schemes. As the next general election loomed the Conservative government became more sensitive to accusations that it was privatising the NHS, and the initiative ran out of steam. Furthermore, NHS trusts and their prospective partners in the private sector were wary of developing schemes which might have to be abandoned with a change of government.

However, during the mid-1990s Labour Party policy on private funding shifted considerably. By 1996 it had accepted that private finance might complement public funds as long as schemes were compatible with NHS priorities. This line was similar to that taken by the House of Commons Treasury Select Committee, which questioned the suitability of the existing scheme to health care (House of Commons, 1996d). Following Labour's victory at the 1997 general election, the government reaffirmed its commitment to PFI. The Department of Health established a new procedure for prioritising and evaluating PFI projects and ensuring their compatibility with NHS priorities. The government also agreed that pathology and radiology would be excluded from PFI projects in future.

During the 1990s interest was also generated in 'managed care' packages operated by the private sector. Under such arrangements private firms, such as drugs companies for example, may provide a package of services on behalf of the NHS (for example, services for asthma patients). Experience from the United States suggests that such schemes may lead to better information for practitioners on treatment and outcomes, and improved coordination of services for patients (Lawrence and Williams, 1996). However, problems have also been noted, in particular that the companies involved could use their role to market their products aggressively and undermine clinical freedom. Within the NHS the scope for 'managed care' schemes is presently limited. It is possible that in future there may be more scope for commercial interests to participate, providing that certain safeguards are introduced to protect the public against conflicts of interest.

Collaborative ventures were encouraged by central government waiting-list initiatives of the late 1980s and early 1990s. Health authorities were instructed to use private facilities as part of the drive to reduce waiting lists. In 1989 alone, over 10 per cent of the funds provided by the waiting list initiative was spent on private hospital care. Further impetus came from the introduction of the internal market, as purchasers of health care began to contract with private facilities. By the 1994–5 financial year the NHS was spending over £580m on health care provided by the private sector, a 170 per cent increase on the 1991–2 figure. Despite this large percentage increase, the proportion of NHS patients treated by the private sector remained relatively low (Williams and Nicholl, 1994). In 1993 less than 5 per cent of private hospital care contracts involved NHS patients (4.4 per cent health authority patients, 0.5 per cent GP fundholders).

The Conservatives also sought to encourage private investment in the NHS and to involve private sector operators in the management of NHS services. One method noted earlier, was market testing. Another policy was the private finance initiative (PFI), and on top of this, a growing interest in 'managed care' schemes. Exhibit 7.1 examines these initiatives.

☐ *The voluntary and informal sectors*

Voluntary and informal provision also grew during the 1980s and 1990s, encouraged by government policy. Currently over £50 million is allocated to voluntary bodies in the field of health and personal social services, most funded by the Department of Health. The voluntary sector also receives funding from local authorities, the NHS and from the general public. There have been specific initiatives to encourage voluntary work, such as the Opportunities for Volunteering scheme funded by the Department of Health where unemployed people are encouraged to participate in voluntary work in the field of social care.

Voluntary organisations have been supported by government in other ways. In 1981 the DHSS urged health authorities to collaborate more closely with the voluntary sector (DHSS, 1981a). Then, in 1986, the voluntary agencies were given a role in the joint planning of services alongside the NHS and local authorities. More recently voluntary organisations have been used as a means of enhancing patient participation in health care decision-making (see Chapter 11).

☐ *Implications of the expansion in private health care*

Private health care is not a new phenomenon. Nor is private involvement necessarily controversial. Indeed, as Salter (1995) observed, the majority of NHS expenditure is on services provided by private sector suppliers (for example drugs, equipment) and independent contractors (such as GPs, dentists). The contemporary debate about private health care focuses on two areas of controversy. First, provision of hospital and community health services, where the private sector was relatively small until the mid-1970s. Secondly, the private funding of health care.

There are two main perspectives on the growth of the private sector. The first sees the private sector as a safety valve for the overstretched NHS. One patient treated privately, it is argued, is one less on a waiting list. The cooperation of the private sector with NHS waiting list initiatives is presented as a further example of this symbiotic relationship. Another benefit claimed for the private sector is that it has provided a useful source of ideas for the NHS in its search for more efficient management systems. The private sector certainly has more experience in areas such as the costing and pricing of treatment, responding to non-clinical needs, and management information systems. A further perceived advantage is that private care provided by the NHS raises revenue which can then be used for the benefit of all patients. A report by National Economic Research Associates (1995) estimated that the NHS benefited financially by £290 per private patient treated. NHS patients may benefit as long as funding is not withdrawn as income from private patients increases, and provided that revenue is not spent purely on private patient facilities.

Yet the growth of the private sector may have had an adverse impact. Some argue that the fundamental principles of the NHS – a comprehensive service for all, free at point of delivery regardless of ability to pay – are undermined by a larger private sector (Iliffe, 1988). Others believe it acts as a parasite, drawing resources out of the NHS (Widgery, 1988). During the 1980s the National Audit Office (NAO, 1989a) found that the cost of treating patients in the private sector was twice as high as the cost of treating them within the NHS. Such arrangements may be criticised as featherbedding the private sector, though it should be pointed out that the higher cost of treating NHS patients privately can be offset to some extent by the savings in overhead costs (such as the building of new facilities) incurred in treating additional patients within the public sector.

The private sector benefits from the NHS in other ways. Private patients requiring emergency treatment on the NHS do not have to draw on their insurance, so the taxpayer rather than the private sector foots the bill. In addition the private sector makes use of staff who have been trained in the NHS, but makes a negligible contribution to training costs (House of Commons, 1990a). Although in recent years some private hospitals have become involved in nurse training their input remains small.

There has also been concern about the lack of monitoring of the private work done by NHS consultants (House of Commons, 1990a). It has also been alleged that some consultants have not been fulfilling their contracts properly and that as a result NHS patients have been neglected. Yates (1995) found that over half of orthopaedic surgeons and ophthalmology consultants were available to see private patients for two sessions a week or more, and were on average spending three half days a week in the private sector, contravening guidance set out by the NHSE in 1990. A link between private practice and lower NHS workloads was identified by the Audit Commission (1995c), which discovered that a quarter of consultants with the heaviest private workload carried out less NHS work than their other colleagues. However, the number of consultants deliberately neglecting NHS duties was thought to be small. This conclusion was shared by the Monopolies and Mergers Commission (1993) which discovered that although on average consultants spent between 6 and 11 hours on private work (the higher figure relating to consultants with maximum part-time contracts), they also exceeded their NHS contractual hours by over 30 per cent. Furthermore, a report by Donaldson (1994) relating specifically to the Northern region found a very low proportion of consultants (around 1 per cent) neglecting their NHS duties by undertaking private practice.

In 1989, the Thatcher government introduced detailed job plans for consultants and closer monitoring of their NHS commitments by health authorities, though this appears to have had limited impact (Audit Commission, 1995c; 1996a). Many have since argued for a proper study of the impact of private medicine on waiting lists, a move supported by the Health Committee (House of Commons, 1991a) and the Welsh Affairs Committee (House of Commons, 1991b) during the 1990s.

☐ *The future of the private sector*

Perhaps the private sector's ability to replace the NHS has been exaggerated. The Institute for Fiscal Studies (Besley *et al.*, 1996) found that even among those with health insurance the vast majority of people supported more spending on the NHS. Many of those insured have high regard for the NHS and continue to use it. Furthermore, it may well be that the private sector is nearing the limits of its expansion. As Nicholl *et al.* (1989b) point out, the private sector is not geared up to perform complex, high-technology procedures on an appropriate scale. Its ability to diversify into these areas in order to compete with the NHS may be limited. Moreover the private health sector has experienced problems of over-capacity conflict and competition. Indeed there are many divisions within the private sector, notably between the commercial (for profit) operators and the provident (non-profit) associations. The expansion of the commercial providers, many of them from overseas, has been well-documented (Higgins, 1988; Laing, 1996). Furthermore there has been conflict between insurers and private hospitals over the pricing of operations and the reimbursement of fees. The private sector has also faced increased competition: insurers from the entrance of life insurance companies into the market, providers from NHS trusts. In addition the whole industry was shaken by the economic recession of the early 1990s as companies and employees cancelled health insurance plans following business failures and redundancies.

Nevertheless, the private sector benefited from the favourable political environment of the 1980s and early 1990s. Future governments may not be so supportive. The Labour government, which came to power in 1997, has a tradition of hostility to private medicine and a far stronger ideological commitment to equity in health care than its predecessor. Even so, as the pay beds issue of the 1970s illustrated, Labour has faced problems when implementing such policies (Higgins, 1988). Despite abolishing tax relief on private health care for the elderly, the Blair government appears less ideologically committed to restricting private practice than previous Labour governments. It also inherited a cautious approach to public expenditure from its Conservative predecessor. Any gap between needs and demands is therefore unlikely to be completely filled by public expenditure (Healthcare 2000, 1995; Besley *et al.*, 1996). In addition, the Blair government endorsed PFI and has considered further charges for health services. So while the private sector may find itself more subject to greater regulation than in the recent past, it is unlikely to find itself without a role.

However, as we shall see shortly, the size of the funding gap is very much open to debate. Some doubt that the level of public funding of health-care has reached its limit. As Baumol (1995) contends, all developed economies may be able to afford higher health expenditures in the future through economic growth and greater productivity. Indeed, increased public funding may well be a more efficient option, acting as a more powerful constraint on health care costs than private-sector led expenditure growth (Wordsworth, Donaldson and Scott, 1996).

■ Public expenditure on health care

The growth of the private sector is influenced by the financial state of the NHS, which in turn is determined by the general economic climate and the government's public expenditure policies (Whynes, 1992). The relatively poor performance of the British economy has often impinged upon the NHS, resulting in periodic financial crises (Webster, 1988, 1996). These crises have produced two kinds of response: a search for alternative sources of finance for health care, and an attempt to control the NHS budget more effectively to make resources go further.

□ *Alternative sources of finance*

There are many alternative ways in which funds can be raised for health care (Bailey and Bruce, 1994; Institute of Health Service Management, 1993). Government can encourage people to take out private insurance, increase charges for health services and encourage the NHS to generate its own revenues (NAO, 1993). Or it may alter the way in which tax revenue is generated. Over the years governments have occasionally explored radical alternatives to the tax-funded system. For example the Conservative government of Harold Macmillan examined the case for a national health insurance system (Webster, 1996). Plans to introduce such a scheme were abandoned in view of the likely public reaction as the 1959 General Election approached.

The Thatcher government considered a number of options during its NHS review of 1988. Various schemes to increase private funding of health care were examined (Green, D. G., 1988; Redwood, 1988) alongside others which proposed a state health insurance system (Brittan, 1988). Other ideas included granting tax relief on private health insurance contributions for the elderly (Brown *et al.*, 1988), later taken up by the government, though general taxation remained the main basis for NHS funding.

Another alternative method of funding is a specific health tax (Field, 1988; Jones and Duncan, 1995; Bailey and Bruce, 1994). This has been considered on a number of occasions, most recently by the Blair government. A specific or earmarked health tax, levied as a percentage of income, has a number of positive features. If fixed over a number of years, and providing the economy is stable, the revenue it generates can provide a firmer basis for financial planning in the NHS. It is also viewed as a more transparent form of funding which enables taxpayers to appreciate the cost of health services and to register their preferences for higher spending with this in mind. On the other hand, it is naive to think that an earmarked tax, could be insulated from the politics surrounding the taxation and public expenditure process. The tax rate would still reflect political expediency. It is by no means certain that it would necessarily generate more resources for health care. Indeed, less funds might be available when tax revenues fell because of a recession or a government commitment to reduced taxation.

One variation on this theme is not to replace tax funding entirely with earmarked taxes, but to introduce new specific taxes to fund increases in health spending. Particular targets include goods which are known to harm health, such as alcohol and tobacco. The idea is to use taxation to discourage consumption of these products at the same time as raising revenue for the NHS, which treats the illnesses related to smoking and alcohol misuse. This sounds ingenious but there are a number of problems. First, taxes on alcohol and tobacco are regressive, they hit the poor harder than the rich. Secondly, these products are already heavily taxed and it is uncertain how much extra revenue would be generated by an added health tax. Third, people who smoke and drink already contribute towards the cost of the health service and would in effect be paying twice, which seems unfair. Finally, there is a great deal of political resistance from the Treasury and from the alcohol and tobacco industries to such taxes.

□ *Controlling the NHS budget*

Successive governments have responded to the financial problems of the NHS by trying to control the spending of resources more effectively. This began under the 1945–51 Labour government and continued in the early 1950s under the Conservatives, with the appointment of the Guillebaud review (see Chapter 4). It will be recalled that instead of providing arguments in favour of cutting back expenditure, the Guillebaud committee reported that the NHS provided good value for money, making it difficult to justify cut-backs.

The squeezing option was used more forcefully twenty years later, by a Labour government. During the mid-1970s, and in the face of a severe economic crisis, government was forced to cut back on public spending. Part of its strategy included the implementation of cash limits which imposed a ceiling on budgets in the public sector, including health authority spending. The incoming Conservative government of Margaret Thatcher retained the system of cash limits and sought to extend it further.

The Thatcher government placed a great deal of emphasis on controlling public expenditure. Indeed this was central both to its economic policy of reducing price inflation, and its political strategy to shift the boundary between the public and private sectors. Initially at least it sought deep cuts in all spending programmes. It also brought in new mechanisms for regulating public spending, including the introduction of 'cash planning', which squeezed public expenditure when inflation was higher than expected. The Thatcher government successfully reduced public expenditure below 40 per cent of national income. Under the Major government a mixture of recession and pre-election spending promises led to increases in public expenditure. However, tighter expenditure controls were imposed after 1993, following a wide-ranging public spending review.

Despite the pressure on overall public spending over the last two decades, the proportion of public spending devoted to the NHS, which remained around 10 per cent in the 1950s and 1960s, actually rose from 11 per cent in 1981 to 14 per cent in 1991 and has since remained at this level (Central Statistical Office, 1996). Furthermore, NHS expenditure increased substantially relative to average prices, rising by 70 per cent in real terms between 1979 and 1995.

There are a number of reasons why the NHS budget continued to grow in spite of curbs on public spending. There was a great deal of public support for more health spending, with almost nine out of ten people in favour of an increase (Taylor-Gooby, 1995). The constant interest of the media in health matters was also a major factor. Any attempt to curb NHS spending took place in the full glare of publicity, putting government on the defensive. Even the Thatcher government was forced to proclaim its commitment to greater rather than less NHS expenditure, particularly in pre-election periods. Meanwhile, the case for increasing health spending was bolstered by a vociferous lobby which included the main professional groups such as the BMA and the Royal Colleges, trade unions, and patients' groups. Further pressure came from Parliament, with widespread cross-party support for higher NHS spending in both the Commons and the Lords.

☐ *Underfunding*

In spite of the growth in the health budget during the 1980s and 1990s, the Conservative governments of Thatcher and Major were nevertheless criticised for not allocating sufficient resources. Indeed, a closer look at public expenditure on health care indicates that the growth rate under the Conservatives was smaller than it appeared (Appleby, 1992; Bloor and Maynard, 1993). First, the growth in health spending was less generous when the rise in the cost of health services was taken into account. Official statements on the increase in NHS spending often ignored the fact that the cost of producing health services (as measured by the Hospital and Community Health Services Pay and Prices Index) usually increased faster than average prices. When this is taken into account, health spending shows a much less spectacular growth rate (Appleby, 1997).

Bloor and Maynard (1993) analysed claims of a 50 per cent increase in NHS spending between 1979–92, and after taking into account the rise in health costs over the same period, estimated that the real increase in spending was much lower at only 22 per cent, an annual average increase of only 1.5 per cent. This was noticeably lower than the Department of Health's estimate of 2 per cent per annum needed to meet the costs of changing disease patterns, new forms of service delivery, demographic changes and developments in medical technology (House of Commons, 1986, p. 26).

On the basis of the adjusted figure, the NHS was seriously underfunded during the 1980s. The cumulative shortfall in spending for this decade was estimated at £4.4 billion (NAHAT, 1990). The underfunding case was also supported by international comparisons. Pritchard (1992) pointed out that compared with mainland Europe the NHS was 'unequivocally under-funded'. He observed that if the NHS were to match the German health budget its allocation would have to rise by a fifth. Figure 7.1 confirms that relative to most other comparable countries, the UK still spends less on health care, both as a proportion of national income and in terms of expenditure per head of population.

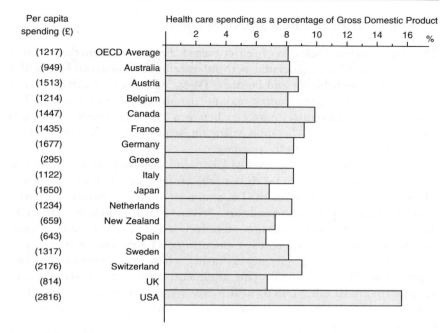

Per capita spending (£)

Health care spending as a percentage of Gross Domestic Product

(1217)	OECD Average	
(949)	Australia	
(1513)	Austria	
(1214)	Belgium	
(1447)	Canada	
(1435)	France	
(1677)	Germany	
(295)	Greece	
(1122)	Italy	
(1650)	Japan	
(1234)	Netherlands	
(659)	New Zealand	
(643)	Spain	
(1317)	Sweden	
(2176)	Switzerland	
(814)	UK	
(2816)	USA	

Source of data: Office of Health Economics, *Compendium of Health Statistics 1995.*

Figure 7.1 *Cross-national comparisons of health expenditure (selected OECD countries), 1995*

Calls for extra funding to redress the accumulated shortfall of the 1980s were rejected. More generous settlements were forthcoming in the early 1990s under the Major government, but these were offset by costly new initiatives, not least the internal market. In the mid-1990s public expenditure plans for health were extremely tight as the Major Government sought demanding efficiency gains. Indeed in the 1996 Budget, the planned level of health expenditure was virtually frozen in real terms.

The Blair government initially declared its intention to work within these strict pre-existing spending plans. However, additional funds were allocated to health for the second financial year after it took office – a 2.25 per cent increase after taking into account the general rate of inflation. On top of this a further £300 m was found to avert a financial crisis in the NHS in the short-term. At the same time the Blair government launched a review of health spending which like previous reviews explored a range of options to generate extra funds including earmarked taxes and additional charges.

☐ *Criticism of the underfunding thesis*

The underfunding thesis has been criticised. First, it is argued that are a number of problems associated with international comparisons of health expenditure (see Schieber and Poullier, 1992). What may be categorised as health spending in one country may not be so regarded in another. The demands on health services may vary between countries. Furthermore, it is widely recognised that the sums spent on health care do not necessarily indicate quality and cost-effectiveness.

Another point is that the level of UK *public* spending on health care (6 per cent of national income) is close to the average for all OECD countries. The main difference between the UK and most other comparable countries is in the area of private expenditure. Private health spending in the UK, despite its recent growth, remains a relatively small proportion of the total. For this reason, some argue, it is more appropriate that the gap be closed by increasing private payments rather than by increasing public expenditure (Whitney, 1988). This argument, however, fails to take into account that most other OECD health care systems are insurance-based. In comparison with similar systems (that is, other national health service models) the UK spends less on health.

The estimates of the year-on-year increases in expenditure required by the NHS have also been criticised. The 2 per cent 'target' increase in funding, based on rough estimates of the costs of new service developments, population changes and so on, is very crude. It takes no account of the extent to which the current budget is being spent effectively and efficiently (Haywood, 1990). Moreover, there is no guarantee that the existing level of resources, the baseline from which target increases are calculated, is appropriate (House of Commons, 1988c, p. ix). A more sophisticated approach is to resource health services on the basis of population needs rather than simply using an historical benchmark.

Critics of the underfunding thesis argue that there should be more emphasis on improving the allocation of resources through better assessment of needs, improved financial management, and by concentrating resources on those treatments and therapies which are most cost-effective. Some go further, arguing that NHS services should be restricted or rationed to cover treatments for which individuals should not be expected to pay; or by limiting NHS services to those individuals who lack the means to pay for treatment.

■ Efficiency, audit and rationing

Over the last two decades the emphasis has been upon making the NHS more efficient, generating resources from within to meet growing demands and promoting greater accountability in the use of resources. These aims lay behind the managerial reforms of the 1980s and 1990s mentioned in the previous chapter. At the same time, bodies such as the Audit Commission and the National Audit Office became more closely involved in auditing and monitoring health services. Meanwhile, greater attention was paid to prioritising and rationing health services.

□ *Efficiency drives*

Efficiency scrutinies, introduced in the NHS in 1982, were used to investigate areas of suspected inefficiency. Such reviews were often called 'Rayner reviews' after the government adviser and businessman who promoted their use. Efficiency scrutinies begin with the appointment of a manager (or in some cases a small inquiry team) seconded from normal duties. The review then examines a particular area of activity with a view to suggesting cost savings. Rayner reviews have been carried out into ambulance services, residential accommodation, storage of supplies, catering and vacancy advertising.

Cost-improvement programmes (CIPs) were introduced in 1984 in an attempt to increase NHS productivity, thereby releasing resources for service improvements. CIPs were initially targeted at broad areas of spending such as supplies and energy costs. During the 1980s the level of cost improvements was around 1.5 per cent of the previous year's budget (NAHAT, 1990). Although the intention was that the money released by CIPs would be used to fund patient services, doubts were raised about whether the reported cost improvements actually took place. CIPs were also criticised for cost-cutting at the expense of efficiency and quality of service. By postponing expenditure in the short term, CIPs could raise costs in the longer term (National Audit Office, 1989b). Subsequently the Audit Commission (1994a) found that only a fifth of potential savings identified by 'value for money' projects had actually been realised.

Efficiency scrutinies were placed on a more systematic basis with the creation of a value for money unit (VFMU) within the NHSE. The VFMU aimed to promote local improvements in efficiency by indicating the potential for savings. For example, it suggested that the boarding costs of patients in hospital wards could be almost halved by developing 'hotels' for post-operative care. Since 1994 the VFMU has concentrated on disseminating good practice, leaving detailed studies of value for money to the Audit Commission.

A broader approach to efficiency gains was pursued in from 1993 onwards. This involved setting of efficiency targets for health authorities to be achieved within the financial year. In 1993–4 the target for cost savings was set at 2 per cent. This was raised to 2.25 per cent in 1994–5 and

3 per cent in following financial years. Subsequently the Blair government, while criticising the narrow measures of efficiency adopted by its predecessor, nevertheless reaffirmed the commitment to release resources mainly through improved cost-effectiveness, particularly in the area of management costs.

Other initiatives of the 1990s focused upon cost-effectiveness in clinical areas. The Conservative government promoted a range of initiatives aimed at monitoring the quality of care, assessing cost-effectiveness and measuring activity levels in relation to resources. The Blair government has since introduced further initiatives in this area (see Chapter 6).

☐ Audit and monitoring

As a national service funded out of taxation NHS expenditure is clearly a matter for Parliamentary scrutiny. The monitoring of NHS expenditure is undertaken by several committees of the House of Commons. Two of these, the Public Accounts Committee (PAC) and the Health Committee (formerly the Social Services Committee), are discussed below. Others include the select committees dealing with Welsh, Scottish and Northern Irish affairs.

PAC is concerned with expenditure, accounting processes and procedures across the government spending programme. Its job is to ensure that public money has been properly spent and has a watching brief against waste and inefficiency in government departments and agencies. PAC has been critical of the Department of Health on issues such as hospital construction (House of Commons, 1993a), GP fundholding (House of Commons, 1995a) and clinical audit (House of Commons, 1996b). The Health Committee monitors government spending plans for health and examines government health polices. For example, it has inquired into issues such as priority setting and community care for mentally-ill people (House of Commons 1995b, 1994).

Two other official bodies monitor health expenditure, policies and services. These are the National Audit Office (NAO) and the Audit Commission. The NAO is a Parliamentary body which prepares the way for enquiries by the PAC, while making its own recommendations to improve value for money. It has reported on issues such as outpatient services and hospital information support systems (NAO, 1995a, 1996a).

The Audit Commission was originally confined to promoting value for money in local government. But even in this capacity it covered health-related issues in its reports on community care, environmental health and housing. Since 1990, when the Audit Commission's brief was expanded to include the NHS, it has investigated efficiency in many areas including the

---

Exhibit 7.2   Financial mismanagement in the NHS

In 1994 the Audit Commission reported 960 cases of fraud over the previous three years, involving £5.9 million. Several cases of financial mismanagement attracted widespread media attention.

1. Wessex Regional Health Authority wasted at least £20m on its computer integration scheme during the 1980s. The contract to provide this service was initially awarded to a private company, but this was reversed and the contract given to a rival bid which was fourth in the original list of possible contractors. Health authority members were not informed of this decision until months after the contract had been signed (House of Commons, 1993c).

2. West Midlands Regional Health Authority was accused of wasting money in connection, ironically, with the hiring of efficiency advisers. Management consultants had been brought in from the private sector to advise on how to promote efficiency in supplies. In all £4m was spent on consultancy fees and other costs. This included annual expenses of £350 000 to cover the cost of high-quality accommodation, the hire of aircraft, and lavish entertainment (House of Commons, 1993b).

3. The Public Accounts Committee (House of Commons, 1995c) was highly critical of the Scottish Office for its role in the Health Care International debacle, where a private hospital subsidised from public funds went into receivership in 1994. £8.4 million of public money was wasted. The committee criticised the failure of the Scottish Office to heed warnings about the viability of the hospital and to evaluate, manage and monitor the risks involved.

4. Managers at the former Yorkshire Regional Health Authority were accused of receiving irregular payments relating to relocation and 'golden handshakes' (National Audit Office, 1996b) There was also evidence of serious conflicts of interest in the letting of contracts, excessive hospitality and the mishandling of loans. The total amount of money involved was around £500 000.

---

work of hospital doctors (Audit Commission, 1995c, 1996a). The Audit Commission also appoints audit teams to examine health authority finances, some of which have uncovered details of inefficiency, mismanagement and fraud within the NHS (see Exhibit 7.2).

One expects bodies such as the PAC and the Health Committee to be critical of the government. After all, they are partly composed of MPs drawn from the opposition parties. However, they also include MPs from the governing party. This is a major strength, particularly when the committee members agree on their recommendations, and in such circumstances its report carries considerable weight. Although MPs from the governing party are supposed to be independent of government influence this is not always the case. For example in the early 1990s the Conservative government was accused of trying to determine the composition of the Health Committee, removing its (Conservative) chairperson and influencing its reports by putting pressure on their MPs on the committee.

The NAO and the Audit Commission are regarded as highly independent bodies. They carry a great deal of authority and have the potential to embarrass the government of the day. For example, both bodies cast a cloud over the Conservative government's internal market reforms by pointing out shortcomings in financial and information management systems (Audit Commission, 1991b; NAO, 1989b).

Increased scrutiny of the NHS and health policy is undoubtedly a positive development. In encouraging audit, the Thatcher and Major governments were to some extent hoist by their own petard, as auditors uncovered evidence of waste and inefficiency, often related to government reforms (see Exhibit 7.1). It is perhaps not surprising to learn that the Department of Health, which has received much of the political fallout from these scandals, opposed independent audit when it was introduced in 1990 (Lawson, 1992).

☐ *Rationing*

There may be overall gains to be made by switching resources away from some treatments and towards others. Few would disagree with reducing resources for ineffective treatments and reinvesting the surplus in those of proven effectiveness (Riley *et al.*, 1995). But the issue becomes much more controversial when it concerns effective treatments which are not considered priorities because the conditions they cure are not life-threatening. These include cosmetic surgery and infertility services, which may not involve the relief of physical pain but nevertheless have important emotional and psychological impact. Conditions such as haemorrhoids, varicose veins and arthritic joints are considered as a relatively low priority, even though such conditions seriously undermine sufferers' quality of life. Finally, certain caring services have been regarded as a low priority and are often identified as a target for diverting resources. One example is continuing care where, as we shall see in Chapter 11, NHS services have been cut back substantially in recent years.

Restricting or eliminating 'low-priority' treatments and services leads to rationing, in a number of ways: on the basis of waiting times, through an explicit assessment of the relative costs and benefits of treating each individual case, or by price. If funding is withdrawn for certain therapies patients have little option but to pay privately. To some extent this has already happened in some areas of elective surgery, such as hip replacements. The restriction or elimination of treatment in so-called low-priority areas will increase this activity. Of course, those who simply cannot afford to pay will be forced to live with painful or emotionally stressful conditions.

The question of rationing was stimulated to some extent by the NHS internal market. However, health commissioners were quite slow off the mark in examining priorities, and were reluctant to rule out funding particular treatments. According to Redmayne's study (1996) only a quarter of health authorities listed services which they would not fund. Common examples included a reversal of sterilisation, breast augmentation and reduction, sex changes. However, a greater proportion listed services which they were reluctant to fund unless clinical need could be demonstrated. This implied the greater use of clinical guidelines and protocols associated with the emphasis on evidence-based medicine (see also Klein, Day and Redmayne, 1996, for a further discussion of rationing in the NHS).

The development of economic techniques such as the QALY (examined in Chapter 3) and other evaluative tools has also generated further controversy. But again commissioners have been relatively slow to adopt such techniques. In the final analysis, narrow economic judgements invariably give way to political pressures. For example, in Cohen's (1994) study only 9 of the 20 investment/disinvestment funding priorities in the field of maternal and child heath identified by economic analysis were actually translated into policy.

Even so, rationing has achieved a higher profile in recent years, largely as a result of publicity given to particular cases. The child B case of 1995 was one of the most prominent (Price, 1996). This case was heard before the High Court following the refusal of the Cambridgeshire Health Authority to pay £75 000 for a second bone-marrow transplant for a young leukaemia sufferer. The health authority received clinical advice that further treatment was not in the child's best interests and later supported its case by claiming that to proceed would not be an effective use of resources. A decision against the health authority in the High Court was subsequently reversed on appeal. Child B did eventually receive further treatment paid for by a private benefactor. Although this initially proved successful she suffered a relapse and died the following year.

Such tragic individual cases illustrate graphically the emotional and ethical dilemmas of rationing. Others raise issues about entire groups of people. Indeed there is much evidence that elderly people are refused treatment on grounds of their age (Royal College of Physicians, 1994). Smokers, heavy drinkers and overweight people also claim to have been disadvantaged by informal rationing procedures

Informal rationing is one thing. Reaching agreement on explicit priorities is entirely different. As Thwaites (1988) has observed, there is a lack of consensus about what constitutes the essential core of the NHS.

Researchers have found widespread disagreements about priorities both among clinicians, and between clinicians and the public (Bowling, Jacobson and Southgate, 1993). Nevertheless, this does mean that one should not strive to reach a consensus. To this end the Royal College of Physicians (1995) called for the establishment of a National Council on Health Care Priorities, including both experts and the public. This body would review methods of determining priorities and the impact of setting priorities while seeking to involve, educate and inform the public, professions and government. Similar sentiments were expressed by the Health Committee of the House of Commons (House of Commons, 1995b), which called for those who commission care to establish procedures that are systematic, transparent, take full account of the views of the public, professions and other interested parties, and, wherever possible, are based on assessments of need, effectiveness and cost-effectiveness.

■ Conclusion

Over the last two decades the private sector has become more important in the allocation of health care resources. This expansion was encouraged by a number of initiatives introduced by the Thatcher and Major governments such as changes in tax relief and market testing. The restrictive approach to health spending, particularly in the 1980s, also played a key role encouraging individuals and employers to take out private health insurance. In addition, efficiency measures and rationing had an impact. Efficiency scrutinies often led to the divestment of functions. Rationing limited the scope of the NHS, forcing individuals to pay for treatment (or draw on insurance), again providing extra business, for the private sector. Finally, waiting list initiatives and later the internal market gave private providers additional work.

But as the private sector grew, the boundary between itself and the NHS became blurred and the relationship between the two more complex. In some respects the private sector is more dependent on the NHS than it was previously. Private providers have always relied on the NHS to bear the costs of training professional staff and to treat high cost cases not covered by insurance. But this independence increased as private operators became involved in joint ventures and the provision of services on behalf of the NHS. This has implications for many, including closer working relationships with the NHS and exposure to the adverse effects of tighter public sector budgets. In addition, private providers faced an increasingly competitive environment as NHS trusts began to market their services far more aggressively.

The blurring of the public and private sectors makes it difficult to evaluate the extent and the impact of privatisation. This absence of evidence prolongs debate. On the one hand it is argued that the overall efficiency of the health care system is impaired by parcelling out various functions to private operators. Others argue that equity principles are breached when the NHS withdraws wholly or partially from the provision of specific treatments. On the other hand, there are doubts about the ability of taxpayers to meet the cost of a modern health service and claims that a cooperative public–private model of health care is more appropriate to the next century.

Yet irrespective of this debate, the trend set by the policies of the Thatcher and Major governments is unlikely to be halted in the immediate future. Wider public–private collaboration in health care was encouraged by the retention of PFI. Although it found additional resources for health care out of existing budgets, the Blair government continued its predecessor's commitment to public expenditure restraint. The new government also began to examine alternative sources of finance, including charges. Finally, it identified efficiency savings and improved clinical effectiveness as key sources for funding future improvements in services, again following a course set by the previous government.

■ *Chapter 8* ■

Commissioning and Providing Health Care

The internal market, devised by the Thatcher government in the late 1980s, represented the most radical reform of the NHS since its creation. It sought to replace a traditional bureaucratic model of planning and resource allocation with a 'quasi-market', in which NHS institutions took on the role of buyer and seller. This chapter examines how this came about, the impact of the changes, and how the reforms were modified by the Major government. The initial efforts of the Blair government to replace the internal market are also discussed.

■ The NHS: crisis and review

The internal market arose from the Thatcher government's review of the NHS in the late 1980s. The review was prompted by a financial crisis in the latter part of 1987 which had been accompanied by pressure from the media, parliament, and the health professions and trade unions to increase NHS funding (Timmins, 1988). The possibility of an NHS review had been floated within government circles before the 1987 General Election, but was considered too controversial (Lawson, 1992). As the political pressure intensified throughout the following autumn and winter, the Prime Minister threw her support behind the idea, primarily to get the NHS off the political agenda.

□ *The Prime Minister's review*

The NHS review bore all the hallmarks of the Thatcher government's policy style: it was speedy, secretive and loyal to the leader (Butler, 1992; Griggs, 1991). The review team consisted of a small group of ministers drawn from the Treasury, the DHSS (later the Department of Health), and the Scottish and Welsh Offices, plus Sir Roy Griffiths the PM's adviser. Thatcher chaired the committee and was able to exert a great deal of control over its direction, particularly during the final stages (Paton, 1992). There were no formal consultations with organised interests likely to be affected by reform. Individual doctors and managers were consulted at special meetings, but not in a representative capacity. Although the review was far from being an open exercise, individuals and organisations were invited to meet health ministers and to submit papers outlining their ideas for reform.

The review focused on two main areas: alternative systems of funding health care, and new mechanisms for allocating resources within the NHS. A number of alternative sources of finance were considered, including insurance-based systems and earmarked taxes. But apart from backing moves to encourage private health insurance, the review decided that the NHS should remain funded mainly out of general taxation.

The advantages of a tax-funded system over other options are well-known. First, it redistributes across the life cycle. People contribute most to the service when they are earning (through indirect taxes on income) and spending (through indirect taxes), and benefit most when their incomes and expenditure levels are relatively low. The system is equitable in that over the average individual's lifetime these contributions and benefits tend to level out.

Second, the tax-funded health care system represents a relatively cheap way of raising resources. Funds are raised as part of a general system of tax assessment and collection. Some of the other alternatives – particularly health insurance systems – involve additional cost and bureaucracy in raising revenue.

The third main advantage is that tax funding is believed to help control the costs of health care. This is reinforced by the reluctance of the public to pay higher taxes, which limits the overall amount of money available for public expenditure. In addition the bids of other public service programmes act as a restraint on the health budget. In other funding systems higher health spending can be more easily generated by raising insurance payments and fees, and it is correspondingly more difficult for government to control the costs of health care.

☐ *Internal markets*

The review then focused on how the NHS could be restructured to improve resource allocation. A number of schemes were put forward to introduce competition into the NHS. Economic incentives were seen by a number of observers, largely on the political right, as the spur for greater cost-efficiency and responsiveness to the consumer (Brown *et al.*, 1988; Butler and Pirie, 1988; Owen, 1988; Redwood, 1988; Whitney, 1988). However, these ideas were not entirely new. Indeed, only a few years earlier an American academic Alain Enthoven (1985) had argued that the NHS was caught in 'gridlock', a condition of general rigidity and inflexibility. He claimed that better value for money could be achieved by rewarding the most efficient providers, and suggested competition as a possible remedy to the problems of the NHS.

☐ Health maintenance organisations

Enthoven's analysis drew heavily on the US experience where greater competition had been introduced in the form of health maintenance organisations (HMOs). Individuals subscribe to an HMO usually on an annual basis. If they become ill the HMO provides care, either directly or by contracting with other providers. By the late 1980s around a fifth of the US population was enrolled in such schemes.

Enthoven himself warned about the dangers of importing the HMO idea direct from the USA. Others argued that the HMO had a mixed record even in its home context, under-providing services for the poor and chronically sick (Petchey, 1987). It was pointed out that many HMOs faced severe financial problems and were forced to merge, resulting in a closure of facilities and a long-term reduction in competition. Subsequently, the policy of introducing competition into US health care attracted criticism for failing to improve efficiency, reducing the quality of health care, and eliminating completely some vital services (Salmon, 1995).

Many of the radical ideas submitted to the NHS review were based upon the HMO model. Goldsmith and Willetts' (1988) plan for a system of 'managed health care organisations' (MHCOs) was a fairly typical example. According to this scheme, MHCOs would take over the role of district health authorities. They would be funded by tax revenues in order to purchase health care on behalf of their resident populations from hospitals, GPs and other health care providers. Subsequently, the private sector would be allowed to compete with the public-sector MHCOs for subscribers. Any difference between the premiums charged by MHCOs and the amount funded by taxation would be met by individuals, generating additional health spending.

The more radical HMO-type schemes did not receive much support from the NHS review. There was more interest in fundholding schemes, which emphasised the gatekeeper role of the GP within the NHS (Bevan *et al.*, 1988; Bosanquet, 1986; Culyer, Brazier and O'Donnell, 1988). Although details varied, these schemes were similar in principle; GP practices receiving a budget would pay directly for hospital and other services, and would compete for patients in order to generate revenue. Practices that used their budgets most effectively would attract patients and expand. Those that were ineffective would contract and eventually go out of business. Eventually the review backed a version of this scheme – GP fundholding – where practices of a certain size could purchase services up to a particular financial limit per patient.

The review also endorsed a division between those who purchased health care and those who provided it. Providers – hospitals and community health services – would be separated from the health authorities who currently managed them and would be expected to generate their own income through service contracts. Providers would also be able to apply for self-governing status, which implied certain freedoms in the management of services and assets.

■ Working for Patients

The NHS review culminated with the publication of a White Paper, *Working for Patients* (Cm 555, 1989). Some of its proposals continued earlier policy themes and initiatives. These included the extension of the Resource Management Initiative (RMI), the formal introduction of medical audit, and changes in the composition of health authorities (all discussed further in Chapter 6). However, the core of the White Paper – an internal market for health care based on a system of contracting for services between purchasers and providers – was new (see Figure 8.1).

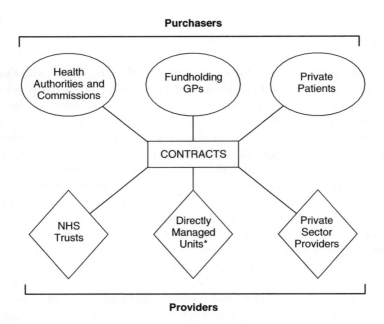

Note: The vast majority of services in mainland Britain are now provided by trusts.

Figure 8.1 *The internal market*

There was a strong feeling, particularly among the health care professions, that the reforms should be piloted and evaluated. One of the main exponents of the internal market, Alain Enthoven, shared this concern. He was critical of the government's proposals, in particular GP fundholding and tax relief on private insurance for the elderly. Nevertheless, the government remained hostile to independent evaluation and refused to back down on its plan to introduce the market within two years.

The reforms required legislation and the main vehicle for this was the NHS and Community Care Act of 1990. Despite the public controversy surrounding the reforms and the hostility of the main organisations representing health professions and workers, the Thatcher government steered its legislation through parliament fairly smoothly. It was helped by a large majority in the House of Commons and by the skilful use of parliamentary rules that curtailed debate.

There were a few concessions, however. The government agreed to establish a statutory Clinical Standards Advisory Group to evaluate the impact of the reforms upon standards of care in the NHS. It conceded that the Audit Commission, which under the new legislation now had a role in auditing the NHS, could examine the impact of ministerial decisions. Furthermore, in Scotland only, ministers agreed that GP fundholding should be independently evaluated.

□ The steady state

Considerable opposition to the government's plans remained, and this did not augur well for the implementation of the reforms. Perhaps realising this ministers sought to reassure the public by playing down the 'market' element in the reforms, using the terminology of 'managed competition' rather than internal markets. At the same time it became clear that the pace of the reforms was slowing, and that important changes in policy were taking place at the implementation stage (Butler, 1992).

It was originally intended that purchasers' budgets would be based on the size of their resident population adjusted to take account of health care needs, a system known as weighted capitation. This was to have been introduced within two years but there were political and practical problems. On a practical level there were difficulties in devising accurate measures of need, essential if purchasers' budgets were to be calculated on a fair basis. Politically, the government realised that a move to weighted capitation would not only reduce resources in London and the South East (where support for the Conservatives was strongest), but would produce a dramatic fall in the demand for some services in this region, particularly those provided by the larger London hospitals.

It was agreed that health authorities in London would receive extra resources in the short term. At the same time an inquiry was established into the future of health services in the capital. This represented an attempt to plan the rationalisation of London hospitals and to develop primary care services, rather than to allow the market to prompt closures directly (see Exhibit 9.1).

There were other changes and delays. Plans to charge providers for their use of assets, buildings and equipment were postponed. Meanwhile official guidance to health authorities stressed that the new contracts should reflect the current pattern of services (DoH, 1990a; 1990b). Health authorities were also encouraged to use block contracts (see Exhibit 8.1) so as to create a more predictable situation.

Exhibit 8.1   Contracts for health care

Three main types of NHS contract were introduced by the internal market reforms:

1. **Block contracts.** The provider receives a fixed payment for services given. The numbers and types of cases treated under the contract are not specifically designated, though upper and lower limits may be set.
2. **Cost and volume contracts.** Providers receive a fixed sum for a basic level of treatment, and receive extra payments for treating patients beyond this level.
3. **Cost per case contracts.** Providers receive an agreed price for each case treated.

Contracts are negotiated between those who commission care and those who provide it. Standard contracts relate to the next financial year, though longer term contracts are now more common. Initially most were block contracts. Subsequently there was a move towards the more flexible types of contract, but this was not as dramatic as envisaged (Ellwood, 1995).

Contracts increasingly began to specify service requirements in some detail: incorporating *Patient Charter* standards (Chapter 11), *Health of the Nation* targets (Chapter 12), clinical audit (Chapter 6), as well as specific requirements relating to the admission, care and discharge of patients. NHS contracts are not enforceable through the courts. Disputes are usually referred to regional offices of the NHS Executive.

In cases where treatment is not covered by a contract, it is classified as an extra contractual referral (ECR). ECRs are authorised by health authorities. In 1996, the Major government attempted to reduce the bureaucracy involved in the approval processes. Following the change of government in 1997 it was announced that contracts would eventually be replaced by long-term service level agreements, and that ECRs and cost per case contracts would be scrapped as soon as possible.

It also became clear that the freedom of the self-governing trusts (SGTs) would be restricted (DoH, 1990c). Central government retained powers to set the financial objectives of trusts, limit borrowing, and control financial surpluses. Ultimately, if ministers wished to do so, they could dissolve a trust. Central government also issued guidance to the trusts on a range of policy and procedural matters. Furthermore, through the appointment of trust chairpersons, non-executive directors, and their influence over senior management posts, ministers and civil servants sought to ensure that a 'steady state' was maintained.

Finally, the introduction of the NHS trusts and GP fundholding was phased in gradually. Only 57 units in England were granted trust status in the so-called 'first wave' beginning in April 1991. These were joined by another 99 in the following year, and a further 137 in 1993. By 1996 virtually all providers on the British mainland had trust status. GP fundholding was also implemented gradually. Only 306 GP practices, covering 6 per cent of the population, adopted fundholding in the first year. Following the second wave of GP fundholders, which became operational in April 1992, around 3000 GPs had fundholding status covering 14 per cent of the population. By 1996 over half the population was covered by fundholders.

☐ *The political context*

Changes at the top provide one possible explanation of why the Conservative government adopted a more cautious approach to reform. In early November 1990, Kenneth Clarke, who had steered through the legislative changes, was succeeded as Secretary of State for Health by William Waldegrave who displayed a more conciliatory approach than his predecessor. The replacement of Margaret Thatcher as Prime Minister by John Major a few weeks later brought a similar change in style at Number 10 Downing Street, with Major at least initially presenting himself more convincingly as a supporter of the NHS, and of public services generally.

Although it is possible that the implementation of the NHS reforms was affected by these changes in political office, it is doubtful that they were crucial. Department of Health guidance slowing down the reforms, mentioned earlier, was issued before Thatcher's resignation. Indeed, it was subsequently revealed that the incumbent Prime Minister was already concerned about the impact of the reforms ahead of the forthcoming General Election. The possibility of delaying the implementation of the NHS reforms was discussed, but in the event only the community care changes were postponed (Timmins, 1995).

There were political reasons for slowing down the reforms. The Conservative government was under pressure from its own MPs who, attributing a number of by-election defeats directly to the NHS reforms, urged Ministers to avoid anything that might further provoke further public hostility. Practical difficulties also constrained the reforms. NHS managers, even those who broadly supported the reforms, told the government that its timetable was unrealistic. In their view the infrastructure of the internal market, the staff, computer systems, procedures and above all the necessary financial management systems could not be in place in time. This view was endorsed by the Social Services Committee (House of Commons, 1989c) the Audit Commission (1991b), and the National Audit Office (NAO, 1989b). One particular problem was the lack of accurate information about health service costs, essential to the effective operation of the market. This problem persisted throughout the 1990s (NAO, 1995b; Ellwood, 1995).

■ The impact of the internal market

Evaluating the impact of the internal market is no easy task. As already mentioned, the Thatcher government was reluctant to pilot its proposals and did not support the idea of an evaluation programme. Some evaluation was subsequently undertaken by official agencies such as the Clinical Standards Advisory Group, the National Audit Office and the Audit Commission, and by other bodies, notably King's Fund which launched an important programme of research (Robinson and Le Grand, 1994). But there was no provision for a systematic evaluation programme on the basis of pilot projects, which meant that the opportunity to have a more open and informed debate about the changes was lost.

This gave short-term advantage to the government, as it would prove difficult to identify any adverse effects at an early stage. However, such problems could not be concealed for ever. The government was therefore forced to alter its policy and intervene in the operation of the market in order to deflect criticism. These shifts in policy represent the second main obstacle to evaluation. One is in effect trying to evaluate something that is constantly changing.

Thirdly, evaluation of the internal market is further complicated by the existence of other policy initiatives. Particular problems arise when trying to evaluate the impact of policies which appear contradictory. The internal market was at odds with other policies, such as *The Patient's Charter* and *The Health of the Nation* strategies. These initiatives sought to impose central standards, while the market approach emphasised decentralisation and entrepreneurialism.

Nevertheless, in spite of these difficulties an attempt must be made to assess the impact of the internal market reforms with regard to key criteria such as efficiency, equity, accountability, the capacity to plan and coordinate services, quality of service and patient choice.

☐ *Efficiency*

Supporters asserted rather than demonstrated the benefits of internal markets in health care (see Hudson, 1992; Le Grand and Bartlett, 1993 for an analysis of these arguments). Meanwhile, critics theorised that the reforms would produce higher transaction costs and would undermine efficiency (Burke and Goddard 1990; Bartlett, 1991).

So what impact did the internal market have on efficiency? Much depends of course on how efficiency is conceptualised and measured (see Chapter 3). The Conservative government's efficiency index – which measured the amount of health care provided in relation to resources – improved by between 2 and 3 per cent annually. However, recorded improvements in the index also reflected factors other than the reforms (such as the use of new technologies, for example). Furthermore, as noted in Chapter 6, the calculation of this index was hotly disputed.

Improved cost-efficiency is indicated by the average cost of hospital services, which fell in a number of sectors: acute services, geriatrics and maternity services. However, this does not necessarily mean that the overall costs of care were reduced – they may simply have been shunted on to others, such as carers, the primary and community health services or social service departments. There is no way of knowing whether or not decisions regarding discharges were more appropriate or efficient: patients prematurely discharged and subsequently readmitted are normally counted as new admissions, giving the impression that the service has delivered efficiency gains when in fact some patients may have spent more time in hospital.

It should be noted that the reduction in capacity – resulting from market pressures to cut costs – may have undermined efficiency in a broader sense. Excessive cost-cutting can mean that services are unable to cope with a sudden upturn in demand. The rising level of emergency admissions in the 1990s subsequently exposed the shortage of capacity in many hospitals (Capewell, 1996).

Even where unambiguous improvements in efficiency were demonstrated, the gains were confined rather experienced throughout the health care system. For example, the price reductions obtained by some GP fundholders (Glennerster, Matsaganis and Owens, 1994, p. 72) were not necessarily available to all, and may have raised prices for others (Webb, 1994). The GP fundholding scheme was credited with limiting the rate of increase in prescribing costs for participants when compared with non-fundholders (Bradlow and Coulter, 1993; Howie, Heaney and Maxwell,

1995; Wilson, Buchan and Whalley, 1995). Others disputed this, suggesting that the impact of the scheme on prescribing costs was short-term and specific (Stewart-Brown *et al.*, 1995).

Even if one accepts that real efficiency gains were achieved as a result of improved costing procedures and changes in working practices stimulated by the market reforms, these gains have to be set against the cost of change. This cost was substantial, possibly as much as £2 billion in start-up costs and a further £0.5 billion a year in running costs (Petchey, 1993). Unsurprisingly official estimates were lower than this, the Department of Health claiming that the start-up costs between 1989–93 amounted to £1179 million (*Hansard*, 1992). As the market evolved, a number of specific areas of concern arose including the high management costs of fundholders (House of Commons, 1995a; Audit Commission 1995e) and trusts (Audit Commission, 1995d) and the cost of extra contractual referrals (see Exhibit 8.1) which in some cases exceeded the cost of treatment (Butler, 1995c).

Following the introduction of the internal market, administrative and management costs increased. Health authority management costs rose from just over £800 million (1988/9 at 1993/4 prices) to £1136 million in 1993/4, a 28 per cent increase in real terms (*Health Care Parliamentary Monitor*, 1995c). Although there is a comparability problem in that the functions of health authorities changed between these dates, the rise is nevertheless significant. In addition, by the mid-1990s management and administrative costs of the trusts in England and Wales represented on average 10.5 per cent of their revenue (Audit Commission, 1995d). Although there are no directly comparable figures for providers' administration costs before the creation of the internal market, calculations on the basis of Department of Health statistics reveal that the administrative costs for hospitals in England in 1990/1 were only 4.2 per cent of the total cost of hospital services (DoH, 1992b; *Hansard*, 1993).

Criticism of the growing costs of administration was associated with the increase in managers, administrative and clerical staff. Between 1989–94, the number of managers increased fourfold and other administrative staff by over 10 per cent. Over the same period the number of nurses and midwives fell by 12.4 per cent (DoH, 1995b). The Department of Health justified the rise in management and administrative staff in terms of job reclassification, and by arguing that the pre-reform NHS was 'under-managed'. However, less than half of the increase in non-clinical staff was attributable to the reclassification of posts (Appleby, 1995; DoH, 1994d).

The internal market was accused of having an adverse effect upon the efficiency of providers, causing particular problems for the providers of specialist services (Mullen, 1995; Clinical Standards Advisory Group, 1993; British Paediatric Association, 1993; Langham and Black, 1995). These problems were attributed to several factors including a lack of knowledge among purchasing authorities about the kind of services required, reluctance to refer patients on grounds of cost, the lack of a fair pricing system which penalised efficient providers, and a failure of resources to match increased workload. Most of these factors were not entirely new, but were exacerbated by the reforms. Others claimed that perverse incentives were not confined to specialist services and throughout the NHS efficient providers were being punished rather than rewarded (Adams, C., 1995; Paton, 1995b).

In summary, the introduction of internal market had a rather ambiguous impact on the efficiency of the NHS. Recorded improvements in efficiency relate to statistical measures which are themselves open to criticism. Changes in efficiency in a wider sense, which include the shifting of costs on to other service providers (individuals, carers and social services), were not systematically measured, though an adverse effect is suggested. When the cost of operating the new regime is added this offsets to a considerable extent the efficiency gains reported.

☐ *Accountability*

Accountability, like efficiency, is open to different interpretations (Day and Klein, 1987; Pyper, 1996). One important aspect of accountability concerns the ability of central government to hold the NHS to account and influence its actions. Accountability in this sense was strengthened to some extent by the Griffiths' management reforms and by the increasing use of central directives, performance agreements and review procedures, as we saw in Chapter 6. The internal market, despite promising a more devolved system, continued the centralist tendencies of these earlier initiatives to some extent (Paton, 1993).

The Conservative government claimed that accountability in the use of resources improved following the internal market, citing the contracting process, new management structures incorporating clinicians, the granting of budget-holding powers to some GPs, and the strengthening of financial audit within the NHS. One notes that paradoxically efforts to strengthen financial audit coincided with revelations of failures of accountability (see Exhibit 7.2). Nevertheless, it is difficult to attribute such cases directly to the internal market reforms. First, important changes to the auditing regime accompanied the introduction of the internal market, with the Audit Commission being given the responsibility for external audit. It is possible that activities uncovered reflected improvements in the auditing system rather than an increasing propensity to commit such misdemeanours. Secondly, most of the major financial scandals originated in the period immediately before the creation of the internal market and cannot therefore be blamed directly on these reforms (Klein, 1994).

Yet it is possible that the internal market may have created even greater opportunities for fraud and financial mismanagement. First, by extending the 'business ethos' of earlier management initiatives it justified actions which were in the past viewed as inappropriate within the public sector. Secondly, by creating more transactions and contracts it made financial conduct more difficult to police, creating more scope for financial misconduct and mismanagement. Thirdly, the commercial secrecy of the new NHS reinforced the reluctance of individuals to 'blow the whistle'. The Audit Commission (1994b) found that one in three of the people its questioned feared the consequences of 'rocking the boat' when the misuse of funds was discovered.

□ *Planning and coordination*

The internal market was heralded as a solution to the past failures of planning and coordination. It was claimed that the market would enable purchasers to concentrate on planning for the health needs of their particular locality free from the responsibilities of operational management. Others agreed that a more appropriate pattern and range of services could emerge, based upon the needs of the community rather than those of the provider (Ham and Matthews, 1991).

Not all shared this sanguine view, suggesting instead that the planning of services and the ability of the different agencies involved in health care to coordinate services would be undermined by the internal market (McLachlan, 1990; Paton, 1992). Certainly a free-market approach, with its numerous buyers and sellers of services and the absence of formal command structures, is the antithesis of planning. This was demonstrated by a simulation exercise undertaken in 1990, before the NHS internal market was launched. The experiment, known as the Rubber Windmill exercise, found that the market failed when individual participants pursued their own self-interests in the absence of a strategic planning framework.

In the period following the introduction of the market, the planning process at local level was largely indicative, with purchasers and providers at best keeping each other informed about purchasing decisions. In some cases there was a lack of communication and a failure to build trust (Ferlie, 1994). At worst there was overt antagonism as the various parties refused to share what they regarded as sensitive information. As a result, planners were denied important information about service provision (Audit Commission, 1993a, 1993b). Similar problems were faced by those seeking to coordinate services and to promote collaboration (Hadley and Goldman, 1995; Rea, 1995). Planning was further complicated by the creation of rival purchasing authorities in the form of GP fundholders who were able to frustrate the planning and coordinating efforts of health authorities. As we shall see later, the Major government responded to this problem by attempting to strengthen the planning framework.

☐ Service quality and patient choice

The internal market was intended as a means of promoting improvements in service quality by creating an incentive to commission health care in a way which maximised health gain and consumer choice. Providers were required to offer greater choice and deliver service improvements, or risk losing contracts and income. But to what extent did quality of service actually improve as a result of the new regime? Did providers become more responsive to the needs of the patient?

Although the internal market was advanced as a means of extending patient choice, patients continued to have little say in the pattern of service delivery. The Organisation for Economic Cooperation and Development (OECD, 1994b), in an otherwise positive report on the impact of reform, failed to find any significant expansion of consumer choice in the early years. Similarly, research by Mahon, Wilkin and Whitehouse (1994) found that the level of patient involvement in the choice of hospital and consultant was low and changed little in the first or the second year of the reforms. Subsequently, there has been little to suggest that patients are displaying 'consumer' qualities or that doctors are competing for patients as envisaged by the architects of the internal market (see Chapter 11).

Instead there were fears that choice was working in the opposite direction and that selection of patients by doctors was becoming a more powerful factor. 78 000 patients were de-listed by GPs in 1992–3 (House of Commons, 1995a) and it is possible that 'cream skimming' – the selection of healthy patients in favour of those who have a propensity to illness – may have been a factor. However, a major study of GP fundholding (Glennerster, Matsaganis and Owens, 1994) did not find evidence of biased selection. This was largely because the method used to set budgets, coupled with the limited range of services purchased by fundholders, reduced the incentives to indulge in cream-skimming. But with the development of total fundholding (where GPs buy the full range of services for their patients) these incentives may well grow.

There was evidence that the purchaser–provider split had a positive impact on the effectiveness of services. In a survey undertaken in 1994, 57 per cent of public health directors believed that this was the case (Marks,

1995). The same survey found that 45 per cent believed GP fundholding had improved the effectiveness of services, though a quarter thought services had deteriorated as a result of the scheme. There is some evidence that fundholders were able to respond more flexibly to patient choice (Glennerster, Matsaganis and Owens, 1994; Howie, Heaney and Maxwell, 1995), but only a minority took full advantage of their status in this respect (Audit Commission, 1996b). Only two-fifths of fundholding GPs demonstrated genuine innovations in the way their practices were run (Whynes, 1997).

The impact of the internal market on quality of service is difficult to measure, partly because of the difficulties of conceptualising and measuring quality in relation to health care (Pollitt, 1993b; Joss and Kogan, 1995). Another problem is that other initiatives accompanied the implementation of the market reforms: such as *The Patient's Charter*, Total Quality Management, clinical audit, and the encouragement of evidence-based medicine through protocols and clinical guidelines. These were to some extent combined with the market approach. For instance standards identified through these processes are increasingly incorporated within contracts. However, this activity is by no means widespread – the Audit Commission (1996b, pp. 23–4) found that only a third of GP fundholders claimed that evidence-based medicine influenced purchasing, and few had access to clinical audit information.

☐ *Equity*

Although the NHS during its lifetime has fallen short of providing an equitable service in many respects, at least these problems were recognised by government during the 1960s and 1970s. The emphasis of policy was to reduce rather than widen inequities. Health reforms in subsequent decades have, according to some, reversed this trend (Mohan, 1995). In particular the internal market was held responsible for creating a 'two-tier system' based on unequal purchasing power between different patients unrelated to clinical need. Hence, patients whose purchaser exerted the most leverage could be 'fast-tracked' in order to obtain quicker or better quality treatment. Interestingly, the survey of public health directors mentioned earlier (Marks, 1995) found that a majority (56 per cent) believed the reforms had undermined the principle of equal access for all patients (18 per cent, however, believed that the reforms strengthened this principle).

GP fundholding was a particular target for criticism. Surveys revealed that up to 40 per cent of units were operating selective admission policies that reflected factors other than clinical need (Association of Community Health Councils, 1993a; Royal College of Surgeons, 1994; Beecham, 1994).

It was also shown that patients of fundholders obtained quicker access to outpatient clinics compared with non-fundholders (Kammerling and Kinnear, 1996). Even so, in the absence of controlled studies measuring the speed of referrals and quality of service among similar cases, it was impossible to prove that non-fundholders' patients were systematically disadvantaged. Furthermore, fundholders' patients could lose out in particular situations, for example where a practice faced severe financial problems or when extra money became available for health authorities to reduce waiting lists (Audit Commission, 1996b, p. 21).

But, as Glennerster, Matsaganis and Owens (1994) pointed out, inequities may have been an indication that the scheme was working and that its benefits should be extended to all practices. Non-fundholders responded by attempting to directly influence health authority priorities and purchasing plans with some success (Graffy and Williams, 1994; Black, Birchall and Trimble, 1994) A significant minority of non-fundholders also developed entrepreneurial skills in developing services for patients (Whynes, 1997).

It is difficult to establish beyond doubt that fundholders were more generously funded than other practices. Some studies indicated that fundholders were relatively generously funded (Dixon *et al.*, 1994). But this may have reflected their higher costs (Spenceley *et al.*, 1994), or different purchasing priorities between fundholders and health authorities (Dixon, 1994). Furthermore, it should be noted that large variations in budgets occurred between fundholders, an issue discussed later.

The introduction of *The Patient's Charter* standards, alongside the internal market, could be seen as an attempt to limit inequalities in health care. But minimum standards do not guarantee equitable access to health care. Potentially, separation of purchaser and provider could also contribute towards a more equitable system by building equity standards into the contracting system. But in practice, contracting seemed to promote wider variations in standards rather than a movement towards universality, with some purchasers (in particular fundholders) being able to insist on special advantages for their patients only.

Finally, it was argued that the internal market undermined equity by stimulating the private health sector. This occurred in two main ways. First, the internal market placed pressure on purchasers (to restrict budgets) and providers (to cut costs) leading to a geographical imbalance in the provision of publicly-funded services (given the variety of local approaches to rationing), and a greater emphasis on the allocation of some services (that is, those no longer available to NHS patients) by ability to pay rather than need. Secondly, it further stimulated the private sector by creating greater incentives to purchase private health care, and for trusts to generate their own private income by expanding pay-bed facilities.

■ The evolution of the internal market

The internal market evolved in a number of ways: by reorganisation and administrative reform; by changes in the planning and regulation of local health services by central government and regional bodies; by changes to the method of resource allocation; and by a range of other developments, encouraged to some extent by the centre but initiated mainly at local level.

☐ *Reorganisation*

The increased administrative costs associated with the internal market were attacked by politicians on the right wing of the Conservative Party as well as by those who had earlier opposed the reforms. The right-wingers argued that the implementation of the reforms had been far too cautious and that there had been excessive regulation. Their solution was to streamline the NHS bureaucracy, first by rationalising the structure of the NHS, and secondly by removing some of the restrictions on the market.

The first proposal attracted much wider support from the government than the latter. The NHS structure indeed looked cumbersome. Two distinct regional structures were being maintained: the RHAs and the NHS Executive regional outposts. At local level there was a strong case for merging district health authorities (whose numbers had fallen substantially as a result of mergers) with the Family Health Service Authorities (FHSAs), which managed family practitioner services. Indeed, some authorities had already begun to integrate their activities on an informal basis by creating joint health commissions. Following a review of the NHS structure (DoH, 1994c), it was proposed that RHAs should merge with the outposts to form new regional offices. Meanwhile, DHAs would be formally merged with FHSAs at local level to form new health authorities.

In addition, health authorities came under pressure to reduce management costs. In 1995 a management costs league table was published enabling the identification of the heaviest spenders. Health authorities were ordered to reduce management costs by 5 per cent and were set an overall benchmark for management costs of £10 per head of population. At the same time the government responded to two efficiency scrutinies which had examined the administrative workload of the NHS. The first inquiry, which examined general practice, recommended a considerable reduction in paperwork and increasing use of information technology (NHSE, 1995c). The second, which examined trusts and health authorities, also demanded a cut in paperwork and a greater use of information technology recommending longer-term service contracts and a simplification of the ECR approvals system (see Exhibit 8.1) (NHSE, 1996b). Although ministers accepted both reports, the extent to which specific recommendations were implemented varied. For example, the simplification of the ECR system was impeded by concerns that health authorities would lose financial control over treatment provided by trusts.

□ *Planning and regulation*

Initially, the Conservative government envisaged a type of business planning for the new NHS with the main participants in the market acting rather like firms in the business sector, developing their own plans in the light of market conditions. However, in spite of the calls for further deregulation it became clear that plans must be reconciled and competition managed within a clear framework of planning, accountability and regulation.

The Department of Health initiated central policy initiatives such as *The Patient's Charter* and *The Health of the Nation* strategy and continued to set priorities and targets for the NHS. It set the lead nationally with regard to particular service developments. For example, in 1995 a national plan for cancer services was devised which was widely seen as an admission that improvements in services could not be achieved by the market alone (DoH, 1995e). The Department of Health also encouraged a more cooperative approach to planning amid evidence of poor communication and collaboration between GPs and health authorities, and between purchasers and providers. Central guidance was introduced to establish accountability arrangements at local level (DoH, 1995d). Fundholders were expected to work with health authorities to achieve national and regional priorities and were urged to share information about their purchasing intentions. In addition the new unitary health authorities sought a more active management role in relation to fundholders than had the FHSAs.

Since the creation of the internal market the Department of Health had intervened to establish various rules and regulations. In 1994 these were superseded by a single document setting out the framework for regulation (DoH, 1994e). These rules, which appeared to be based on the US Federal Trade Commission/Department of Justice guidelines for the health care industry (Dawson, 1995), outlined areas where intervention in the market could be undertaken, including mergers, closure of services and anti-competitive behaviour. By laying down ground-rules for central intervention, the government had openly accepted that the market, left to its own devices, threatened wider policy objectives. Some observers believed this move was a step in the right direction (Le Grand, 1994). Others were more critical, arguing that the idea of central intervention to correct market failure raised fundamental questions about the whole purpose of the market mechanism in health care, and that the guidance merely added to the confusion surrounding the policy (Paton, 1995a). Other criticisms focused on the potential for inefficiency implied by the new rules and the lack of independent enforcement of the regulations (Dawson, 1995).

Finally, the restructuring of the NHS, described earlier, was widely interpreted as a move in the direction of greater central intervention. The regional tier was in effect absorbed into the Department of Health by the abolition of the RHAs. Despite the government's claims that the regional offices would have a 'light touch', they retained considerable powers not only to shape local health strategies and monitor performance but to regulate and manage local NHS markets.

☐ *Resource allocation*

It was originally intended that health authorities and GP fundholders would receive funds in relation to the size of their relevant populations (the resident population for health authorities; for fundholders the number of patients on the practice list) adjusted to reflect variations in the level of need. This weighted capitation approach seemed both equitable and uncontroversial. Indeed it seemed to follow on naturally from RAWP – the needs-based funding formula introduced by the Labour government during the 1970s, which the Conservatives had retained (see Chapter 4).

In practice, however, the new weighted capitation policy raised many objections and was slow to develop. First of all, as with RAWP, there were disputes about how population need should be measured. The Department of Health was heavily criticised for rejecting the use of social indicators, such as measures of deprivation, as a basis for allocating health authority funds at regional level. Some RHAs did use such indicators when allocating resources to districts.

Another issue highlighted by critics was the variation in fundholders' budgets. Day and Klein (1991) found that the highest spending fundholders had twice the level of funding per patient of the lowest spenders. Although the Department of Health expressed its intention to move towards weighted capitation funding for fundholders, enormous practical problems meant that these budgets were largely determined by previous referral activity.

In 1993, in view of continuing concern about the fairness of the funding system, the availability of new data on population needs, and with the prospect of a further reorganisation of the structure of the NHS, the Department of Health began to explore the options for change. Studies commissioned by the department concluded that it would be impracticable to move towards a capitation formula for the allocation of GP budgets based on measures of health and socio-economic needs (Sheldon *et al.*, 1994). However, the research programme did find that as a short-term measure, age and sex weighted capitation was a more equitable basis for funding than the present system based on past activity levels. The department in turn proposed that fundholder budgets should be set with regard to capitation benchmarks, reflecting the variation in the age and sex composition of GP lists, while not entirely excluding historical or local factors.

At the same time a new formula was proposed for allocating resources to health authorities. This included an element for social factors such as unemployment, illness rates, and the proportion of single carers. But far from resolving disputes surrounding the allocation of resources, this merely fuelled controversy. This was because like most alterations to funding regimes it produced winners and losers. The Department of Health eventually decided on a less-risky strategy which involved phasing in the changes and retaining a 'market forces factor' within the formula (in effect giving protection to London and the South East, high cost areas which would otherwise lose funds). Finally, it was decided to 'zero-weight' a quarter of the health and community health services budget. This last move was justified by the Department of Health on technical grounds – that certain services such as health promotion and services for people with learning difficulties were not linked to social factors. This was not regarded by most as a convincing argument for zero weighting. However, political reasons were also evident, the decision not to weight this element benefiting the Conservative-dominated London and the South East at the expense of the North (Hacking, 1995, 1996).

Concern about the fairness of the funding formula remained (House of Commons, 1996e). It may be technically possible in the future to improve resource allocation on the basis of formulae which reflect need more accurately. However, given that re-allocation of resources will always produce controversy, these issues will never be ruled by purely technical considerations.

☐ *Commissioning*

As the internal market began to evolve, it became clear that there was a great deal of variation in the interaction of purchasers and providers at a local level. Despite the conceptual simplicity of the division between the two, in practice a variety of local arrangements for the commissioning of services were established. The main models are outlined in Exhibit 8.2.

Some models clearly reflected the Conservatives' policy – for example the progressive extension of fundholding. Others, however, were generated

Exhibit 8.2   *Commissioning health services*

■ GP fundholding

Following its introduction, GPs fundholding expanded not only in terms of the proportion of population covered by the scheme, but also with respect to the range of services purchased. A new, limited form of fundholding – community fundholding – was introduced in 1995 to encourage smaller practices to join the scheme. The advent of multifunds – where individual practices combine under a single management structure – also attracted smaller practices. The scope of the standard scheme meanwhile expanded beyond the original list of hospital services to include the purchasing of virtually all elective and community health services by 1996. A number of schemes were piloted, allowing selected fundholders to purchase particular services outside the standard scheme (such as in-patient mental health services). In addition, experimental 'total purchasing' schemes were established which involved purchasing all hospital and community health services including emergency services and maternity care. The Blair government intends to end GP fundholding in 1999 (see below).

■ Joint commissioning

This term was used mainly to describe informal arrangements between the former FHSAs and DHAs prior to the creation of the unitary health authorities. But it was later applied to any form of joint working between commissioners of care. It may relate to the formation of a consortium, to commission services that benefit more than one health authority. Or it can refer to relationships and mechanisms for coordinating the activities of GP budget holders and health authorities (see below). Alternatively it may be applied to collaboration between health authorities, GPs and social services departments.

■ Locality commissioning

In many localities health authorities have sought to improve links with GPs by creating commissioning groups which discuss service priorities. In some, separate groups exist for fundholders and non-fundholding GPs; in others there is a more integrated approach where all GPs are represented in the same forum. Increasingly, attempts are being made to decentralise management on the basis of smaller localities within health authority boundaries. This involves the development of closer working relationships between GPs and managers or professionals employed by health authorities. These arrangements may be accompanied by a devolution of management responsibility and budgets to those operating at the local level. The Labour government, elected in 1997, signalled its support for locality commissioning schemes. It is intended that in future all GPs along with community nurses will form Primary Care Groups. These will hold budgets for hospital and community health services, cash-limited general medical services and prescribing, for a defined population.

Sources and further reading: Shapiro (1994), Balogh (1996).

at the local level. Some, such as joint commissioning arrangements between district health authorities and FHSAs, began as informal links and initially went against the grain of government policy. Eventually, as part of the reorganisation plan mentioned earlier, the case for formal mergers was accepted.

As the market developed, an emphasis on collaboration rather than competition became evident. In some parts of the country competition was never really an option because of the lack of alternative providers (this was particularly the case in rural areas). But even where competition was possible, purchasers and providers began to realise that it was much easier and less costly to build up a dialogue and collaborate with each other rather than to move contracts. In some areas the contracting process was used as an opportunity to improve the quality of care, rather than to simply cut costs.

Increasing emphasis was placed upon assessing and responding to local needs. In a growing number of areas various models of local commissioning were adopted in an effort to make planning more sensitive to local needs and to coordinate the various interests on the commissioning side (see Exhibit 8.2). This offset to some extent the impact of mergers which followed the introduction of the internal market and which led to the creation of larger and potentially more remote health authorities. Meanwhile, the Conservative government itself urged health authorities to listen more carefully to users and to 'local voices' (NHSME, 1992). Although the emphasis initially was mainly upon market research techniques rather than encouraging real participation, some health authorities became active in seeking to elicit the public's preferences (see Chapter 11).

■ Reversing the reforms?

The Labour Party (and the Liberal Democrats) campaigned against the internal market reforms during and following their introduction. However, as the reforms became entrenched both began to realise the impracticality of reversing the changes. Total abolition would absorb valuable parliamentary time. Many of the changes would be very costly to unravel, such as replacing contracting, demerging health authorities and trusts for example. Moreover, while the reforms still continued to attract hostility, the new system was underpinned by new vested interests (such as fundholders and private operators) and by significant and growing sections of the public (including fundholders' patients and privately-insured people) who could possibly be mobilised to resist attempts to reverse the reforms.

Consequently, both Labour and Liberal Democrat health policies began to move closer to that of the Conservatives (Labour Party, 1995; Liberal Democrats, 1995). They accepted the purchaser–provider split (though preferring the term commissioning to purchasing), and the principle of delegated management by trusts. However, Labour remained committed to abolishing the internal market and GP fundholding, while the Liberals opted for reform.

In 1997 the new Labour government announced plans for replacing the internal market (Cm 3807, 1997). It proposed the end of the fundholding scheme, the replacement of contracts with service level agreements, and a reduction in the number of commissioning and providing bodies. In addition Primary Care Groups (PCGs) involving all GPs and community nurses would commission services on behalf of defined populations, taking one of four forms: advisory bodies to health authorities; bodies holding devolved budget powers; freestanding commissioning bodies; commissioning bodies with added responsibility for providing community health services. It was envisaged that PCGs would evolve towards the third and fourth models. Meanwhile, it was intended that competitive forces would be reduced by a stronger planning role for health authorities coupled with a duty on all local agencies involved in health and social care to cooperate with one another.

■ Conclusion

Despite the initial radical zeal, the internal market gave way to a more tightly regulated and cautious approach. But this is not to say that the reform turned out to be insignificant. On the contrary it had wide-ranging implications in conjunction with other reforms of the 1980s and 1990s. The supporters of internal markets identify a number of achievements and improvements since 1991, but it is unclear whether these were directly the result of the internal market changes. In addition one must consider the costs and negative consequences attributed to the reforms.

The experience of the NHS internal market demonstrates that reforms often have a dynamic of their own. This often makes it difficult for their creators to remain in complete control. Moreover, incoming governments find it difficult to reverse changes once they have been implemented. This certainly occurred with the internal market, continuing reform of the purchaser–provider split being the only realistic course available, at least in the short term.

■ *Chapter 9* ■

Primary Health Care

Until relatively recently primary health care services attracted little attention from policy-makers. This is perhaps surprising given that for most people the first point of contact with the health service is through a primary care professional, such as a GP, pharmacist, dentist, optician or community nurse. Furthermore, the vast majority of episodes of illness are managed by those working in the primary care sector. This chapter explores the main problems and challenges facing primary health care, along with the efforts made by policy-makers to address these problems in recent years. It seeks to explain why the contribution of primary care has been recognised at last, and discusses possible future developments in this sector.

■ What is primary care?

One of the most confusing things about primary care is that the term is interpreted in a variety of ways. Broadly speaking, primary care is a philosophy that emphasises the need to move care out of large institutions and into community-based settings. The underlying aim is to make health services, and other interventions, more responsive to the needs of the community. The World Health Organisation (WHO, 1978) set out a number of practical ways in which policy should develop, including the promotion of self-help, the integration of medical care with other social services, environmental improvements, the promotion of good health rather than simply good quality health services, meeting the needs of underprivileged and under-served groups in the community, and allowing the wider community to participate in the planning and delivery of health services.

The setting of health care is seen by many as the defining characteristic of primary care. Hicks (1976), for example, defines primary care as those services which are delivered in doctor's surgeries, clinics, special institutions for the handicapped and disabled, and in patients' own homes. Alternatively, the term can be used to refer to specific services provided by the NHS. In this sense primary care covers a huge range of services including health maintenance, prevention of illness, diagnosis and treatment, rehabilitation, pastoral care and the certification of illness (Pritchard, 1978). Finally, primary care relates to services provided by specific professional groups based in the community. These include GPs, dentists, pharmacists, opticians, district nurses, midwives, health visitors, chiropodists and speech therapists.

The various definitions of primary health care reveal different degrees of ambition about the possibility, and the desirability, of changing the focus of health care. In addition, as this chapter will reveal, there are conflicting perspectives that reflect wider professional rivalries among health professionals working in community settings. These conflicts interact with other factors, including the hostility of hospital-based interests to a radical shift towards primary care.

■ The problems of primary care

Throughout the postwar period, at least up until the 1980s, the primary care sector was regarded as a relatively neglected area, with considerable scope for improvement (Marks, 1988; Taylor, 1988). But the sector was not given priority (Stowe 1989). Politicians realised that building a new hospital was far more popular than extending primary care services. This mentality reinforced decisions about resources, with the hospital sector increasing its share of the NHS budget up to the 1980s (see Figure 5.5).

The reasons for this relative neglect are not difficult to discover. At the time the NHS was created, the status of those working in primary care was much lower than their colleagues in the hospital sector, as reflected for example in the relationship between hospital consultants and GPs (see Chapter 2). In addition, professionals working in the hospital sector tended to have more political influence than those in primary care. The differences in status and political influence persisted to a considerable extent over the postwar period.

A further problem for the primary care services was their lack of visibility. With the possible exception of the family doctor service, the public never seemed to regard them with the same kind of importance as hospital services. This continues today, posing particular problems for those seeking to adjust the balance between primary and secondary care.

Differences in prestige, political influence and political visibility provide only a partial explanation of why primary care was neglected by policy makers. To some extent, central government did not have the means to forge new directions in primary care. Until 1974 community health services were largely in the hands of the local authorities (see Chapter 4), and central government faced considerable difficulties in developing a national vision for these highly fragmented local services. Furthermore, primary care services provided by the NHS structure were delivered largely by independent contractors: GPs, dentists, pharmacists and opticians. Beyond altering these contracts, government could not compel the professions to support particular policy initiatives. Even when contracts were altered, it was mainly a response to the grievances of the professions rather than to public concern about the quality of services. But, by the end of the 1970s reform could not be avoided any longer. Three main problems were increasingly evident: professional rivalries; poor management and coordination; and, in some areas, poor quality services.

The primary health care team (PHCT) had been encouraged in the 1960s to improve professional cooperation (Ministry of Health, 1963). This involved the attachment of nurses, health visitors, midwives (and sometimes other professionals, such as social workers) to GP practices. While the PHCT was regarded as a step forward, such arrangements sometimes failed (DHSS, 1981b). GPs tended to dominate, much to the annoyance of the other professions, thus undermining cooperation. In addition, PHCTs were rarely based on explicit agreements about each participant's role and this led to poor coordination and a failure to recognise mutual responsibilities.

Primary care also suffered from a fragmented management system. An opportunity was missed in 1974 when Family Practitioner Committees (FPCs) replaced the old Executive Councils in England and Wales. The FPCs' main task, like their predecessors, was to administer the contracts of GPs, dentists, pharmacists and opticians. But they lacked a clear management role. To complicate matters further, other primary care professions such as district nurses were from 1974 onwards managed by District Health Authorities (DHAs). Collaboration between DHAs and FPCs was poor, with neither willing to accept overall management responsibility (see Ottewill and Wall, 1990). To make matters worse, primary health care services were poorly coordinated with community care provided by local government. Attempts to improve coordination of health and social services through joint planning had a limited impact, as will be shown in the next chapter.

Finally, there was increasing concern about the quality and effectiveness of primary care services. The Royal College of General Practitioners, in its evidence to the Royal Commission on the NHS in the late 1970s, mentioned unacceptably low standards in a minority of practices. There was particular criticism of primary care in inner cities where needs were often complex and services limited (Cmnd 7615, 1979). Initially, worries about effectiveness and quality of service were confined to specific areas or practices. However, the increasing demands being placed on the primary care sector began to generate more fundamental concerns about its ability to deliver high-quality services.

■ Primary health care in the 1980s

The Thatcher government believed that by providing alternative forms of care and support, primary care reform could restrict demands on the hospital service and thereby limit the financial burden of the NHS on the taxpayer. It focused on the gatekeeper function of the primary care services, and in particular the GPs who played a major role in regulating access to other forms of care provided by the NHS, such as hospital services and medicines. At the same time the government recognised that primary care expenditure – notably the spending on family practitioner services – was difficult to control. Spending patterns reflected the clinical decisions of practitioners, and unlike hospital spending was not subject to overall 'cash limits' imposed on health authority expenditure. The main fear within government circles was that spending restraint in the hospital sector would be offset by increased expenditure on primary care.

The Thatcher government also focused on the problems of managing primary care, in particular the lack of financial and managerial accountability in the sector, the independence of the family practitioners, and the inability of FPCs to influence their performance. Other considerations drew the government towards primary care reform. There was much scope for increasing charges. Ministers argued that this encouraged individuals to take responsibility for their own health, while discouraging unnecessary and excessive use of NHS services. Primary care, which already depended on a range of independent contractors, was recognised as having considerable potential for the development of private provision, greater competition and wider consumer choice.

□ *The Thatcher government's policy*

The Thatcher government's approach to primary care reform was initially piecemeal. During the early 1980s the opticians' monopoly over the supply of spectacles was abolished and entitlement to NHS spectacles was subsequently removed and replaced by a voucher system. Meanwhile, the pharmacists' contract was renegotiated in an attempt to reduce costs. A selected list of NHS medicines was introduced. This restricted the freedom of GPs to prescribe medicines in seven categories, including laxatives, tonics and cough remedies (further categories – including drugs for skin conditions, allergic disorders and certain anti-rheumatic medicines – were added later). Furthermore, the government sought to drive down the cost of prescription medicines while raising prescription charges substantially year by year.

In 1986, however, the government decided to press ahead with comprehensive reform. It published two documents as a basis for discussion about future reforms. These were the Green Paper *Primary Health Care: An Agenda for Discussion* (Cmnd 9771, 1986), and the report of a review into community nursing *Neighbourhood Nursing: A Focus For Care* (DHSS, 1986b) also known as the Cumberlege report.

The Green Paper contained a number of highly controversial proposals. It proposed a good practice allowance (GPA) for GPs who satisfied certain criteria. In the event GPA was dropped, and a range of financial incentives introduced instead. The eligibility criteria for the GP's Basic Practice Allowance (BPA) was also tightened up with regard to practice list size and doctors' availability to patients. In an effort to promote competition among GPs it was proposed that they should in future receive a higher proportion of their income from capitation fees (the fee received for each patient on their list). The Green Paper also suggested making it easier to change doctors and this was later implemented, patients wishing to change no longer requiring permission from their current GP.

A controversial measure that was not taken forward would have allowed outside organisations to provide primary care services (an idea which resurfaced again in a White Paper of 1996). This was heavily criticised by the professions and by the Opposition parties. Similarly a proposal to relate prescription charges more closely to the cost of medicines was dropped, replaced by new charges on eye and dental checks which proved equally controversial.

The Cumberlege report, too, was controversial, though in a different way. By defining primary care in terms of community nursing, its recommendations represented a challenge to the GPs' domination of this sector. The report noted the familiar problems of poor collaboration and fragmentation in primary care, which had persisted into the 1980s (see Bond, Cartlidge and Gregson, 1987). It also identified a failure to maximise the contribution of nurses in the community.

To remedy these problems, the Cumberlege report recommended re-organising the community nursing service on the basis of small local areas or 'neighbourhoods' which would plan services on the basis of local needs. It argued for a more equal relationship between GPs and community nurses, with explicit agreements between neighbourhood nursing services and GP practices, and clearer objectives and roles for the primary health care team. It also called for the ending of subsidies to GPs, which enabled them to employ nurses, and called for nurses in the community to be given greater responsibilities including the power to prescribe drugs.

Mindful of the opposition of GPs (already upset at some of the proposals in the Green Paper), the Department of Health did not openly back the Cumberlege report. However, it did support some of the proposals, such as nurse prescribing, which was supported by the medical profession. In spite of the lack of official support the report did have some impact. Many health authorities began to reorganise services along the lines recommended by Cumberlege (Martin, 1992). Subsequently, community health trusts introduced decentralised management structures based on small localities, which in some areas, facilitated closer cooperation between GPs and community nurses (Ottewill and Wall, 1990, p. 361; White, Leach and Christensen, 1996).

The government's policy was subsequently outlined in a White Paper, *Promoting Better Health* (Cm 249, 1987). The principles of the Green Paper – competition, economic incentives, clearer accountability, a more interventionist management style and an increase in private expenditure on primary care – survived, though some of the detailed proposals, as noted, were amended.

■ The implementation of *Promoting Better Health*

The White Paper was challenged on a number of grounds (Marks, 1988). There were three main areas of contention: charges, management reform and new contracts for the primary care professions.

□ *Charges*

The decision to impose charges on sight tests and dental checks was heavily criticised. A number of further concessions resulted. As a result children under 16, students aged 16–18, and those receiving social security benefits (such as income support and family credit) were exempted from both charges; expectant and recent mothers and young people aged 16–18, from the dental charge only. Those already suffering from severely impaired eyesight, or who had been diagnosed with diabetes or glaucoma, or had a family history of glaucoma, were exempted from the eye test charge.

Ministers argued that the charges were modest – initially £3 for a dental examination and £10 for the eye test – and would not discourage the use of services. They claimed that charges reflected the principle that individuals should take responsibility for their own health, and did not represent a radical departure from the existing policy of charging for prescriptions, dental treatment, spectacles and appliances.

Dentists and opticians disputed this. They claimed that charges would discourage individuals from having such tests, and that serious illnesses such as oral cancer and glaucoma might go undetected. They also pointed out that delayed treatment would be less cost-effective than early intervention. Following the imposition of the charges, the number of eye tests fell by 30 per cent within a year. This may have been due partly to patients bringing forward their tests to avoid the charge. Yet two years after the charge was imposed, the number of eye tests was still well below the 1989 level. However, the proportion of the population claiming to have had a sight test in the previous twelve months actually increased from 29 per cent to 32 per cent of the adult population between 1987 and 1994 (OPCS, 1996, p. 76), suggesting that the longer term impact of the charge has been less dramatic.

The number of people having dental examinations also fell following the imposition of charges. Two years after the introduction of the charge, dental checks were just under 10 per cent down on the 1988/9 baseline. The number of courses of adult dental treatment also declined significantly over this period. However, in the following year this figure surged above the original baseline, indicating that the impact of the dental charge was weaker in the longer term. An alternative measure – the percentage of adult population having dental checks – fell from 49 per cent to 48 per cent between 1989–91, but rose to 51 per cent in 1993 (OPCS, 1995).

Although people appeared less discouraged by the charges in the longer term, no one knows how they would have behaved in the absence of charges. The recorded rise in the proportion having annual checks may have been even higher had the service remained free. Furthermore, the impact of the charges on low income groups who do not claim benefits is unknown. Finally, the extent to which the treatment of illnesses has been delayed is difficult to calculate: though in one case study, referrals for glaucoma were shown to have fallen by almost one fifth following the introduction of the sight test fee (Laidlaw *et al.*, 1994).

Finally, the imposition of charges raised fears about the privatisation of services in this sector. Increased charges for appliances, medicines and dental treatment, coupled with the introduction of charges for eye and dental checks, were seen as the thin end of the wedge leading eventually to payment for medical and nursing services.

□ *The management of primary care*

Promoting Better Health sought to extend the role of the FPCs in the management of primary care. Doubts had been cast upon their ability to perform such a role (Allsop and May, 1986; NAO, 1988), and there were specific concerns about inadequate levels of staffing, training and a general lack of resources. FPCs also lacked clear objectives and had few sanctions with which to influence practitioners.

Following *Promoting Better Health,* FPCs were given new financial powers. They exercised more discretion over the allocation of funds for GP staff and the development of premises giving them added leverage over family practices, though the extent to which practices could be held accountable in this respect depended on their need for such resources

(Huntington, 1993). The management role of FPCs was strengthened by the appointment of general managers in 1989. Subsequently, the FPCs were reconstructed and renamed Family Health Service Authorities (FHSAs). These were smaller and contained fewer representatives drawn from the professions.

Working for Patients – discussed in the previous chapter – reiterated the importance of FHSAs in relation to the monitoring of family practitioner contracts, quality of service and GP drug budgets. Yet at the same time their independent role was undermined. FHSAs were brought under the wing of the regional health authorities rather than being directly accountable to the Department of Health. Furthermore, the internal market appeared to threaten the FHSAs' role. They lacked the purchasing power of the DHAs, and increasingly entered into joint commissioning arrangements with them. Following a review of the NHS structure in 1993, FHSAs were formally merged with district health authorities (DoH, 1994c).

☐ *Professional contracts*

Under the terms of the new contract, which came into force in 1990, the government intended that GPs would receive a larger proportion of their income from capitation fees. Originally it was believed that this proportion would rise from 46 per cent to 60 per cent of the GPs' average income, though by the 1994/5 financial year just under 52 per cent actually came from capitalisation fees (NHSE, 1995c). A range of specific financial incentives and targets was also introduced in the 1990 contract to encourage doctors to perform certain tasks such as screening, immunisation, health checks, minor surgery, health promotion and child health surveillance.

The 1990 contract was imposed on GPs against their will. They supported the movement towards prevention, health promotion and improvements in the quality of care, but were concerned about how the new contract sought to achieve these aims, believing that competition and financial incentives would undermine clinical judgement. They further believed that the extra workload would impede rather than enhance the effectiveness of the family doctor service. Finally, some GPs – notably those working in rural areas and in the inner cities – thought their location and the size and composition of their lists would make it difficult for them to reach the targets set by the contract.

The government responded with additional lower threshold targets for immunisation and cervical cancer screening. These increased incentives to GPs who had little hope of reaching the higher targets of 90 per cent of children immunised and 80 per cent of female patients screened. New payments were also introduced for GPs working in rural areas and in inner cities, but these concessions did not address doubts regarding service effectiveness and GPs' workload.

The impact of the 1990 GP contract is difficult to evaluate, partly because of other reforms introduced around the same time – notably GP fundholding – and partly because of other trends affecting the quality of service – such as the decline in the number of GPs working alone, for example. The overall picture is one of improving quality of service, but substantial inequalities persisting between rural and suburban areas, and urban and inner city areas. According to Leese and Bosanquet (1995a and 1995b), whose detailed study supported these conclusions, practices demonstrated a strong response to the new incentives. Between 1987 and 1993 computerisation of group practices rose from 38 per cent to 94 per cent. The percentage of practices employing practice managers increased from 61 per cent to 88 per cent. Those employing practice nurses went up from 60 per cent to 96 per cent. There was a high uptake of specific disease management programmes for patients with asthma and diabetes. Immunisation rates and cervical screening rates rose following the introduction of the contract. Between 1990 and 1995 the proportion of two-year-olds immunised against measles increased from 84 to 91 per cent in England, with similar rises in diphtheria, tetanus, whooping cough and polio immunisation. Cervical screening rates in England also increased, from 80 to 86 per cent between 1991 and 1995.

In the 1990s, GPs began to undertake more minor surgery. They also became more heavily involved in health promotion and monitoring. However, the efficacy and cost-effectiveness of these developments has been challenged. Early results showed that the increase in minor surgery undertaken by GPs did not produce the expected fall in hospital workload (Lowy *et al.*, 1993). Even more worrying was evidence that GPs lacked expertise in this field (Centre for Health Economics, 1995).

Other doubts centred on the health promotion activities of GPs. Health checks were criticised for catering for the 'worried well' rather than those in genuine need (Waller *et al.*, 1990). Subsequently, large-scale studies found that although health checks did have some effect, they were not an efficient approach to promoting health and preventing illness (Family Heart Study Group, 1994; Imperial Cancer Research Fund Oxcheck Study Group, 1995). It was accordingly suggested that other strategies, such as targeting high-risk populations, would bring far greater benefits (Field *et al.*, 1995). Following some modifications to the method of allocating health promotion payments in 1993, the Major government eventually abolished the regime in 1996, replacing it with a more streamlined system which paid GPs on the basis of locally-agreed health promotion activities.

The issue of workload remained at the forefront of GPs' concerns following the implementation of the 1990 contract. Leese and Bosanquet (1995a) found that the workload increased sharply. Time spent on administration rose on average from 2.48 hours a week in 1989/90 to 3.53 hours in 1992/3 (*Hansard*, 1994). This was associated with the extra form-filling and bureaucracy associated with the new contract as well as other reforms such as *The Patient's Charter* and GP fundholding. In 1996 the Major government responded to GPs' complaints about their administrative workload by reducing their reporting requirements and simplifying the system of claiming fees and allowances.

The other contentious issue was 'out of hours' visits. The 1990 contract placed greater pressure on GPs to be directly available to patients. This, coupled with the rise in requests for visits outside normal hours, added considerably to their workload. In protest, family doctors voted in 1992 to end their contractual duty to provide 24 hour cover for patients. Eventually a solution was negotiated. In 1995 the Department of Health agreed to increase the night call fee and permitted new arrangements whereby GPs could hand over responsibility for 'out of hours' visits to a named and fully-qualified family doctor. The deal also pledged funds for the development of 'out of hours' services involving the development of a network of emergency care centres based on health centres and GPs' surgeries.

Other primary care professions negotiated changes to their contracts in the aftermath of *Promoting Better Health*. In contrast to the acrimony surrounding the GPs' contract, these changes were negotiated in a more relaxed atmosphere, though in the case of the dentists the implementation of the new contract subsequently produced much controversy.

The 1990 contract moved dentists towards a capitation-based system. It introduced capitation fees for children and retention payments for adults registered with a practice. The aim was to encourage continuing care and prevention, a move widely supported by the profession. However in 1991/2 there was a dispute with the Department of Health over the level of payments. The department claimed it had overpaid dentists and that NHS fees should therefore be reduced. Many dentists protested by refusing to admit new NHS patients to their lists and, in some cases, removing those currently registered with them.

The Department of Health initiated a review of NHS dentistry, followed by the publication of a consultative document in 1994. This suggested relating payments more closely to the costs of treatment, and altering fees to place even greater emphasis on prevention. The document set out the longer-term possibility of moving towards a commissioner–provider model for NHS dentistry (Cm 2625, 1994).

Meanwhile, the problems facing NHS dentistry remained. Large numbers of NHS patients were removed from dentists' lists. Between June 1994 and May 1995 alone, 941 000 NHS patients were deregistered (Jackman, 1995). According to the General Dental Practitioners' Association, NHS treatment fell from 89 per cent of 57 per cent of dentists' workload between 1990 and 1995 (*Independent*, 1995).

In 1995 a two-stage solution to the problem was proposed. In the short term there would be changes to the payments system – the flat rate child capitation system would in future reflect the higher cost of specific treatments. Also, the amounts received by dentists for each adult patient on their list was to be reduced. In addition a new prior approval procedure for expensive dental treatment was proposed. To address the problems of access to NHS dentists a small amount of extra funding was given to health authorities to enable them to pay for dental work where local shortages were particularly acute. Looking to the longer term, the Department of Health announced it would seek to introduce a commissioner–provider system between health authorities and dentists as outlined in the earlier consultative document, with local pilot schemes to assess viability.

■ Further developments

The pressure on primary care providers intensified considerably in the first half of the 1990s. In England the number of GP consultations rose by 16 per cent between 1990 and 1994. Over the same period the number of prescriptions issued increased by 15 per cent. Between 1991/2 and 1994/5 the number of initial contacts by community nurses in England rose by 8 per cent (from 2 468 000 to 2 665 000). Health visitors also faced a growing workload, the number of persons visited at home rising from 3 643 000 to 3 711 000 between 1990/1 and 1994/5.

Increasing workloads have been partly due to changing demographic and disease patterns. Rising expectations about services is another factor. Furthermore, broader changes in the pattern of health care provision – inspired by other reforms – added to the workload of the primary care sector. Finally, government policy in the 1990s increasingly emphasised the development of primary care as the pivotal sector in the NHS, adding further to its responsibilities.

□ *Commissioning health services*

The granting of fundholder status to GPs had far-reaching consequences for primary and secondary care. The scheme gave participating GPs financial leverage over hospitals and, subsequently, community health services. Although initially GP budgets were relatively small, representing on average as little as 2 per cent of a local hospital's budget, the threat of losing income was still very real. Consequently hospitals began to respond to the requests of fundholders for changes in services. This gave rise to allegations of unequal treatment through the fast-tracking of fundholders' patients (see Chapter 8). But fundholding was credited with stimulating broader changes in the pattern of service provision, such as direct access to hospital services and outreach clinics (see below).

As the fundholding scheme expanded, GPs began to control a larger proportion of resources. By 1995 fundholders purchased a fifth of their patients' health care by value. Furthermore they could influence an even wider range of services through other commissioning arrangements involving non-fundholding GPs (see Exhibit 8.2).

GP fundholding became the central component of the Major government's strategy to create a primary care-led NHS. The rationale was that GPs were closer to the patient and could identify needs more effectively. It was assumed that they were extremely knowledgeable about the individual patient's needs, and that fundholding would promote a more responsive service on the patient's behalf. However, there was little evidence that GP practices were developing a systematic approach to needs assessment (Audit Commission, 1996b). Few actively consulted patients and hardly any involved them in decision-making.

The Department of Health urged both GPs and health authorities to be more responsive to the needs of patients and the wider public. In 1992 it called upon health authorities to listen more carefully to the public and to establish ways of assessing local views (NHSME, 1992). The role of the health authority in setting overall strategies in the light of local needs was reiterated following the extension of the fundholding scheme in 1994. Health authorities and fundholders were urged to work together to ensure that commissioning was undertaken with regard to the needs of the local community (NHSE, 1995b).

A further consequence of fundholding was that it explicitly promoted GP-led primary care. In April 1993 fundholding was extended to cover community health services. Increasingly, other members of the primary health care team were either directly employed by or contracted to GPs. The main worry here was that effective teamworking could be undermined by the domination of one perspective, to the detriment of patient care. Yet it will be recalled that the operation of the primary health care team has often been the focus of criticism. A more optimistic view was that fundholding created the opportunity for a more coherent form of teamworking, more closely geared to the needs of patients. Certainly the evidence points to an expansion of the range of community health services offered by fundholding practices (Audit Commission, 1996b), but the extent to which this actually satisfied the needs of patients was never fully evaluated.

The promotion of GP-led primary care in the 1990s continued a policy initiated in the previous decade. In the 1980s, GPs had been given incentives to increase the employment of nursing staff in their practices. The number of practice nurses in England and Wales subsequently doubled from 4600 to 9600 in England between 1990 and 1994. There was some criticism of this trend, largely on the grounds that the distribution of these new posts occurred in a haphazard fashion without regard to need (Audit Commission, 1993b).

☐ *Changing patterns of provision*

The focus upon primary care intensified during the 1990s as a result of changing patterns of provision, stimulated partly by the internal market and other reforms. The fundholding scheme allowed GPs to purchase a range of diagnostic tests, giving them greater direct access to hospital-based services (Bish *et al.*, 1996). In some areas GPs were given responsibility for managing non-urgent waiting lists on behalf of consultants. In addition, fundholding encouraged the provision of 'outreach' clinics (Bailey, Black and Wilkin, 1994) where hospital-based specialists hold clinics in GPs' surgeries.

Commissioning authorities also began to show a greater interest in other community-based care, such as 'hospital at home' schemes. Hospital at home can be broadly defined as services which prevent hospital admission or facilitate early discharge (Shepperd and Iliffe, 1996). Examples include kidney dialysis, parenteral feeding (for patients who cannot digest food), and mechanical ventilation (to assist patients with breathing difficulties) as well as post-operative aftercare schemes for patients discharged from hospital. Although there are a wide range of schemes in practice, two main types are distinguished. Those based in the community where care is provided by GPs, district nurses and other members of the primary care team, and those provided on an outreach basis under the supervision of consultants with varying degrees of community health services involvement.

The increase in day surgery, stimulated by new technology and the cost pressures to reduce hospital stays, has further added to the pressure on the primary care sector (Barrow *et al.*, 1994). By 1995 day cases represented over half of all elective surgical cases, double the proportion of the mid-1980s. However, this implies a much larger role for primary care services in the pre-operative assessment of potential day cases, post-operative care

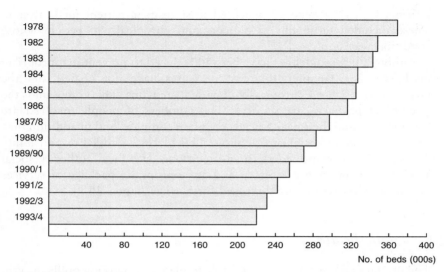

Source: Department of Health.

Figure 9.1 *Hospital beds: average number available daily (all specialties, 1978–94), England*

and support, management of post-operative complications and assessment of the effectiveness of treatment.

Increasing workloads have been generated by the tendency for hospitals to discharge in-patients much earlier than used to be the case. Average lengths of stay fell dramatically in the 1980s and 1990s. For acute patients the average length of stay fell from 9.8 days in 1978 to 7.1 days in 1989 and 4.4 days in 1993. There are a number of reasons for this. First, a belief among professionals that patients recover from illness better at home. Second, the premium on hospital beds arising from the decline in their number (see Figure 9.1) resulting from efforts to rationalise hospital care (see Exhibit 9.1). Third, government policies on community care and NHS continuing care which have promoted the care and treatment of patients outside hospital.

☐ *Community care and continuing care*

For many years government policy has emphasised the treatment of people wherever possible in the community, on the grounds that it is both efficient and humane to do so (see Chapter 10). Initially this policy applied mainly to mentally-ill and handicapped people, and social care for elderly people. In recent years this policy has been extended. The cost pressures on hospitals during the 1980s and 1990s gave them an incentive to discharge patients who they believed benefited least from in-patient medical care. These included terminally-ill patients and chronically-ill people whose condition was stable.

Although new guidelines have been introduced to prevent inappropriate discharges (see Chapter 10), cost pressures have not abated and the incentive to discharge chronically-ill patients remains. This compounds the burden on primary care services. The numbers of people involved are considerable and their health needs are often complex, and in addition they require a range of social care services. This places an added responsibility upon primary care providers to ensure, along with local authority social services, that needs are assessed and an appropriate package of services provided. These issues are discussed further in Chapter 10.

☐ Public health

The primary care sector has a vital role to play in promoting public health. Those involved in primary care, in view of their proximity to the public, have many opportunities to improve the health of the whole population. Their day-to-day contact with patients enables them to detect illnesses at an early stage, either on an informal basis or through systematic screening programmes. They can help to improve health by giving advice about lifestyles. They also generate an enormous amount of information about health needs which can facilitate local health strategies.

Increasingly, the work of primary care professions is shaped by public health considerations. All are expected to operate within the national, regional and local priorities and targets for the reduction of illness. But attempts to encourage the primary care sector to become more pro-active, though highly desirable from a public health point of view, are unlikely to achieve much in isolation. Without extra resources, the focus on public health priorities is likely to become another distraction from the everyday business of dealing with patients. Moreover, as we shall see in Chapter 12, action by primary health workers is largely ineffective in the absence of broader socio-economic policies aimed at promoting health.

■ Toward a primary care-led NHS?

There is no single vision of the future of primary care. This message was underlined by the Institute for Public Policy Research (1995a) which argued for an experimental plurality of commissioning models so that the most effective method might be discovered. It suggested the creation of primary health agencies and local authority-led purchasing as alternatives to GP fundholding.

The themes of diversity and experimentation were found also in the Major government's consultation document (DoH, 1996c) and White Paper on primary care published during the following year (Cm 3390, 1996). Some proposals were potentially radical including: allowing trusts and others (including private companies) to develop primary care services, practice-based contracts (allowing non-medical professionals to hold primary care contracts) and unified budgets for general medical services, prescribing, hospital and community health services. Some of the proposed developments reflected changes that were already taking place in some localities, such as integrated health and social care projects (Coulter and Mays, 1997). The White Paper reaffirmed the commitment to fundholding as the preferred method of change, but at the same time emphasised the importance of proceeding on the basis of properly-evaluated pilot projects.

One of the last pieces of legislation passed by the Major government was the NHS (Primary Care) Act of 1997, which introduced the provisions set out in the White Paper. The Blair government did not seek to repeal this legislation, but instead used it to pilot a number of primary care projects. Moreover, the importance of a primary care-led NHS was further emphasised in its White Paper of 1997 (CM 3807, 1997). This document proposed the abolition of GP fundholding and the creation of Primary Care Groups (PCGs) to commission care for patients (see p. 209). It was also suggested that in the longer term these bodies could take over the running of community health services including community hospitals.

The view that the NHS should become increasingly oriented toward primary care has not gone unchallenged. Consultants have moved to defend their specialist role, arguing that more primary care will not reduce the need for large hospital units (Royal College of Physicians, 1996). Their arguments have coincided with increasing doubts about the cost-effectiveness of new forms of primary care, such as outreach clinics (Leese, 1996), minor surgery (Lowy *et al.*, 1993) and direct access to hospital services (Bish *et al.*, 1996).

Finally, as can be seen in Exhibit 9.1, there are often enormous political difficulties in shifting resources from secondary to primary care, particularly where this involves the rationalisation and closure of hospitals. It appears, then, that a much more gradual, evolutionary mode of reform will prevail. Primary care is no longer the backwater of the NHS. The balance between the two sectors is less unequal and the boundary increasingly flexible, but the pace and extent to which hospital-based care will decline in the years ahead should not be exaggerated.

Exhibit 9.1   Acute hospital reviews in London and other cities

The move towards primary care can be impeded when the implications of shifting resources from hospital-based care become evident. During the 1990s, most cities have undertaken reviews of acute services, and for similar reasons. First, concern about under-resourcing of primary care and the desire of health service planners to shift resources into this sector. Secondly, the internal market in health care, which in principle enabled commissioners to move contracts away from high to low cost services, threatening the viability of some providers. Thirdly, financial pressures which forced providers of acute services to explore mergers as a way of reducing costs. Fourthly, long-standing concerns about the duplication of hospital services within a locality.

Between 1991 and 1995, 304 hospital units closed in the UK, including 60 general acute units. This was advanced as evidence that the hospital sector was in decline. However, in many cities – including London, Liverpool, Birmingham, Bristol, Glasgow, Sheffield, Manchester and Leeds – plans to rationalise hospital services were delayed, scaled down considerably and in some cases, abandoned (Institute of Health Service Management, 1995; Butler 1995a). Local pressure groups and the media successfully promoted a lack of public confidence in reorganisation plans. This happened in London, for example, with the campaigns of hospital support groups supported by the *Evening Standard*. In addition, local political networks were invariably mobilised against such proposals – as in the case of the planned rationalisation of children's hospitals in Manchester, where local MPs and local authority councillors united in opposition. Local medical opinion is also a key factor. In many areas this has inhibited change, but not always. For example in the case of the Leeds acute services review, senior medical opinion was believed to be largely in favour of rationalisation. Local opinion was, however, very much opposed to the plans and they were subsequently shelved.

The technical, financial and even the clinical case for reconfiguration of services can be undermined by political pressure. However, as the London case demonstrates, even when proposals are put forward, there is no guarantee that it will be effectively implemented.

The London case is not typical – the problems of health care in the capital are complex and long standing (Benzeval, Judge and New, 1991; King's Fund, 1992) – yet it does contain some valuable lessons. Following the introduction of the internal market, the Major government realised that a number of London hospitals faced financial collapse. In an effort to avoid such an embarrassing outcome so soon after the launch of the new policy, ministers side-tracked reform by setting up an inquiry into London's health service,

$\longrightarrow$

Exhibit 9.1 continued

→

headed by Sir Bernard Tomlinson. Tomlinson (1992) recommended the expansion of primary care and a planned rationalisation of acute services. Improvements in primary care were widely welcomed, as standards were regarded as relatively poor in the capital.

Tomlinson's recommendations for acute services were, in contrast, very unpopular. They involved the closure of at least ten hospitals and a reduction by 2500 in the number of hospital beds. The concentration of hospital services in London implied that it was relatively generously provided for in terms of acute services. However, this was disputed (Jarman, 1993; Edwards and Raftery, 1995). London has complex health needs as a result of social deprivation, the diverse ethnic composition of its population, and its transient population of visitors and workers.

The government accepted Tomlinson's recommendations on primary care, committing £170m to the development of these services (DoH, 1993c). It also accepted the case for a hospital closure and merger programme which threatened the future of some of London's most famous hospitals including Bart's (St Bartholomew's). To diffuse the campaigns which had been launched to save these hospitals the government delegated implementation to a special group, while specialist services were subjected to a further review.

Some specific campaigns, notably to save Bart's as a free standing institution, proved initially unsuccessful. Others did secure some concessions. Guy's Hospital, for example, obtained a limited reprieve for its casualty unit, while Great Ormond Street Children's Hospital successfully resisted proposals that it should merge with the University College London Hospital (UCLH). The government also manipulated the market to prevent or delay closures – as in 1995 when purchasers were instructed not to move contracts to other cheaper providers in an attempt to bolster the finances of UCLH.

Criticism of the changes continues. Even the King's Fund (1995), which had produced an earlier report calling for the rationalisation of hospital services, was later critical of the pace of change and the failure of primary care services to develop alongside the rationalisation of hospital services. Notably, the Blair government ordered another inquiry into London's health services shortly after taking office in 1997, and further closures were halted for the time being. The new government also signalled its support for other schemes to reshape services. For example, Health Improvement Plans (and in particular areas, Health Action Zones – see Exhibit 13.1) were proposed as a means of securing agreement among all the agencies involved on ways to improve health and health care locally.

■ *Chapter 10* ■

Care in the Community

The heaviest users of health services include the elderly, mentally-ill and handicapped people, physically disabled people, and children. Together, elderly people and children account for 60 per cent of the expenditure on NHS hospital and community health services (HCHS). Just over a tenth of HCHS expenditure is allocated to services for mentally-ill people and a further 5 per cent for people with learning difficulties. In addition, these client groups require a wide range of social care and support, including income maintenance, appropriate accommodation, practical assistance and advice.

Although it has long been recognised that these groups require special attention, the problems involved in developing an adequate network of services for them are equally long-standing. They often have complex health needs and many are vulnerable and dependent. To make matters worse, services have often failed to match these needs. The NHS has traditionally been geared to the provision of acute services. Meanwhile other key services and means of support, such as social services, social security and housing provision, have often been poorly coordinated. Furthermore, the services provided for the elderly, the mentally-ill and the mentally handicapped were labelled the 'Cinderella services' as a reflection of their low status, lack of resources, and, in some respects, poor quality (Means and Smith, 1994). Although this term is used less often today, the relative inferiority of these services persists to a considerable extent, in spite of efforts of successive governments to develop and improve them.

■ Community care policies

Community care is open to a variety of interpretations (Higgins, 1989). Yet most recognise its fundamental principles: an emphasis on care and support in the home, a reliance on caring professions practising outside large institutions, and the mobilisation of the community itself through both individual and collective effort to care for those in need. Government policy on community care is often traced back to a speech in 1961 by the then Health Minister, Enoch Powell, in which he announced plans to close down the large mental hospitals. However, official thinking had been moving in this direction for some years. In 1954, for example, a government report had favoured community care for the elderly (Ministry of Health, 1954). The Guillebaud Committee also set out the case for community care on both humanitarian and economic grounds (Cmd 9663, 1956).

☐ *Arguments for community care*

Throughout the 1960s a broad consensus developed in which care in the community for certain client groups was seen as a more appropriate and effective option than institutional care. The poor standards of care for institutionalised patients became increasingly evident. This was confirmed by a series of cases that emerged during the late 1960s and early 1970s involving the maltreatment of patients in long-stay hospitals (Robb, 1967; Martin, 1984). These were, perhaps unfairly, perceived as being typical of the standard of institutional care and reinforced the notion that community care was a more humane policy.

Community care was also favoured because it seemed to avoid the dependency which patients experienced even in the most benign institutions. By integrating individuals within the community it was believed they could achieve their full potential with a degree of independence. Another argument was that community care made it more difficult for society to ignore the needs of groups such as the mentally-ill, handicapped and disabled people, as they would no longer be hidden away from public view. Finally, community care was believed to be cheaper than institutional care. This argument became more forceful during the 1970s and 1980s as pressure on public sector spending increased.

☐ *Community care in the 1960s and 1970s*

Despite the growing support for community care during the 1960s it remained largely a paper policy. The policy was re-emphasised in the early 1970s with the publication of White Papers on services for the mentally handicapped (Cmnd 4683, 1971) and the mentally ill (Cmnd 6233, 1975). It was accepted by this time that for community care to become a reality, the NHS and local authorities would have to collaborate far more effectively. To this end a system of joint planning was introduced in 1974, involving the creation of Joint Consultative Committees (JCCs) composed of health authority members and local authority councillors. These were later supplemented by Joint Care Planning Teams involving officers drawn from both authorities. In a further development financial incentives were introduced in 1976 in an attempt to promote collaborative projects. Joint finance became available enabling health authorities to make annual grants to local authorities or voluntary organisations wishing to establish community-based schemes.

In addition, the government signalled its intention to shift resources towards community services used by the elderly, the mentally ill, the mentally handicapped, the physically handicapped, and children (DHSS, 1976a). However, these expansionary commitments were later toned down largely as a result of public expenditure constraints and protests from the acute sector (DHSS, 1977).

The squeeze on public spending by both the Labour government of the late 1970s and its Conservative successor inhibited the development of community care services. Health authority budgets maintained the existing pattern of services rather expanding community-based services. The impact of expenditure constraints squeezed cost-effective forms of community care, such as home help services, which were relatively easy to prune.

■ Community care policy from the 1980s

The Thatcher government was particularly attracted to the concept of community care in view of its potential for reducing public expenditure on health and social care (Audit Commission, 1986). The policy fitted in well with the government's philosophy by creating opportunities to shift the burden of care from the state to the individual and stimulating the independent sector. During the early 1980s community care was promoted in a number of policy documents (DHSS, 1981a, 1981c; Cmnd 8173, 1981) New programmes were devised such as the Care in the Community Initiative under which the NHS allocated funds to local authorities and voluntary organisations caring for long-term patients in the community. The joint finance scheme was also revamped and attempts were made to strengthen joint planning. However, in spite of these initiatives it soon became clear that the policy was failing.

□ *The failure of joint planning*

An effort was made to improve joint planning, bringing the Family Practitioner Committees and the voluntary sector into the planning process. Yet it became clear that more was needed to promote effective collaboration. Collaboration often failed because of the contrasting organisational cultures and structures of the NHS and local authorities, which meant that needs were often defined in different ways. For example, the majority of health authorities regarded the elderly mentally ill as part of the psychiatric service, while local authorities saw them primarily as clients of its elderly services (Health Advisory Service, 1987). Related to these different perspectives were professional rivalries between NHS and local government staff (Green, 1986).

The NHS and local authorities had different planning timescales, accountability and management structures (NAO, 1987). In many localities difficulties arose because local authorities and health authorities did not have coterminous boundaries. Some observers, however, were less convinced that the establishment of common organisational structures and boundaries would necessarily improve the situation (Challis, Klein and Webb, 1988).

The poor quality of joint planning persisted into the 1990s (Audit Commission, 1992a). Discussion at Joint Consultative Committees (JCCs) tended to be dominated by marginal issues and specific projects rather than strategic issues. Important areas of concern, including policies for people with disabilities, were not covered sufficiently and in some cases not discussed at all.

The weaknesses of joint planning led to poor coordination of services. A study of elderly people showed that social services and health authorities liaised regularly in only 7 per cent of cases where individuals were receiving care from both agencies (Davies, Bebbington and Charnley 1990). Similar problems of coordination at grassroots level were experienced by other client groups such as the mentally ill, mentally handicapped people, and the physically disabled (Audit Commission, 1989; Beardshaw, 1988; Health Advisory Service, 1987; House of Commons, 1985). The result in many localities was piecemeal, fragmented and incoherent services.

Inadequate levels of collaboration were reflected in the low take-up of joint finance. Local authorities feared the longer-term financial burden implied in the acceptance of such grants which only supported projects for a limited period (Green, 1986). It was later discovered that the funds were mainly used for NHS schemes, rather than promoting an expansion of local authority social services (Wistow, Hardy and Turrell, 1990; NAO, 1987).

Inquiries into the problems of coordination and collaboration urged greater clarification of responsibilities. In 1985 the Social Services Committee called for social care for mentally handicapped people to be financed and administered by local authorities (House of Commons, 1985). The Audit Commission (1986) argued that local authorities should be responsible for mentally and physically handicapped people, with the NHS being responsible for the mentally ill, and the elderly remaining a joint responsibility. These plans did not appeal to the Thatcher government, which chose instead to clarify the existing responsibilities for joint planning and collaborative programmes.

□   *The voluntary and commercial sectors*

Problems of collaboration were complicated further by the expansion in the role of the independent sector. The Thatcher government sought to promote the independent provision of community care by increasing funding to voluntary organisations emphasising their role in policy documents, and urging health authorities to cooperate and consult with them (DHSS, 1981a). The increasing emphasis upon voluntary provision began to arouse strong suspicions that the government was intending to privatise health and social services, or at the very least cut public expenditure by substituting state provision with voluntary activity (see Johnson, 1989; Deakin, 1991). Critics pointed out that the voluntary sector was ill-equipped to take over large areas of service delivery and lacked the capacity to provide a comprehensive set of services. There was concern that voluntary organisations were not directly accountable to Parliament. There were also fears that voluntary organisations were being drawn into a closer relationship with the government, compromising their independence.

Voluntary bodies did not relish the prospect of displacing public sector provision, preferring instead a partnership model. Nonetheless, fears about the substitution of statutory services by the voluntary sector created an unhelpful atmosphere. In addition there was often a mutual lack of understanding about roles and working practices that on occasion impeded effective partnerships between the two sectors. Effective working relationships were further undermined by the sheer size and diversity of the voluntary sector (NAHA and NCVO, 1987).

Another key feature of the government's policy in the 1980s was to promote private long-term care for the elderly, the chronically ill, and people with physical handicaps. Figure 10.1 illustrates the growth of the private residential care sector. When nursing home places are also taken into account, the commercial sector's share grew from 46 per cent (1989) to 64 per cent (1996), and the voluntary sector from 10 to 12 per cent. Over the same period the public-sector supply of long-term institutional care fell from 43 per cent to 23 per cent (Laing, 1996).

The expansion of commercially-provided care was boosted by changes in 1980 which allowed social security claims to cover the costs of residential care. As a result, the amount of social security expenditure on residential care for the elderly rose dramatically, from less than £20m in 1980 to around £700m by the end of the decade. Ironically, the Thatcher government's encouragement of commercial care frustrated at least two other policy objectives: to encourage domiciliary rather than residential care, and to reduce the burden of care on the public finances.

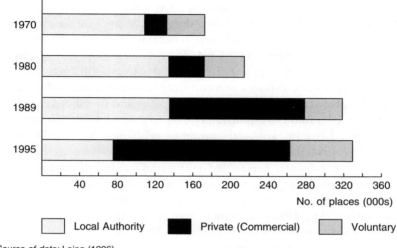

Source of data: Laing (1996).

Figure 10.1   *Places in residential homes, by sector (UK)*

☐ *Service standards*

Worries about standards in private residential care homes during the early 1980s led to new legislation. Under the Registered Homes Act 1984, local authorities were given powers to register and inspect residential care homes in the private sector. Later in 1991, 'arms length' inspection units were created to inspect standards in local authority homes as well as private residential care. However, local authorities were not responsible for standards in nursing homes, which remained a health authority function. Although an increasing number of health and local authorities established joint inspection units, central government resisted calls for the regulation of the two sectors to be integrated in a single body at local level (DHSS, 1988; National Institute for Social Work, 1988). Eventually in 1997 the Major government accepted that health and local authorities should have joint responsibility for regulating all residential and domiciliary services, a move endorsed by the Blair government.

There was also particular concern in the 1980s about the lack of community facilities for mentally-ill and mentally-handicapped people. Most observers agreed with the Social Services Committee that the removal of hospital facilities had outrun the provision of services in the community (House of Commons, 1985, p. xviii). Nearly 100 000 long-stay patients were discharged into the community between the 1950s and 1980s, while only 4000 places were created in local authority hostels (Groves, 1990). As these discharges were not monitored, no one knows what happened to these people, though many became homeless, destitute, or ended up in prison (Weller, 1989; Coid, 1984).

Another issue was the plight of informal carers. Informal care by families, friends and neighbours was encouraged by government during the 1980s, which stressed that the care of the elderly and of other vulnerable groups was a community responsibility and that 'care in the community must increasingly mean care by the community' (Cmnd 8173, 1981, p. 3). For many, this brought heavy responsibilities indeed. There are currently over six million informal carers in Great Britain regularly looking after sick, disabled or elderly persons. A quarter of carers spend at least twenty hours a week caring for someone. The majority – almost 60 per cent – are women (Green, H., 1988), and their unpaid efforts save the taxpayer approximately £34 billion a year (Travers, 1996).

Many carers have needs which are rarely met. Support services are poorly developed and there is a chronic shortage of respite care. According to a survey by the charity Scope, less than a third have access to respite care (Scope, 1995). Of those who care for someone for twenty hours a week or more, only 5 per cent find it relatively easy to arrange for alternative care of two days' duration. A fifth find it difficult or very difficult to arrange such cover, while over two fifths find it impossible to make such arrangements (Adams, 1991).

The burden of caring, often without outside help, damages the health of carers. A third spend 24 hours a day caring, and a further 40 per cent care for between eight and 24 hours (Scope, 1995). Not surprisingly, approximately a tenth of men and a quarter of women who care for the elderly suffer from fatigue. It has been estimated that around 10 per cent of carers have serious health problems of their own (Green, H., 1988; Adams, 1991). Three-quarters admit their health has been affected as a result of caring (Scope, 1995). A survey of the Carers' National Association membership revealed that two-thirds became ill after caring for sick, elderly or disabled friends or relatives (*Guardian*, 1992). The same survey found half had financial problems which added to the level of stress. Only a third of carers have paid employment, and over half of the rest cannot work because of their caring responsibilities (Scope, 1995). Other research has confirmed that of those who look after sick or disabled relatives for over 10 years (a third of carers fall into this category), many are financially disadvantaged (Hancock and Jarvis, 1995). All of which confirms the point made by the Royal College of Nursing (1990) that 'the quality of life for the carer can be more impaired than the person for whom they are caring'.

Although the carer's perspective on community care reform is far from sanguine, there have been some positive changes more recently including the passage of legislation in 1995 in the form of the Carers' Act – which places an obligation upon local authorities to assess the needs of carers. However, no obligation to meet these needs was imposed.

□ Funding

Much controversy has surrounded the resourcing of community care. One of the main arguments in favour of community care was its potential to generate savings by replacing 'high cost' institutional care with 'low cost' community services. During the 1980s this became increasingly contested. A 1981 study found that community care was not always a cheaper or more effective option and that in some cases low-cost care in the community was inadequate (DHSS, 1981d). Others, too, thought it unsafe to assume that community care was a cheaper option. The Social Services Committee (House of Commons, 1985) directly questioned the principle of cost neutrality – that the shift towards community care could be achieved without adding to public expenditure. It argued that a community care policy based on a cost-neutral assumption was not merely naive, but positively inhumane.

At the same time it was accepted that the budget for long-term care was spent inefficiently. According to the Audit Commission (1986), £500m was spent on care funded through the social security system, most financing residential care. Two-thirds of the government budget for the care of the elderly, the mentally ill, and people with mental and physical handicaps was spent on residential care. The Audit Commission believed that many more could be cared for in their own homes at lower cost.

There was, and still is, some uncertainty about the extent to which individuals can be moved into the community. The Public Accounts Committee (House of Commons, 1988b) suggested that 77 per cent of those in institutions could be cared for in the community if appropriate domiciliary services were available. However, others doubted that large numbers of people were being inappropriately admitted (Henwood, 1992). In one study, Bradshaw and Gibbs (1988) found only 7 per cent of a sample of elderly people had been inappropriately admitted to residential care. However, they did concede that a further 10 per cent of residents would not have required admission had there been adequate support services in the community. Meanwhile, more recently, research into nursing-home care has suggested a high level of inappropriate admissions. An audit by the Department of Geriatric Medicine, St George's Hospital Medical School found only 11 per cent of nursing home residents were 'definitely appropriate' for such care, with a further 54 per cent classed as 'possibly appropriate' (Bennet, Smith and Millard, 1995).

■ Griffiths' community care reforms

□ *The report*

By 1986, the Thatcher government had become convinced of the need to reform community care. Mrs Thatcher's policy advisor, Sir Roy Griffiths, was invited to examine the issue. His report set out three guiding principles (DHSS, 1988): that the right services should be provided early enough, to the people who need them most; that individuals should have more choice and a greater say over services; that people should be cared for wherever possible in their own homes, or in as near a domestic environment as possible.

Griffiths sought to give clear responsibilities for services at all levels. At the top, a minister responsible for community care. Local authority social service departments would identify needs, set priorities, and develop plans for community care. At the individual level, case managers would coordinate the assessment of needs and arrange appropriate packages of care. Griffiths believed that the perverse incentives in favour of residential care should be removed by reducing social security payments for those in residential homes to a basic level. The balance (the care element) would then be paid by local authorities on behalf of those requiring residential care. For those who did not need this, the care element could be used to purchase an alternative package of community services from local authorities, the NHS and the private sector.

Griffiths envisaged that central government would provide a substantial chunk of the resources for community care. However, such resources would be allocated on the basis of approved local authority community care plans, drawn up in consultation with other interested parties, such as health authorities, voluntary organisations and the commercial sector. Griffiths also recommended that central funds allocated to community care should be ring-fenced, so that they could not be put to other uses.

□ *The implementation of the Griffiths reforms*

Griffiths' recommendations came as something of shock to the government. Throughout the 1980s, the Thatcher government had been hostile towards local government and was particularly suspicious of its spending ambitions. The Prime Minister and her senior colleagues were therefore extremely unhappy at the recommendation to grant local authorities a key role in the new regime. After some delay the government's response was eventually published as a White Paper, *Caring for People* (Cm 849, 1989). This upheld Griffiths' central idea that the lead responsibility for community care should be given to local authorities, while backing the widely supported principle of individual case management. However, it did not create a minister for community care as Griffiths recommended. The government also refused to grant specific 'ring-fenced' community care funds for all client groups. Only services for the mentally-ill were intended to receive earmarked grants channelled through health authorities. However, three years later the Major government imposed wider restrictions on the use of funds for community care.

The White Paper stressed privatisation far more heavily than Griffiths. Although the Griffiths report encouraged private provision where this was more economic and efficient than direct provision by the public sector, it did not openly advocate the widespread replacement of statutory services. Subsequently the Thatcher and Major governments made it clear that maximum use should be made of commercial and voluntary providers. At the same time it was decided that council-run homes would not receive the residential allowance – a housing cost element for each resident. This placed them at a disadvantage compared with commercial and voluntary homes, and provided an incentive for councils to privatise their homes and place residents in the private sector.

The importance of the private sector was further underlined during the implementation of the reforms. The Department of Health required local authorities to allocate 85 per cent of any new money received from central government towards services provided by the private sector. This '85 per cent rule' was designed to protect the private residential sector from the loss of 'new business' and to promote the gradual expansion of private community-based services. In practice only 70 per cent of the new money was actually earmarked because of the failure to uprate earlier allocations in line with inflation (see Laing, 1996, p. 184).

In spite of criticism about the pace of change (House of Commons, 1990b–f) the government pressed ahead with the necessary legislation, in the form of the NHS and Community Care Act of 1990. However, the implementation of most of the community care provisions was subsequently postponed until April 1993 (Cm 1343, 1990). The government had miscalculated the impact of the reforms on local tax levels. Had the community care reforms been implemented as planned, around £15 would have been added to each community charge bill in 1991/2. Given the proximity to the forthcoming general election, political expediency dictated that the reforms must be delayed.

■ The impact of the Griffiths reforms

It is not surprising that little in the way of positive change was perceived in the period immediately following the reforms. A survey of GPs in 1995 found that three-quarters perceived no improvement in community care under the new regime, though over half believed that services had actually deteriorated (BMA, 1995a). Another survey that same year revealed that three out of four carers did not perceive any differences since the introduction of the reforms (Carers' National Association, 1995).

Community care reform, though a national policy, was implemented at different speeds and with varying degrees of success in different localities (see NHSE/SSI, 1995; Audit Commission, 1996c; Social Services Inspectorate, 1996; Wistow *et al.*, 1994). Some social service departments decided not to create a purchaser–provider division in social care (Leadbeater, 1996). Many were reluctant to devolve budgets (Audit Commission, 1996c), while the development of care plans for individuals did not occur to the extent originally envisaged by Griffiths (Hawley and Hudson, 1996; Social Services Inspectorate, 1996). It is therefore difficult to generalise about the specific impact of the community care reforms. Nevertheless, one can draw a number of tentative conclusions.

☐ *Resources, rationing and privatisation*

Under the new regime, central government re-allocated resources for community care from the social security budget to local authorities on the basis of a special transitional grant (STG) phased in over a four-year period, beginning in the 1993/4 financial year. The transfers totalled over £2 billion, yet local authorities maintained that resources were insufficient to meet the demand for community care. Although this was interpreted by some as special pleading, these claims attracted support from some independent analysts (Laing, 1996, p. 182; Audit Commission 1994c, 1996c).

A genuine lack of resources was further suggested by an increase in both rationing and charging for social services. Local authorities, like health authorities, began to take a much greater interest in priority-setting and rationing (Audit Commission, 1996c). This involved ranking groups of people on the basis of need (as indicated by risk and dependency). Each authority tended to develop its own unique system of assessing priorities, defining eligibility and allocating resources. Moreover, the public was largely ignorant of the criteria involved.

Rationing by price also increased (National Consumer Council, 1995). Although local authorities had always been able to charge for services, the scope for charging expanded as a direct result of the financial pressures on local authorities following the community care reforms (Baldwin and

Lunt, 1996). New and higher charges discouraged the take-up of services and affected low-income groups and those with high levels of disability (Scope, 1995; Baldwin and Lunt, 1996) in spite of the fact that local authorities increasingly used means tests as a basis for such charges.

The community care legislation placed an onus on local authorities to assess need. However, there was no obligation to provide or commission services which met the assessed level of need (Ellis, 1993). Both central government and the local authorities argued that the availability of care must reflect resources. But the legal position remained unclear and was tested in the courts. In June 1996, in a landmark judgement, the Appeal Court ruled that councils could not withdraw services for elderly and disabled people on the basis of resource shortages without first undertaking a reassessment of needs. This was subsequently overturned by the Law Lords in March 1997.

The community care reforms were intended as a means of expanding the role of the independent sector, and the majority of residential and nursing homes are now run by commercial and voluntary organisations. The independent sector also has a growing role in the provision of domiciliary services. In England in 1992, only 2 per cent of home-care contact hours funded by local authorities was provided by independent contractors. By 1995 this had risen to 29 per cent (Laing, 1996, p. 172).

However, these trends do not tell the whole story. The growth in the independent residential care sector was partly stimulated by the transfer of local authority homes to voluntary bodies. Meanwhile, parts of the independent care sector faced severe problems. Residential care homes endured a financial squeeze following the reforms. Local authorities drove a harder bargain when placing residents in care, making it more difficult for homes to raise prices as much as they wished. In addition, a fall in the numbers entering residential care post-reform (Laing, 1995) affected costs as well as revenues. As less dependent people were diverted away from residential care, homes found themselves dealing with a higher proportion of people with complex needs, who were more costly to care for (Fitzhugh, 1995).

Another problem which particularly affected the independent domiciliary providers was the preference of local authorities for 'spot contracts' (where services are negotiated and paid for when required). This made it difficult for the independent sector to plan long term and develop new services (Audit Commission, 1996c; Lewis *et al.*, 1996). Finally, independent providers, whether in the residential or domiciliary sector, articulated a range of grievances about the new system, including the failure of local authorities to consult them about service developments (Scottish Council for Independent Care, 1995).

☐ *Service standards and efficiency*

The publication of *Caring for People* implied greater central monitoring of community care. Under the new regime, funding is linked to the monitoring of local authority community care plans by the Department of Health. The Social Services Inspectorate (SSI), located within the department, plays an important role here through its programme of national monitoring, which includes detailed studies of progress in particular authorities and in-depth thematic studies into aspects of community care (for example, services for carers, mentally-ill people and so on).

Other bodies are also involved. The Audit Commission has a key role in relation to the comparative performance of community care services. Meanwhile, the NHSE is responsible for monitoring health authority performance in relation to primary care, long-term care and community care. In the light of criticisms of regulatory overload and a lack of coordination between the various inspecting and monitoring agencies (Day and Klein 1990), efforts have been made to achieve closer working links. For example, the Audit Commission and the SSI now undertake joint inspections, and the SSI and the NHSE have developed a joint approach to monitoring community care (Henwood and Wistow, 1995)

There has been little agreement on the impact of central monitoring. Salter and Salter (1993) claimed that central government exerted little influence over local implementation and that the new regime merely gave an illusion of greater central control. However, Davies (1994) took a different view, arguing that there was greater central direction in recent years and that the combination of the Audit Commission and the Department of Health (through the SSI and NHSE) held a powerful influence over community care at a local level. Henwood and Wistow (1995) similarly emphasised the positive aspects of central monitoring, identifying it as a valuable means of checking local progress. But they observed that the system was far from perfect, being geared to processes rather than outcomes, and that it should involve users and carers to a greater extent (see also Davies, 1994; Henwood, 1995; and Henwood *et al.*, 1996). Meanwhile, some studies found that central regulation had prompted positive changes in patterns of service (Lewis *et al.*, 1996).

Central monitoring has generated information about standards and the efficiency of community care provision. However, critics were right in suggesting that the primary focus of performance monitoring has been upon process rather than outcome-based measures. This has made it difficult to assess the impact of the changes upon those who receive services. An added problem, according to some, has been the deliberate repression of criticism by the dominant management culture (Hadley and Clough, 1996).

Evidence post-reform regarding the quality of service experienced by users and carers suggested a considerable variation in standards (Henwood, 1995). Some local authorities offered more choice and were more responsive to users and carers than others (Social Services Inspectorate, 1996; Lewis *et al.*, 1996). Although service providers appeared more responsive than in the past, their interests were still perceived as dominant (Henwood, 1995). There was also a tendency to fit existing services to needs, rather than rearrange services to meet assessed need (Hawley and Hudson, 1996).

The new regime, by introducing greater central direction and monitoring, sought to standardise procedures and promote 'good practice'. However, central government refused to set national standards of service in the field of community care. National guidance was issued, but only to providers of NHS services that impinged on community care, such as continuing care and mental health services (see Exhibits 10.1 and 10.2). Central government pressured local authorities to establish local community care charters, while rejecting calls (supported by a wide range of organisations including MIND, the BMA, the Health Committee, and Help the Aged) for national standards relating to community care services, eligibility criteria, and charges for social services.

Furthermore, there has been some variation in the efficiency of different local authorities with regard to community care (Audit Commission, 1996c). Beyond this lie broader concerns about the impact of competition and the commissioner–provider split on the efficiency of social care provision. Although competition appeared to produce some productivity gains, at least initially, there was a growing perception that high transaction costs and increased spending on management and administration was undermining the efficiency of services (Wistow *et al.*, 1994; Lewis *et al.*, 1996; Hawley and Hudson, 1996).

☐ Collaboration and coordination

Effective community care has often been undermined in the past by poor coordination between health authorities and local authorities. These problems persisted to some extent following the 1993 reforms. Reorganisations both in the NHS and in local government during the 1990s added to the difficulties of collaboration.

First, the new regime created an added incentive for the agencies involved to shift costs on to each other (Salter, 1994). This was particularly

---

Exhibit 10.1 *The continuing care debate*

The funding and provision of long-term care reached the top of the political agenda in 1994 with revelations about discharging chronically-ill individuals from hospital. In one case the health service ombudsman ruled the NHS had a duty to provide care for a severely brain-damaged stroke victim who had been discharged to nursing home care (Health Service Commissioner, 1994. See also Health Service Commissioner 1996c, 1996d).

The controversy centred upon the movement of patients from NHS 'continuing care' – which is free of charge – to means-tested care purchased by local authorities. Other issues included inconsistency of discharge arrangements, lack of clarity about eligibility for NHS care, variations in the availability of NHS continuing care in different localities, and the wide discretion exercised by social service departments with regard to imposing charges for social care.

The Major government was particularly concerned about the impact on middle-class voters who stood to lose inheritances if elderly relatives sold assets to pay for care. But when in 1994 the Department of Health attempted to clarify NHS responsibilities, its draft guidance received a hostile reception (NHSE, 1994b). This was largely because it appeared to override existing guidance, which stated that patients should not to be discharged to a residential or nursing home against their wishes or where this would result in a financial penalty being imposed on them. Others attacked the guidance for its emphasis on local policies, believing this to be an abdication of central government's responsibility to set national standards.

When the final version of the new guidelines appeared, a number of concessions were evident (DoH, 1995f). Although refusing to set national standards for continuing care, central government did set out local responsibilities in greater detail. In addition, health authorities were required to establish a system for reviewing decisions regarding eligibility for NHS

$\longrightarrow$

---

evident in home care, where disputes about which agency should fund or provide care became ever more protracted (Social Services Inspectorate 1996; Henwood, 1995). The early discharge of people from hospital increased the financial burden upon social services departments, as well as NHS primary care services, exacerbating disputes over costs.

Secondly, the internal market in health care had some unforeseen effects on collaboration. The extension of fundholding to community health services in some localities undermined collaboration by introducing new priorities at odds with those of the NHS community trusts and social service departments (Henwood, 1995).

Third, the reorganisation process both in health and social care sapped efforts to improve collaboration (Charlesworth, Clarke and Cochrane, 1996; Wistow *et al.*, 1994). This was viewed mainly as a short-term problem. Indeed, some believed that the dislocation of old, flawed patterns

> ### Exhibit 10.1 continued

→

care. Furthermore, health authorities that had withdrawn from providing continuing care were required to reinvest in this area.

The Major government sought to stimulate individuals to invest in long-term care insurance plans. From April 1996 all pre-funded benefits paid under such schemes became tax free. A Green Paper was also introduced in 1996 aimed at encouraging care plans by offering people protection for their assets if they took out private insurance (Cm 3242, 1996; see also Institute for Public Policy Research, 1996). This was taken forward by a further White Paper in 1997, though Labour's victory at the 1997 General Election put an end to this initiative for the time being.

In 1996 the threshold at which individuals were expected to make a contribution to the cost of residential and nursing home care was raised. Previously individuals could be charged in full if they had capital over £8000. Individuals with less than this amount but with over £3000 in capital paid charges on a sliding scale. These thresholds were raised to £16 000 and £10 000 respectively. A court ruling in March 1997 allowed councils discretion to charge individuals with savings below this lower threshold in situations where their original savings had been above £16 000, though this was later overturned on appeal.

The Health Committee, among others, called for national criteria on eligibility for continuing care (House of Commons, 1995d). It concluded that guidance to health authorities remained unclear and inadequate. In a later report (House of Commons, 1996a), it endorsed a proposal (originally made by the Royal College of Nursing) that the costs of nursing care in nursing homes should be met by the NHS. Meanwhile, others called for a compulsory insurance scheme for long-term care (Joseph Rowntree Foundation, 1996; see also Institute for Public Policy Research, 1996). These and other proposals were subsequently considered by a Royal Commission on Long Term Care established in 1997 by the Blair government.

of collaboration was no bad thing. However, the organisational turbulence in health and social care persisted over a number of years, causing further disruption (Charlesworth *et al.*, 1996).

Post-Griffiths, efforts to promote joint working were renewed. Under the new regime, health and local authorities were expected to reach agreements on hospital discharge arrangements and continuing care packages. For local authorities this became a precondition for receiving the STG funding. Meanwhile, as shown in Exhibit 10.1, new national guidelines on continuing care were developed to limit inappropriate discharges. However, implementation remained a problem. Monitoring exercises undertaken following the reforms indicated that success in joint working at the individual case level was patchy and depended greatly on the commitment of managers and the staff involved (Social Services Inspectorate, 1996). Moreover, the dreadful consequences of poor

---

Exhibit 10.2   *Policy initiatives for mental illness*

During the 1990s a number of important policy developments occurred with regard to community care for mentally-ill people. This was prompted by public concern arising from a series of high-profile cases of suicide and homicide committed by individuals suffering from mental illness. It was also reinforced by pressure from mental health charities, professional bodies and individuals directly affected by such incidents, highlighting the inadequacy of services for the mentally ill (Mental Health Foundation, 1994; Royal College of Psychiatrists, 1994). Furthermore, a series of official inquiries and investigations exposed the shortcomings of care in the community for mentally-ill people (Audit Commission, 1994d; House of Commons, 1994; North West London Mental Health Trust, 1994; Ritchie, Dick and Lingham, 1994; Blom-Cooper, 1994) and underlined the link between inadequate care, homicide and suicide (Royal College of Psychiatrists, 1995).

In addition to the community care reforms discussed in this chapter, the Major government responded with a 'ten point plan' in August 1993. The highlights were:

1. Fresh guidance from the Department of Health on the discharge of mentally-ill people into the community.
2. Supervised discharge arrangements, allowing those responsible for the care of mentally-ill people to take and convey patients to a hospital for treatment against their will. These measures became law in 1995.
3. Supervision registers. Introduced in 1994, this measure required hospitals and community health units to set up registers of seriously mentally-ill people discharged into the community.
4. Other measures included: guidance to health authorities to ensure that adequate levels of mental health services were included in their plans, clarification of the Mental Health Act Code of Practice, better training, and new programmes monitoring standards of mental health services.

In 1994, the government stated that mental hospitals would only close when community services were available (Waterhouse, 1994a). Following an

$\longrightarrow$

---

collaboration for the individual were graphically highlighted by the media (BBC, 1994).

One of the more positive aspects of the new regime was the move towards joint commissioning between health and social services. Ideally this involves health and social services entering into joint working arrangements to ensure a shared sense of purpose over what services should be available and who should receive them. As a result, contracts and resources should reflect the pattern of needs identified (Hudson, 1995; Poxton, 1994).

Joint commissioning covers a variety of arrangements. An early example was the Easington Joint Commissioning Board (JCB) in County Durham,

---

Exhibit 10.2 continued

→

earlier announcement, a Mental Health Services Charter (which relates to NHS services, not those provided by local authorities) was finally published in January 1997 (DoH, 1997a).

These initiatives did not dispel public concern, particularly about the lack of resources. Despite increases in central grants to local authorities and efforts to persuade health authorities to plan for mental health needs, it was shown that funds were still tied up in hospital care with community services being relatively under-resourced (Audit Commission, 1994d; House of Commons, 1993d, 1994). In addition, concern was expressed by those caring for mentally-ill people about the unworkability of the new measures, namely supervised discharge arrangements and supervision registers (Eastman, 1995; Harrison and Bartlett, 1994). There has also been further evidence of poor quality care (Mental Health Act Commission, 1995) and a failure to learn from previous service failures of the past (Royal College of Psychiatrists, 1995).

Policy implementation has been poor as indicated by two official reports in 1995 (Social Services Inspectorate, 1995; Clinical Standards Advisory Group 1995). They revealed a failure to implement the Care Programme Approach – under which the mentally-ill have a personal care package and liaise with a named 'key worker'. Continuing problems of joint working between health and local authorities in relation to services for mentally-ill people were also identified.

Fresh guidance on joint working was issued in 1995 (DoH, 1995g). Central government later detailed the range of services that it believed should be available for the mentally ill – including the provision of smaller residential facilities (DoH, 1996d). Subsequently, in the final months of the Major government a Green Paper on mental health was issued (Cm 3555, 1997) which set out a number of options for structural change. This including the possibility of a new mental health and social care authority at local level to commission health and social care services for severely mentally-ill adults of working age. These and other options were subsequently reviewed by the incoming Labour government.

---

which included representatives from the health authority, local authorities and local GPs. The JCB worked with local planning groups (LPGs) covering smaller geographical areas which identified needs, feeding this back into the commissioning process. Initially such schemes operated mainly as planning bodies. They increasingly began to involve the transfer of resources, in some cases between health and local authority budgets, on the basis of agreed initiatives. Innovative schemes have been developed involving the transfer of funds from health authorities to social services departments to pay for community care and residential care. Alternatively, in other cases, local authorities have commissioned health authorities to provide social care.

A number of problems have impeded the development of joint commissioning arrangements in addition to the traditional problems of joint working discussed earlier (Hudson, 1995; Nocon, 1994). For example, there are legal difficulties involved in pooling budgets and establishing joint organisations between local authorities and NHS bodies. Aside from such specific difficulties, it appears that joint commissioning in its present form is not a simple solution to the problems of inter-agency collaboration. At best these initiatives build on good relationships in particular localities. At worst, they are largely a continuation of unsuccessful modes of joint working under a new name (Hawley and Hudson, 1996).

■ Conclusion

Griffiths observed that community care was a poor relation, 'everybody's distant relative but nobody's baby' (DHSS, 1988). Ten years on, community care issues have a much higher profile, particularly with regard to long-term care and the care of mentally-ill people. This rise to prominence may well have occurred for the wrong reasons; the Thatcher and Major governments were mainly concerned to shift the burden of care from the state to individuals and reduce public expenditure (Langan, 1990). Nevertheless, these actions had some positive effect by encouraging debate and focusing public concern on a number of key issues that had been neglected for too long. For example, access to and availability of community care, funding and the mechanisms for allocating resources, and the need to improve the quality of services.

Hence the Conservatives' reforms of community care have been portrayed as an opportunity for improvement and expansion of services (Levick, 1992). Joint commissioning is seen by some as a way of breaking down the barriers between health and social services; the commissioner–provider split as a means of improving the quality and responsiveness of services. Meanwhile, needs assessment, while not guaranteeing access to services, has been applauded for making explicit the gap between needs and resources and encouraging debate about how such deficits should be met. Yet, as has been noted, some of the optimism about these developments may be exaggerated. Considerable problems remain, particularly with regard to collaboration, variations in standards of service, and inconsistencies in policies regarding access and charges.

The Griffiths' community care reforms have been largely accepted and there is no real prospect of them being reversed. The Blair government established a Royal Commission on long-term care, while plans to extend private insurance for social care, initiated by the Major government, were shelved for the moment. Meanwhile, the search continues for ways of improving collaboration between health and social services. For example, in 1997 local authorities were invited to nominate potential candidates for appointment to NHS authorities and boards. The government has also proposed that local authority chief executives should participate in health authority meetings. Cooperation may be strengthened further by the proposed statutory duty of partnership to be imposed on NHS bodies and local authorities, and by the development of health action zones in particular areas (see Exhibit 13.1). Finally, health and local authorities have been asked to produce joint investment plans for continuing and community care services, and there is a possibility that in future budgets for health and social services may become more fully integrated.

■ Chapter 11 ■

Health Care Users

Over the last two decades, the belief that health services should be more responsive to the needs and requirements of users has grown (Kennedy, 1981; Williamson, 1992). In addition, the value of lay perspectives in judging the standard of services is increasingly recognised. Those responsible for health services are under greater pressure to listen more carefully to the individual patient and to encourage wider participation in health care decision-making.

This chapter examines how the NHS has responded to these pressures. It begins with an examination of earlier efforts to represent and safeguard patients' interests and how these traditional mechanisms have altered in recent years. This is followed by an analysis of *The Patient's Charter* reforms, introduced by the Major government during the 1990s. Finally, the chapter explores a range of mechanisms adopted by the NHS to involve users and the wider community in health care decisions.

■ Watchdogs and complaints procedures

During the early 1970s attempts were made to improve patient accountability and representation within the NHS. These arose out of public concern that patients' interests were being disregarded, exemplified by several scandals in long-stay hospitals (see Chapter 10). On top of this there was a general feeling that a 'democratic deficit' existed in the NHS and that the interests of patients and the general public should be represented more effectively within the decision-making process. New measures included the creation in 1974 of Community Health Councils (CHCs). In the previous year a Health Service Commissioner (also known as the health ombudsman) was appointed to investigate public complaints about maladministration. Complaints procedures were also reviewed in this period.

□ Community Health Councils (CHCs)

The creation of CHCs in effect institutionalised the voice of the community within the NHS (Klein and Lewis, 1976). As well as representing the views of the public, CHCs began to undertake a range of other tasks, such as monitoring local services, informing the public and assisting patients with complaints. Their role remains much the same today. Apart from changes to management and funding arrangements they have emerged largely unscathed from successive NHS reorganisations.

However, CHCs have not been immune from the wider changes taking place within the NHS. Indeed a question mark hung over the future of CHCs following the introduction of the internal market. They survived largely because government needed to reassure the public and saw an opportunity for CHCs to play a greater role in monitoring services and in identifying local needs. However, efforts to incorporate them within the commissioning side of the internal market raised questions about their independence and their effectiveness in articulating public preferences. Meanwhile, CHCs feared that an emphasis on commissioning would distance them from the main focus of their work, the provider units.

Concern about the independence of CHCs was not new (Hogg, 1986), but CHCs themselves believed that the public increasingly saw them as part of the NHS establishment, rather than as an independent voice In addition, the early 1990s brought explicit challenges to their independence as some regional health authorities threatened to cut CHC budgets following campaigns against hospital closures (Hunter, 1995). The replacement of RHAs by NHSE regional offices raised further fears. A compromise was eventually reached on new funding arrangements, with CHCs now financed out of a central budget.

Meanwhile, criticism of the effectiveness of CHCs continued. Ironically this was partly due to a growing interest in other methods of gauging the patient's perspective, such as opinion surveys, focus groups and citizen's juries, discussed in detail later. This raised the prospect that CHCs might be bypassed or replaced by the use of such techniques. Yet CHCs were reluctant to alter their role. They were particularly wary of being involved in priority-setting and rationing, believing that such procedures lacked public legitimacy. Some CHCs were also reluctant to get involved in quality assurance projects, even where commissioners and providers requested their help. This was largely because they felt their independence was compromised by participation in schemes outside their direct control (Moon and Lupton, 1995).

CHCs were right to be concerned about threats to their independence. It is perhaps their most valuable asset and without it their credibility is much reduced. As far as their effectiveness is concerned, CHCs are perhaps more vulnerable to criticism, though it should be recognised that their effectiveness is strongly influenced to matters outside their control. They are undoubtedly under-resourced relative to their workload, which in recent years has increased dramatically (Moon and Lupton, 1995). Their effectiveness is further constrained by their limited powers. CHCs' efforts to work with GPs and local authorities have often been impeded by the fact that they do not have a clear statutory role in relation to these agencies.

CHCs have also experienced problems with regard to NHS hospital and community health services, where their statutory role is more clearly defined. As Moon and Lupton (1995) have shown, these problems are particularly evident in the acute sector where trusts tended to exclude CHCs from all but the annual statutory meetings. In contrast, they found much more openness in community trusts which saw the CHCs as allies in their battle for resources. However, new regulations introduced by the Department of Health in 1997 may change this. Under this new regime, all trusts are required to liaise more closely with CHCs, and more trust meetings will be held in public, increasing the opportunities for CHCs to participate.

The future of CHCs is open to debate. Notably, a Department of Health-commissioned study in 1996 called for a radical reappraisal of their role (Insight Management Consulting, 1996). One recommendation was that CHCs should move away from monitoring health services and providing information to the public, and should instead carry out specific evaluation projects on behalf of health authorities. In addition, the report proposed that CHCs should advise patients on how to complain rather than assist directly. The report was not explicitly endorsed by the Major government and was rejected by its Labour successor. Even so, its essential message, that the role of CHCs should be clarified, has attracted some support.

☐ *The Health Service Commissioner*

The role of the health service commissioner (or ombudsman) has expanded since the creation of the office in 1973 (Giddings, 1993). The commissioner can investigate complaints from members of the public about NHS services. He may also respond to complaints from the public about the withholding of information by health authorities and trusts. He cannot, however, examine cases that are before a tribunal or which are the subject of legal action in the courts.

The health ombudsman represents the third stage of the new integrated complaints procedure established in 1996, which is discussed in more detail below. Prior to this, he could only investigate complaints of a non-clinical nature and was prevented from examining complaints against GPs. The ombudsman is also permitted to look at the failure of the NHS to provide services. In one notable case the ombudsman criticised a health authority for discharging a chronically sick patient into a nursing home (see Exhibit 10.1).

The ombudsman can recommend compensation and redress. He cannot force a health authority or hospital to take action, but may revisit cases where the response has been inadequate. His main weapon is publicity. Extracts of investigations are published in twice-yearly volumes. These are well-publicised in the media and are circulated to health service managers by the NHSE. The ombudsman's reports are scrutinised by a select committee of MPs which may give added publicity to particular cases and can recommend changes in the ombudsman's powers. The committee can be effective in promoting a more positive response from health authorities which do not act on the ombudsman's initial report. It has the power to summon and cross-examine senior managers – which for those concerned can be an unpleasant experience.

Generally, the health ombudsman has been regarded as a success (Klein, 1977; Giddings, 1993), the only criticisms being his restricted brief and lack of powers to compel those guilty of maladministration and service failure to correct the situation. However, the brief of the health ombudsman was extended by the new complaints procedure introduced in 1996. It is to this development we now turn.

☐ *Complaints procedures*

The number of complaints about NHS services rose sharply during the 1980s, and by the early 1990s there were over 50 000 complaints a year. These statistics, though reflecting perhaps an increased willingness to complain and a greater awareness of complaints procedures, nevertheless indicated considerable dissatisfaction. The Major government was particularly concerned about the rising level of complaints which gave political opponents plenty of ammunition. It was keen to devise a new scheme whereby more complaints could be resolved informally at a local level. At the same time there was a growing belief within the NHS that complaints could be used more positively as a means of improving services. Rather than simply a way of registering discontent, a complaint could be fed back into the process of service delivery possibly and prevent a re-occurrence.

The main professional bodies were also concerned about complaints procedures and in particular the adversarial nature of investigations (see Allsop and Mulcahy, 1996). Meanwhile, consumer and patients' groups had long campaigned for a simpler and user-friendly system with a strong independent element (National Consumer Council, 1992; Association of Community Health Councils, 1993b).

There was widespread consensus that reform was necessary. However, as previous attempts revealed, little could be achieved without the consent of the professions, in particular the doctors. Earlier efforts to extend the brief of the health ombudsman to clinical complaints had failed. Similarly, proposals to introduce an element of independent investigation into the complaints process – as recommended by the Davies committee in 1973 – were considered too controversial (DHSS and Welsh Office, 1973). As a result, only limited changes to complaints procedures were introduced, including a new system for clinical complaints in hospitals (1981), and the creation of designated complaints officers in health authorities (1985).

Failure to undertake comprehensive reform meant that those wishing to complain were faced with a 'patchwork quilt' of procedures which included the disciplinary procedures of the GMC, the health ombudsman, and the complaints systems run by hospitals and family health services. Furthermore, to add to the confusion there was a distinction between systems handling clinical judgement and those established for non-clinical complaints.

In 1993 the Wilson Committee was appointed to examine complaints procedures (DoH, 1994f). Its recommendations, accepted almost in their entirety by the Major government, created an integrated three-stage system for all types of complaint about family health services, hospital and community health services. In addition, new complaints procedures were applied to externally-provided services, including those supplied by private hospitals on behalf of the NHS. The new system was introduced in April 1996 and is described below (DoH, 1996e).

Stage one of the procedure is *local resolution*. An attempt must be made to resolve the complaint at the level where it occurred, and in a way which is fair, flexible and conciliatory. In the case of family health services the practice is responsible for establishing a resolution procedure. In health authorities and trusts, minor complaints may be resolved by front-line staff. Matters of a more serious nature are referred to a designated complaints manager or to the chief executive. It is a requirement that a written complaint must elicit a written response from the chief executive concerned, though as the health ombudsman's reports have indicated this requirement is not always observed. A further point is that if the complainant suggests legal action is forthcoming, no further action can be taken with regard to the complaint.

Complainants dissatisfied with the efforts of the health authority, trust or family practice to resolve the issue locally may request an *independent review* of their case – the second stage of the complaints procedure. This request is dealt with by a non-executive member of the health authority or trust who has been nominated as the convenor. The convenor must then consult with an independent lay person (drawn from a list of suitable persons held by the regional office). Together they must decide if local resolution procedures have been fully exhausted and, if so, whether an independent review panel could play a useful role in resolving the complaint. The complainant does not have an automatic right to independent review. The convenor may at this point send the complaint back for local resolution.

If it is decided that an independent review is necessary, the independent lay person consulted by the convenor is usually nominated as the chairman of the review panel. Other members include the convenor and a third member (for trust panels this will be a GP fundholder or a health authority non-executive director; for health authority panels it will be another lay person drawn from the regional list). Where the complaint involves clinical judgement, appropriate advice must be sought from an appropriately qualified assessor. At the independent review stage this person will be drawn from outside the area and nominated by the regional office. At earlier stages clinical advice may be taken from someone within the health authority or trust concerned, but this person must not be connected with the complaint in any way.

The panel may conduct its inquiry as it sees fit, with the independent chairperson having the final say on procedure. It must, however, operate on a confidential basis and all parties involved must have the opportunity to express their view. A further proviso is that assessors must be present when clinical issues are being discussed. The panel produces a final report setting out its conclusions and recommendations, a copy of which is received by the complainant and the chief executive. The latter must then write to the complainant stating any action, if any, that will be taken.

In the case of a health authority or trust complaint, the panel must report within 12 weeks. No more than 120 working days must elapse between the request for independent review and the response to the report by the health authority or trust concerned. These time limits are even shorter for family health services complaints (the report must be completed in only 8 weeks). Local resolution for health authority and trust complaints must take place within four weeks (10 working days for practice-based complaints). There are time limits for complainants, too. The complaint must be made within six months of the event (or within six months of becoming aware of a cause for complaint, providing this is within a year of the event), though this time limit can be waived. Complainants seeking independent review must request this within 28 days of being informed of the outcome of local resolution.

Should the complainant not be satisfied, either by the decision to refuse independent resolution or by the response to the independent panel's report, he or she may ask the *health ombudsman* to investigate. This represents the third stage of the procedure. It will be recalled that the ombudsman now has the power to investigate clinical complaints and complaints against family practitioners as well as other NHS services. In addition, staff have the right to complain to the ombudsman if they feel that they have been treated unjustly by complaints procedures.

The success of the new system depends on a variety of factors. First, the public must be properly informed of the procedures for making a complaint and what they can reasonably expect when a complaint is made. If this is not done, the confusion and cynicism that will result could bring the new system into the same sort of disrepute as the procedures it replaced. Second, the effectiveness of the local resolution stage is crucial in view of its implications for the later stages of the complaints process. If first-stage procedures are inadequate, the later stages will become overloaded and their effectiveness undermined. Finally, much depends on the independence of the external review process and the responsiveness of managers and the professions to panel reports.

It is too early to draw any conclusions about the operation of the new system, though there is evidence available. On a positive note, the health ombudsman in a report shortly after the new procedures were introduced found signs of a new willingness by managers and professionals to value complaints (Health Service Commissioner, 1996a). However, the same report did find cases where managers had unfairly blocked patients' requests for independent review, in breach of guidance from the Department of Health.

■ The Patients' Charter

The introduction of *The Patient's Charter* in 1992 was heralded as an attempt to redress the balance in favour of health service users (DoH, 1991). It was part of a wider government initiative – *The Citizen's Charter* – to make public sector institutions more consumer-orientated (Cm 1599, 1992).

The original *Patient's Charter* set out ten national rights and nine service standards that patients could expect from the NHS. Three rights were new, including the right to detailed information on local health services; guaranteed admission for virtually all treatments within two years of being placed on a waiting list; and the right to have any complaint investigated, with a full and prompt reply from the chief executive of the health authority or the general manager of the hospital. The nine service standards included: respect for privacy, dignity and religious beliefs; a named nurse (or midwife, or health visitor) to be responsible for care; patients to be seen within 30 minutes of specified outpatient appointment time; and patients to be seen immediately and assessed for treatment when attending at accident and emergency departments. Other standards related to access to services for those with special needs, information about treatment, ambulance arrival times, cancellation of operations, and hospital discharge arrangements.

The Patient's Charter was revised and extended in 1995 (DoH, 1996f), and will be revised again following the change of government in 1997 (see Exhibit 11.1). Specific charters have been introduced for particular client groups such as children and young people (DoH, 1996g), expectant mothers (DoH, 1994g) and mental health service users (DoH, 1997a). In addition, commissioners and providers at local level have been encouraged to develop their own charters. Efforts have also been made to introduce charters in general practice – over half of practices now have their own charter – and in community care at local level (DoH/DOE, 1994).

☐ *Reaction to The Patient's Charter*

The idea of a charter for health service users was supported by the Labour and Liberal Democrat parties well before the Conservative government decided to introduce *The Patient's Charter*. Patients and consumer groups had also pressed for a clearer statement of rights and standards. The professions, too, welcomed moves to clarify responsibilities and rights, provided that these reflected professionally-defined good practice, reinforced the self-regulation of service standards and did not impose excessive and unrealistic demands on service providers.

☐ *The impact of The Patient's Charter on standards*

The Patient's Charter was credited by its supporters with promoting improvements in professional and managerial performance. Its impact on standards was complicated by other factors, including the internal market reforms, reorganisation and managerial changes, waiting list initiatives, changes in the level of funding, new technologies and working practices, all of which affected service provision in the years following its introduction.

A further problem is that many of the rights and standards set by *The Patient's Charter* are difficult to evaluate – 'respecting patient's privacy', for example. Others are more concrete, such as waiting times, and it is here where the success of the *Charter* has been loudly proclaimed. Waiting time indicators fell prior to its introduction and in the following period, between March 1990 and 1995, the number of patients waiting more than twelve months for admission fell from over 200 000 to 32 000. The largest fall occurred between September 1991 and March 1992, the period immediately before the *Charter* came into force (interestingly, a month before the 1992 General Election). By March 1996, only 4600 people had been waiting over twelve months for admission.

Exhibit 11.1   Patients' Charters

The Patient's Charter, revised in 1995, sets out a range of rights, guarantees and expectations. These will be modified further in 1998 (see below).

Access to services

Rights

The patient has the right to:

- receive health care on the basis of clinical need, not on ability to pay, lifestyle or other factors;
- be registered with a GP and to able to change GP easily and quickly;
- be offered a health check when joining a GP practice. Patients aged 16–74 have the right to ask for a health check if they have not seen their GP for three years. Those aged 75 and over have the right to be offered a health check by their GP once a year;
- be prescribed appropriate drugs and medicines (and for particular groups, for example patients 60 and over, to get prescribed medicines free of charge);
- receive emergency medical treatment;
- be referred to a consultant who is acceptable to the patient, when the GP thinks it necessary. The patient also has a right to be referred for a second opinion subject to agreement between the patient and GP.

Guarantees

- patients will not wait more than 18 months for admission for treatment.

Expected standards

- it should be made easy for everyone to use NHS services;
- children should be cared for in a children's ward;
- health authorities should find patients a GP within two working days;
- health authorities should send medical records to a patient's new GP within two working days for urgent cases and six weeks in other cases;
- admission for treatment for coronary artery bypass grafts within one year;
- an operation should not be cancelled on the day it is due, or after admission. If it is the patient can expect to be admitted again within one month;
- when a patient is referred by a GP or dentist to a hospital, nine out ten can expect to be seen within 13 weeks and all within 26 weeks. However, if a patient prefers to see a consultant who is in great demand, outpatient appointments may be delayed beyond these times;

→

Exhibit 11.1 continued

→

- when a patient goes into an accident and emergency department they can expect to be seen immediately and have their need for treatment assessed;
- when going to an outpatient clinic, patients can expect to be given a specific appointment time and be seen within 30 minutes of that time;
- when admitted through accident and emergency units, patients can expect to be given a bed as soon as possible and at least within two hours;
- before discharge, patient can expect a decision to be made regarding their continuing needs for care.

Personal consideration and respect

Rights

- the patient can choose whether or not they want to take part in medical training and research;
- the patient has the right to be told before going into hospital whether they will be admitted to a mixed-sex ward, except in emergency cases.

Expected standards

- staff who deal with patients should wear name badges;
- the NHS should respect the patient's privacy, dignity, religious and cultural beliefs at all times and in all places;
- where the patient is admitted to a mixed-sex ward, separate washing and toilet facilities should be available;
- patients can expect to be given a written explanation of a hospital's food, nutrition and health policy, and the catering service standards which can be expected;
- the hospital environment should be clean and safe. Reasonable measures should be taken to protect the personal safety of patients. Facilities should be available to keep money and belongings safe. Hospitals should be clearly signposted and enquiry points available.

Information

Rights

The patient has the right to:

- have any proposed treatment, including risks involved, clearly explained;
- have access to their own health records and to know that the NHS has a legal duty to ensure patient records are confidential;

→

Exhibit 11.1   *Patients' Charters continued*

→

- have any complaint about NHS services (whoever provides them) investigated and to receive a written reply from the chief executive or general manager within four weeks;
- receive detailed information about local health services, including information about waiting times and GP services.

Expected standards

- a qualified nurse or midwife should be identified as responsible for each patient's nursing and midwifery care, and the patient should be informed of the name of this individual;
- if the patient wishes, relatives and friends should be kept up to date with the progress of treatment.

Community health services

Expected standards

- a patient requiring a home visit from a health visitor, nurse or midwife should be consulted about convenient times and be visited within a two-hour time band. Providing 48 hours notice is given, the patient should be given an appointment on the day they ask for;
- patients can expect to receive a visit from someone in the district nursing team within four hours of an urgent referral being made and within two days in non-urgent cases;
- expectant mothers should receive a visit from a midwife both before and after the baby is born, if both agree this is necessary. They can expect to receive a visit from a health visitor within 10 to 14 days after the birth of a baby;
- a visit from a health visitor can be expected within five working days if the patient is newly registered with a GP and has a child under five years.

Other services

Rights

- if the patient is registered with an NHS dentist, they have the right to receive advice in an emergency and treatment if the dentist considers this to be necessary;
- patients have a right to receive a written prescription and to take this to an optician of their choice. They also have the right to a written statement telling them that no prescription is necessary;
- patients have a right to decide which pharmacist they wish to use for their prescriptions and to have their prescriptions dispensed promptly.

→

Exhibit 11.1 continued

$\longrightarrow$

Expected standards

- ambulance services will work towards achieving an emergency response to 999 calls within eight minutes for incidents identified as 'immediately life threatening'. The public can expect services to achieve a 75 per cent success rate by 2001. For other incidents, the emergency responses are 14 minutes (urban areas), 19 minutes (rural areas);
- patients can expect their health authority to respond to a request to help them find an NHS dentist within five working days;
- patients should be told of the expected cost of dental treatment in advance;
- patients can expect to receive advice from optometrists on whether they can get NHS sight tests and about vouchers to help pay for glasses or contact lenses;
- patients should receive a thorough eye examination which includes checks for disease and abnormality;
- optometrists should inform the patient if they find that further medical treatment is necessary and refer the patient accordingly;
- patients fitted with contact lenses should be given all the necessary information and instruction about cost, use and maintenance and should receive the necessary aftercare for at least six months, and advice on how frequently they should be seen afterwards;
- patients can expect medicines and appliances to be supplied in suitable containers and labelled with clear instructions, and when unsure can expect pharmacists to explain these instructions;
- patients can expect to be given an explanation for any delay in seeing a pharmacist and to be told when a prescription will be ready. When a medicine is not in stock, the patient can expect to be told when it will be available. If a pharmacy is not open, information about out-of-hours arrangements should be displayed on the door or window.

Local standards and charters

Health authorities, trusts, GPs and local authorities are encouraged to devise their own charters. Health authorities are expected to set local standards on waiting times in accident emergency departments. Hospitals should also display information on *The Patient's Charter* and publish details about the number of complaints received and the time taken to deal with them.

Further changes to *The Patient's Charter*

The Blair government, while committed to retaining a patient's charter, announced its intention to modify certain rights and standards. In particular it sought to alter the standards relating to treatment in Accident and Emergency units and to place emphasis on patients' responsibilities. It was expected that the new NHS Charter would be published in the Summer of 1998.

Source: DoH (1996f) *The Patient's Charter and You.* Crown copyright is reproduced with the permission of the Controller of Her Majesty's Stationery Office.

In other areas of the charter, NHS performance measures came close to target. By 1996, nine out of ten patients were seen within 30 minutes of the appointment time. 90 per cent were assessed within five minutes of arrival at accident and emergency units. In other areas performance was less impressive, for example, the performance of ambulance services in urban areas fell short of the national standard. In 1995 only 84 per cent of ambulances met the target response time (the figure was 96 per cent in rural areas). The performance of the London Ambulance Service was particularly poor (House of Commons, 1995e), though there has since been some improvement.

National averages can be misleading. They conceal extremely poor performance in particular localities, units and specialities. Performance indicators published by the Department of Health (DoH, 1995c; 1996b; 1997b) identify under-performance against national standards. Yet, even when relatively poor performance is identified against national benchmarks, the relevant factors may lie outside the control of the health authority or provider concerned.

Even where official figures show that standards are being achieved, critics have questioned the accuracy of the measures. Much depends on how performance is measured and how the figures are presented. During the late 1980s the Thatcher government began to focus on waiting times rather than waiting lists as an indicator of performance. This seemed logical given that the individual patient was concerned mainly about the length of time spent waiting, but there was an important political dimension to this shift in emphasis. Waiting times proved easier to manipulate. As waiting lists – the traditional measure of NHS under-performance – continued to grow (reaching the one million mark in November 1996), waiting time measures, as noted earlier, fell.

How did this happen? For the purpose of performance measurement, people were divided into categories waiting for particular time periods: up to 12 months, 12 to 18 months, 18 months to 2 years, and so on. Hence it was possible for those waiting over 12 months – a relatively small proportion of the total waiting for treatment – to fall, while the overall number of people waiting rose. Meanwhile, median waiting times – the average length of time a patient spends on a waiting list – remained roughly the same (Radical Statistics Health Group, 1995).

Furthermore, official waiting times did not reflect the actual length of time patients spent awaiting treatment (Radical Statistics Health Group, 1995). Until 1995 waiting times were recorded from when a patient was placed on a waiting list by a consultant; the time elapsing between GP referral and the first appointment with a consultant was not counted. Subsequently, a new indicator covering this period was introduced (see Exhibit 11.1). However, other evidence suggests that waiting times were manipulated by removing patients from lists (Newton, Henderson and Goldacre, 1995). The accuracy of data on waiting times in outpatients (House of Commons, 1995f) and in accident and emergency departments (Audit Commission, 1996d) were also questioned.

Statistical manipulation not only misleads the public, it distorts clinical priorities. As Frankel and West (1993, p. 131) conclude, long waiting times are not the consequence of a mismatch between supply and demand, but an expression of implicit priorities. Although these priorities have not always been appropriate, urgent cases have usually received the priority they deserved. In contrast, the new standards set alternative priorities based on administrative targets such as waiting times. Hence the allegations that administrative targets in effect determine who should be treated and when, resulting in non-urgent cases being treated ahead of those where clinical need is greater.

A narrow focus on performance standards has also distorted resource allocation. In an effort to reduce waiting times, central government has often in the past launched special funding initiatives. However, as research into the impact of waiting time initiatives has shown, targeted funding often failed to achieve its objectives and represented an ineffective use of resources (Newton, Henderson and Goldacre, 1995).

Studies of patients' views of *The Patient's Charter* standards contrast sharply with official statistics on performance. For example, research by Bruster *et al.* (1994) found that *Charter* standards were not being met in five areas: respect for privacy, dignity, religious and cultural beliefs (problems reported by up to 9 per cent of respondents); relatives and friends being informed of progress (problems reported by between 14 and 28 per cent); cancelled operations (reported by 11 per cent); named nurse (two-thirds were unaware that a named nurse was responsible for their care); and continuing care (half of respondents were concerned that they had not received help regarding discharge and continuing care). In addition, almost a fifth of patients felt that the standards on signposting premises were not being met.

☐ *Rights*

Patient surveys have also revealed that the rights set out in the *The Patients Charter* are not always upheld. The survey by Bruster *et al.* (1994) revealed that in four areas — a clear explanation of proposed treatment, access to health records, choice about participation in medical education and training, and guaranteed admission within two years, *Charter* standards were not being met.

Moreover, it has been argued that *The Patient's Charter* rights are rather limited. Even if upheld in practice, patients would still be in a weak position. Some of the rights are deliberately vague, for example the right to emergency dental treatment and to a second opinion are restricted by professional judgements. Furthermore, the rights are really conventions rather than rights. They are not enshrined and, apart from any action that might be taken by the NHS Executive to reward or punish performance, there is no guarantee that they will be upheld.

The weakness of *The Patient's Charter* is illustrated by the difficulties patients face when seeking information about themselves and about NHS services generally. The *Charter* states that patients have a right to information. To support this tables are published comparing the performance of local health authorities and providers against national standards. The Major government introduced a number of consumer hotlines (such as the health literature line and the health information line) to provide basic information about health and health services. A Code of Openness was also introduced setting out the conditions and criteria for access to information in the NHS, and which is policed by the health ombudsman (NHSE, 1995a). This (along with another code on the subject of confidentiality) builds on the statutory requirements regarding patient information and records.

Changes in the law in the 1980s and 1990s permitted patients to gain access to their medical records. In 1990 the Access to Health Records Act allowed patients to see manual records compiled after 1 November 1991. Subject to agreement of the relevant health professionals, patients may have access to earlier manual records. Access to computer based records was granted earlier by the Data Protection Act of 1984.

Nevertheless, several obstacles to access have been revealed (Association of Community Health Councils, 1994). Some patients have been deterred by excessive charges and obstructive staff. Particular difficulties were faced by those seeking legitimate access to records on behalf of next of kin. Other patients experienced problems trying to persuade professionals to correct what they believed were errors in their records.

Nevertheless, the number of recorded complaints about the lack of openness in the NHS is small. The health ombudsman received only 21 complaints about non-compliance in 1996 (Health Service Commissioner, 1996b). This certainly underestimates the scale of the problem. As the ombudsman himself observed, the code remains a well-kept secret attracting little publicity either within the NHS or among the general public. Most of those who have experienced problems in obtaining access to information seem to be unaware that a complaints procedure exists.

It is further suggested that rather than providing more information, a *disinformation* campaign was waged in the NHS during the 1990s (see Radical Statistics Health Group, 1995; Waterhouse, 1994b). According to this view, performance tables, literature lines and charters formed part of a broader marketing strategy designed to bolster support for government health policies. In other words, by disseminating 'good news' about the NHS and by promoting rights which largely exist on paper only, government sought to delude people into believing that they were being empowered and services improved.

☐ *Consumerism*

The emphasis of *The Patient's Charter* on the rights of the individual 'consumer' was challenged by some, who argued that models of consumer power were inappropriate to health care. There are a number of reasons why this was held to be so.

First, there is little to support the belief that health service users act like conventional consumers of commodities (Leavey, Wilkin and Metcalfe, 1989; Salisbury, 1989; Shackley and Ryan, 1994; Thomas, Nicholl and Coleman, 1995), even in the realm of private health care (Calnan, Cant and Gabe, 1993) and in pluralist health care systems (Hibbard and Weekes, 1987).

Secondly, the balance of knowledge, expertise and status favours the professions over the user. This acts as a powerful constraint on consumer sovereignty (Shackley and Ryan, 1994). Ultimately, the professions can deal with the 'awkward customer' by transferring the responsibility for treatment to someone else, as illustrated by the removal of patients from GPs' lists, noted in Chapter 8.

Thirdly, the consumer model is too crude and adversarial in its application to health care. According to this view, an emphasis on developing and supporting trusting partnerships between patients and doctors is more appropriate than giving the former a list of rights and standards that are difficult to enforce and which in some circumstances may undermine such relationships (Lupton, Donaldson and Lloyd, 1991).

Finally, the focus on the 'supermarket' model of consumerism is too narrow. Winkler (1987) argued that there was too much emphasis on customer relations and not enough on reducing the disparities in power between users and providers of health services. She set out a number of alternative models (see Exhibit 11.2) that provide a sounder basis for effective public participation and professional accountability.

Notwithstanding the limitations of *The Patient's Charter*, the NHS has in recent years experimented with different ways of involving patients. Patients are becoming involved in the assessment of service quality. They are being asked for their opinions on service development and resourcing decisions. These initiatives are not directly the product of *The Patient's Charter*, though it perhaps created a favourable climate for such developments.

Exhibit 11.2   *Models of consumer power*

1. *The Community Health Councils model*   Consumers are represented by an organisation which monitors local services on their behalf and which may take up individual cases.
2. *The Democratic Accountability model*   Consumers elect representatives on to the bodies which manage local services.
3. *User Power model*   The consumers decide for themselves the care they require. Health professionals then supply the necessary pattern of care.
4. *Partnership*   Health professionals and consumers of health come together to decide what action is best. This can operate at an individual level (doctor and patient) or at an institutional level (between health agencies and patient representatives).

■ Participation by patients and the general public

During the 1970s some practitioners, mainly in the field of general practice, established participation groups as a means of eliciting patients' views about services (Pritchard, 1981). Though providing a useful dialogue between practitioner and user, these initiatives were regarded as a very limited form of participation. Indeed, aside from the opportunity provided by statutory consultation procedures and the activities of CHCs, the patient's voice was largely absent from the arena of health care decision-making. Patients had no role in relation to the monitoring of service quality, either. Indeed, the professions were particularly hostile to such moves on the grounds that their traditional autonomy would be undermined and that patients did not possess the capacity, knowledge or expertise to make judgements regarding the quality of care.

As the inadequacy of these arguments was exposed (Kennedy, 1981; Williamson, 1992) practitioners became increasingly uneasy about the suppression of the patient's perspective. Some were attracted to the view that health care could be improved by listening more carefully to patients. A number of professional groups introduced new mechanisms to facilitate better communication between patients and practitioners. For example, the Royal College of General Practitioners established a patients' liaison group in the early 1980s and other professional bodies have since followed suit.

Interest in the patient's perspective was further stimulated by other policy initiatives in the 1980s and 1990s. *The Patient's Charter*, as has been shown, did not directly empower patients, but at least it placed their minimum requirements on the agenda. Furthermore, local schemes were stimulated as it became clear that the *Charter*'s stated aims could not be achieved without some form of user-involvement in the setting of standards and the evaluation of services (Hart, 1996; Steele, 1992).

Meanwhile, the commissioner–provider split placed an explicit responsibility on health authorities and GPs fundholders to assess needs. They began to devise ways of measuring needs taking into account the views of patients and the wider public. This was bolstered by other changes – such as the reorganisation of health authorities in the 1990s which reinforced their role in identifying local needs. Furthermore, the NHS Management Executive had earlier emphasised that authorities and other purchasers should listen to 'local voices' when making decisions about service priorities (NHSME, 1992). This was later reinforced by central government guidance. The 1996/7 NHS Priorities and Planning Guidance included as a medium-term priority the need to give greater voice and influence to users of NHS services and their carers, in their own care, the development and definition of standards set for NHS services locally, and the development of NHS policy both locally and nationally (NHSE, 1995b, p. 5).

Furthermore, the potential contribution of service users to improvements in standards was highlighted by the range of quality initiatives in the NHS in the late 1980s and 1990s. Many of these, discussed in Chapter 6, focus on the consumer. An example is TQM – which in its pure form takes the consumer perspective as the ultimate test of quality of service. In practice, such initiatives have been bolted on to the existing power relations in health care – where the consumer is in rather a weak position. However, at the very least they have legitimised the patient's perspective and, where managers and professions are united in supporting such initiatives, have encouraged moves towards a more patient-focused service.

☐ *Promoting participation*

While the policy environment has been broadly favourable to the incorporation of user and public perspectives, the establishment of mechanisms and procedures to achieve this has depended largely on local initiative and support. As a result, there is considerable diversity in arrangements established at local level.

There are several ways in which patient perspectives about service standards are sought (McIver, 1991). First, public opinion and satisfaction surveys. These are used to measure public views on priorities (Bowling, Jacobson and Southgate, 1993; Bowling, 1996), local opinion about service provision generally, and levels of satisfaction among users of services and carers (Popay and Williams, 1994). Surveys can be undertaken directly by commissioners and providers, or may be contracted out to market research agencies, academic researchers and voluntary organisations.

A second method involves the establishment of a forum to discuss issues including priorities, access to services and quality issues. On general issues such as priority-setting or broad changes in patterns of service provision, the body needs to represent a wide range of opinion and should be composed of people from a variety of backgrounds, including users and carers as well as the general public. On highly specific issues, perhaps to elicit the views of users or carers on service standards, a small focus group is regarded as more appropriate.

There are many different ways of establishing and operating a forum. One particular model that has attracted interest in recent years is the citizens' jury (Stewart, Kendall and Coote, 1996). This arrangement is used in other countries, such as the USA and Germany, as a means of sounding out public opinion. It involves the formation of a small 'jury' (usually around 20–25 people) drawn from the local community to discuss a particular issue. The jury considers evidence presented by experts and witnesses, and delivers its verdict following a period of discussion. In the UK a number of health authorities, including Cambridge and Huntingdon, Kensington and Chelsea, and Sunderland have piloted the citizens' juries on issues such as hospital closures, priority-setting and alternative means of service provision.

Some health authorities have ongoing systems of consultation. Somerset Health Authority established a number of panels representing local people to discuss priorities in the early 1990s. The conclusions of these panels were then considered by the health authority when it set priorities (Bowie, Richardson and Sykes, 1995). Hospitals, too, have established their own ongoing consultation arrangements, sometimes in conjunction with local CHCs. The Basildon and Thurrock Trust, for example, established a patient representative body in 1993, its membership consisting of people having recent experience of acute hospital services (*Health Rights*, 1995, p. 5).

The third type of arrangement is where patients' and carers' organisations are consulted directly about services. As Pickard, Williams and Flynn (1995) observe, these groups are important channels through which local opinions can be heard. They include local branches of national patient groups, such as the Multiple Sclerosis Society, as well as 'free-standing' local organisations.

There are two main types of patients' group. Those that campaign across the broad range of issues affecting patients, such as CHCs (and their national body, the Association of Community Health Councils for England and Wales), the Patients' Association, and general consumer groups such as the National Consumer Council and the Consumers' Association. The second type is focused around a specific issue (such as mental health), or a particular service, illness or type of patient. These groups often play an important 'self-help' role (Lock, 1986; Temple and Wilson, 1988; Kelleher, 1994). They also have an important representative function, and can contribute to the monitoring and improvement of standards of care (Kirkness, 1996). Surprisingly little is known about how these organisations interact with the NHS. It is assumed that compared with professional groups they are much less influential, but the growing activism of these groups and their participation in debates such as long-term care and rationing underlines the need for a comprehensive study of their role in the policy-making process.

The main types of patient involvement discussed above can be found in community care as well as health care (Bewley and Glendinning, 1994; Hoyes *et al.*, 1994; Wistow and Barnes, 1993). In this sector, too, efforts have been made in recent years to improve participation by users and their carers. Similar issues regarding empowerment are raised here, and similar problems – particularly with regard to the obstacles impeding participation – are identified.

☐ *Problems of participation*

Efforts to incorporate user and public perspectives have attracted criticism, relating both to the use of particular techniques and to the broader difficulties of promoting effective public involvement.

The reliability of opinion surveys has been questioned. In the case of patient satisfaction surveys the wording of questions can affect responses and may influence the results (Cohen, Forbes and Garraway, 1996). Furthermore, surveys are essentially producer-led and can be used to support their case rather than improve the responsiveness of services to users (Hart, 1996). Similar considerations apply to larger-scale surveys of public opinion on priority-setting and service developments. There is also the added danger that the views of an important minority may be submerged in the majority opinion. Carefully-designed surveys can enrich the debate about priorities, though it must be remembered that different sections of the community often have different preferences about rationing (Bowling, 1996).

Other market research techniques such as focus groups and citizen's juries have been criticised; the means of selection and the representativeness of such arrangements have been questioned (Edwards, 1996). Some doubt whether qualitative methods such as in-depth interviews, panels, forums and so on actually elicit the personal ideas of respondents. One study found that participants lacked confidence in making judgements and felt ill-equipped to play a role in decisions about prioritisation (Dicker and Armstrong, 1995).

The role of patients' groups has been challenged. Like many voluntary organisations they are often run by highly-committed individuals, and there is always a danger that they will not accurately represent the diverse views of service users. Some organisations are quite good at seeking out the views of members using questionnaires and local focus groups to gauge opinion, and the larger patient organisations have national and local conferences to raise issues and endorse policies. But, notwithstanding these efforts, there is no evidence available on the extent to which patients' groups accurately reflect the views of their members.

Another problem is that not all service users will join a group, and their interests may be indirectly represented by an organisation claiming to act on their behalf. But if they are not members or do not participate actively in the group, the link between their preferences and the policies of the organisation becomes tenuous. Furthermore, in some cases no organisation exists to represent the views of users, and as a result their interests may be ignored by decision-makers and service providers. Some patients lack the necessary resources, knowledge and information to establish a group. Or it may be that – particularly in the case of acute patients – their interests are short-term and they have less incentive to organise. This perhaps explains partly why most patient organisations seem to focus on issues relating to chronic illness and long-term care.

Added to concerns about the techniques and mechanisms of patient involvement are doubts about their impact on policies and services. At national level, user organisations are politically weak. They do not have the same stature as the professional bodies or the organisations representing health authorities and trusts. User groups are increasingly represented on official committees established by the Department of Health to consider policy and service developments, but remain out-numbered by representatives of producer interests.

At the local level participation seems to be increasing, but on the terms set by health authorities and service providers (Leonard *et al.*, 1997). Despite a willingness to involve users, there is a fear among managers and the professions that this might lead to a loss of control over services (Pickard, Williams and Flynn, 1995). Moreover, to seek out views does not mean they will actually be heeded (Popay and Williams, 1994). In practice, user views are often used selectively by commissioners and providers to support a particular case rather than to promote a more responsive service.

Finally, efforts to extend user participation have ironically coincided with a growing 'democratic deficit' in health care (Institute for Public Policy Research, 1995b). In the 1980s and 1990s the NHS became more centralised politically and adopted a more 'managerialist' style of decision-making (see Chapter 6). This trend was at odds with the notion of increasing public participation which requires a more democratic structure of decision-making (Pollock, 1992; Popay and Williams, 1994).

■ Conclusion

More attention is being paid to the patient's perspective, not just in the UK but internationally. In 1994, 36 European nations endorsed the *Declaration on the Promotion of Patient's Rights in Europe*. This set out a number of principles relating to medical records, accurate information for patients, and the right to be treated on the basis of medical criteria. Though not legally binding, the declaration adds further weight to national efforts to improve patients' rights. The patient's perspective was further emphasised in a subsequent international agreement in 1996. *The Ljubljana Charter* stressed the importance of the citizen's voice in shaping health care services. The contribution of the public was mentioned specifically in the context of contracting, quality of services, waiting lists and complaints. The importance of timely information and education in enhancing patient's rights was also emphasised.

In the UK, *The Patient's Charter* and other reforms have highlighted the patient's perspective. Although the balance of power between users and service providers has not significantly altered, these reforms have at least provided a favourable climate for the development of initiatives to incorporate the views of users and the wider public. Such initiatives have been encouraged further by a growing realisation among the health professions that patient involvement can improve the quality and effectiveness of services.

However, doubts about particular mechanisms of public participation and involvement remain. The user perspective still lacks weight in national decision-making and at local level. Moreover, the NHS remains an undemocratic institution and in several respects became more so during the 1980s and 1990s. This democratic deficit in health care must be tackled if the 'supermarket model' of health care consumerism is to be transcended.

■ *Chapter 12* ■

The Health of the Nation

Action to promote the health of the whole community dates back to the earliest civilisations (Rosen, 1993). The Ancient Greeks recognised the links between location, environment, lifestyles, nutrition and the health of the community. The Romans too were aware of these factors, and sought to improve public health through large-scale engineering works such as water supply systems and sewers. Centuries later, the Victorians established a legislative and administrative framework which led to improvements in health through better housing, sanitation and a cleaner environment. But for most of the twentieth century, health policy has been mainly concerned with the provision of health care rather than with the promotion and maintenance of good health. This reflected to some extent the dominance of the biomedical approach over public health medicine (see Chapter 2).

In recent decades there has been a revival of interest in the public health approach. It is now realised that many of the challenges facing the health system, outlined in Chapter 1, require something more than an expansion of health services. Governments around the world have responded by developing strategies aimed at improving the health of their populations.

This chapter is divided into three main parts. First, there is a discussion of the decline of the public health approach in the twentieth century and the roots of its recent regeneration. This is followed by an account of the Thatcher government's approach to public health during the 1980s. Finally, there is an analysis of the national health strategy devised by the Major government in the early 1990s and how this might develop in the future under a Labour government.

■ The fall and rise of the public health approach

□ *The decline of public health*

During the first part of the twentieth century, the emphasis of policy began to shift from public health towards the provision of health care and, in particular, the development of hospital services. This reflected the growing role of the state in promoting, financing and providing health care services, culminating in the creation of the NHS after the Second World War (Brand, 1965). Subsequent reorganisation of responsibilities within central government further sharpened this focus. By the 1950s the main government department responsible for health policy, the Ministry of Health, had lost many of its wider public health responsibilities including housing and sanitation to other departments. Health policy at national level became increasingly concerned with the development of services. In Klein's (1980) words, 'Britain had a health service but no policy for health.'

As the century progressed, health policy at a local level similarly focused on service provision. The Medical Officers of Health (MOHs), created by the Victorians to act as guardians of the public health at local level, became more service-orientated. Moreover, their status deteriorated as local authorities lost some of their health service functions after the Second World war (Ottewill and Wall, 1990). Later, the reorganisation of social services in 1970 removed their responsibility for these services as well. Shortly afterwards, the NHS reorganisation of 1974 transferred all but environmental health and personal social services from local government to the new health authorities.

The post of MOH was abolished in the 1974 reorganisation. MOHs were replaced by community physicians, mainly concerned with service planning and employed by district health authorities. Though it was intended that their status would be higher than the MOHs they replaced, this move did not halt the long-term decline of the public health doctor (Lewis, 1987). Further decline was prompted by the Griffiths management reforms which led to the abolition of many community physician posts.

☐ The need for a public health strategy

The continued decline in the status of public health medicine was accompanied paradoxically by a growing recognition that the burden of illness in modern societies required something more than an expansion of health services. In the UK, as in other industrialised countries, much illness is in the form of chronic disease. Many of these diseases, including heart and circulatory diseases, cancers and respiratory diseases, can be prevented to some extent by action at the community level. But the value of preventive action is not confined to chronic disease. Acute health problems are also preventable; including deaths, illness and injuries caused by accidents, violence, drug abuse and infectious diseases.

Many significant causes of mortality and morbidity can be prevented at the community level. These can be divided into three categories: lifestyle, environment and deprivation.

☐ *Lifestyle*

Smoking, poor diet, alcohol and drug abuse and 'unsafe' sexual habits are among the most important lifestyle factors affecting health.

- Smoking-related diseases kill approximately 100 000 people each year (Royal College of Physicians, 1983b). In addition to its role in heart disease, smoking is a causal factor in respiratory illnesses such as emphysema, bronchitis and cancers of the throat and lung; lung cancer alone kills 37 000 people a year in the UK (Cancer Research Campaign, 1996). In addition, smoking during pregnancy can damage the foetus and is a risk factor in sudden infant death syndrome (Blair, Fleming and Bensley, 1996). Evidence on the impact of passive smoking suggests that non-smokers may also be at risk (Independent Scientific Committee on Smoking and Health, 1988). Smoking-related diseases are relatively difficult to cure – lung cancer survival rates are quite low – and therefore the most cost-effective strategy to deal with the health problems associated with smoking is prevention: to persuade people not to smoke.

- Diet is an important lifestyle factor affecting health, (BMA, 1986a; WHO, 1988), and dietary factors are associated with at least 35 per cent of all cancers (Doll and Peto, 1981), and perhaps more (Austoker, 1994). The evidence linking diet to particular cancers varies considerably. There is quite strong evidence of a link between diet and bowel cancer, the second largest cause of death from cancer in the UK (Royal College of Physicians, 1981). Increased consumption of fruit, vegetables and fibre in the diet is associated with a reduced risk of this form of cancer.

  Diet is also implicated in heart and circulatory disease (British Cardiac Society, 1987; COMA, 1994; Key *et al.*, 1996). High blood cholesterol is recognised as a major risk factor for heart disease, and a 10 per cent reduction in cholesterol concentration is associated with a 30 per cent reduction in heart disease at age 60 (Law, Thompson and Wald, 1994). Blood cholesterol can be reduced by increasing dietary fibre, reducing total fat consumption (particularly saturated fat, derived mainly from animals) and by drugs. However, there is evidence linking low cholesterol levels to other causes of morbidity and mortality, implying that a lowering of cholesterol levels across the board may exacerbate other health problems (Jacobs *et al.*, 1992; Dunnigan, 1993). Other studies, however, found that the increased risk associated with low or reduced cholesterol was small and was outweighed by the benefits of a reduced risk of heart disease (Law *et al.*, 1994). High blood pressure, another major risk factor in heart disease and strokes, is also related to diet. Excess consumption of salt is associated with higher blood pressure (Elliott *et al.*, 1996). Furthermore, obesity has been identified as a risk factor in heart disease, stroke and cancers (Garrow, 1991; DoH, 1995i; Office of Health Economics, 1994).

- Alcohol is implicated in a wide range of health and social problems including accidents, violent assaults, mental illness, and a range of physical disorders and illnesses (Faculty of Public Health Medicine, 1991a). The Royal College of General Practitioners (1986) put the annual number of deaths from alcohol abuse at 40 000. There appears to be a general relationship between the level of alcohol consumption in a society and the level of alcohol-related problems (Edwards, 1994). The doubling of the amount of alcohol consumed per adult in the UK over the past thirty years has been matched by a growth in alcohol problems over the same period. Around 13 per cent of women and 27 per cent of men drink above the government's own safe limits (OPCS, 1996). However, recent evidence has suggested that in moderation alcohol consumption may help to reduce the risk of coronary heart disease among some groups (Rimm *et al.*, 1996)

- Drug abuse has wide-ranging social consequences far beyond its effects on health. It is difficult to quantify the health effects of drug-taking, largely because of the huge range of substances that can be classified as recreational drugs. Some drugs can be taken legally for recreational reasons, such as alcohol and nicotine. Others are used illegally for recreation but have a legal use as medication (anti-depressants, steroids, morphine) or have some other legitimate use (solvents). Others are outlawed in view of their use primarily as mood-altering recreational drugs (ecstasy, cocaine, cannabis, heroin). Aside from the psychological impact of drug addiction, a range of diseases and other physical consequences (accidents, injury, poisoning) are associated with drug abuse, causing a high level of morbidity as well as premature mortality. Furthermore, drug abuse can interact with other health and social problems (for example, the link between HIV infection, prostitution and drug abuse). Drug taking is far from being a minority activity – the 34 000 or so notified drug addicts in the UK being only the tip of the iceberg (Home Office, 1995). There is particular concern about the scale of drug taking among the young – surveys of teenagers under 16 reveal that between 40 per cent (Miller and Plant, 1996) and half (Parker, Measham and Aldridge, 1995) claim to have tried drugs. Most activity seems to involve experimentation with 'soft' drugs, particular those closely connected with contemporary youth culture, such as ecstasy. Nevertheless, the consequences for users can be serious and occasionally fatal, as tragic individual cases have graphically illustrated.

- The number of reported cases of sexually transmitted diseases (STD), as noted in Chapter 1, has risen dramatically during the postwar period. However, it was the emergence of AIDS that made the prevention of STDs a high-profile issue (Hancock and Carim, 1987). As there is no cure at present for those infected, prevention remains the only effective way of tackling the disease.

☐ *Environment*

- Accidents are a major cause of illness and death. As we saw in Chapter 1, much of this toll involves young people and is road-traffic related. Around 5000 deaths every year in Britain result from road accidents, with a further 4500 caused by accidents in the home, and 300 from accidents at work. Most are preventable by altering the environment within which people live and work, and by educating individuals about risks. The working environment can pose a wider threat to health over and above the level of illness and premature mortality caused by accidents in the workplace (Watterson, 1994; Health and Safety Executive, 1990; Snashall, 1996). Occupational diseases, including dermatitis, asthma and deafness, are a significant burden on health services accounting for 7 per cent of general practice consultations (McCormick, Fleming and Charlton, 1995). In addition, increasing stress levels in the workplace have been linked to a range of physical and mental health problems (Jenkins, 1993). The total annual cost of work-related illness, injury and accidents in the UK has been estimated at between £11 billion and £16 billion (Health and Safety Executive, 1994). Finally, it should be noted that the workplace provides a setting in which to promote health in a positive way, rather than simply being a focus for the prevention of occupational injury and illness (Dugdill and Springett, 1994)
- Environment pollution is linked to major health problems (Hall, 1990; WHO, 1986). Air and water pollution can have a significant detrimental effect on the health of the population, particularly upon vulnerable groups such as children and the elderly. However, the impact of environmental pollution is often complex and it is not always possible to identify a simple causal process. For example, the relationship between pollution and asthma (Parliamentary Office of Science and Technology, 1994; COMEAP, 1995) is based on circumstantial evidence. Yet in such cases preventive action may be judged necessary because the potential consequences of inaction are so serious.

Further sources of pollution arise from contamination in the agricultural and food industries (Cannon, 1987; Millstone, 1986). Pesticides, food additives and modern food production techniques have been associated with a wide range of health problems. In addition, the growth in food poisoning and the rise of other food-borne infections (notably the link between BSE and CJD) have been attributed in part to food technologies and processes (House of Commons, 1989a; Lacey, 1994).

☐ Deprivation

• As shown in Chapter 1, there are wide variations between social classes in terms of relative mortality and morbidity. However, the relationship between social conditions and health variations is often the subject of controversial debate. It is widely accepted that specific social conditions such as poor housing (Arblaster and Hawtin, 1993; Lowry, 1991), unemployment and job insecurity (Ferrie *et al.*, 1995; Smith, R., 1987) are associated with ill-health. Limited educational opportunities are also believed to have an impact on social deprivation and may contribute to variations in ill-health (BMA, 1987). Low income is linked to poor health status, and income inequality has been associated with variations in health and illness in society. Later in this chapter there is a closer examination of the impact of inequality and deprivation on health in the context of socio-economic policies pursued by the UK government in the 1980s and 1990s.

Although it is useful to categorise possible causes of ill-health, the distinctions blur in practice. Health problems rooted in deprivation, for example, are often linked to unhealthy lifestyles. For example, those on low incomes are less able to afford a wholesome diet, and environmental factors are similarly related to lifestyles. The use of the motor car, a major cause of pollution and accidents, is clearly related to the individualistic and materialistic lifestyle of modern industrialised countries. Furthermore much ill-health, notably mental illnesses such as anxiety and depression, is influenced by a combination of factors relating to lifestyles, environments and material conditions.

☐ Public health strategies

Governments have pursued strategies aimed at preventing health problems and identifying illness at a stage where treatment is more likely to be effective. Essentially, these strategies have three main elements (Jacobson, Smith and Whitehead, 1991).

First, *education* – to persuade individuals to adopt healthy lifestyles and reject or moderate habits harmful to health – such as smoking and heavy drinking. Education may also be aimed at groups and private institutions in an attempt to encourage collective action to prevent ill-health. Examples include the promotion of alcohol awareness, and smoke-free zones.

Second, *clinical prevention*. This includes services to monitor health and detect illness at an early stage. For example, the provision of screening facilities to detect the early signs of breast and cervical cancer. Also included in this category are other preventive interventions such as immunisation against diseases such as mumps, measles, whooping cough and rubella (German measles).

A third component of a public health strategy is *intervention at the social and environmental level*. This involves adopting policies to tackle the root causes of ill-health in society. The state has considerable legislative and financial powers to promote health. It can ban or restrict activities harmful to health, or impose penal taxation upon such activities. It has the capacity to coordinate national and local policies to ensure that health objectives are not compromised, and has the strength and legitimacy to regulate powerful vested interests whose activities may undermine public health, such as the alcohol, tobacco and food industries. Furthermore, it can arbitrate between individuals' rights and liberties. Some individuals in a liberal society may choose to indulge in health-damaging behaviour even when fully informed. These rights, however, impinge on others. The issue of smoking restrictions in public places exemplifies how the state must balance the conflicting rights of its citizens.

Policy-makers in many countries began to turn their attention to public health strategies during the mid-1970s. This was a period of severe economic crisis which led to a squeeze on publicly-funded health services, and a search for more cost-effective health strategies. Prevention was seen as a way of saving funds, though it is now increasingly recognised that higher rather than lower costs may be incurred by a preventive strategy as people live longer (Normand, 1991).

The UK government published a consultative document (DHSS, 1976c) which identified key areas for future action: inequalities in health status; heart disease; road accidents; smoking-related diseases; alcoholism and mental illness; drugs; diet; and venereal disease. The tone of this document was not prescriptive, it aimed to promote discussion rather than to outline a programme of action.

It was expected that the subsequent White Paper (Cmnd 7047, 1977) would set out such a programme. In the event this was a rather cautious document which failed to articulate a coherent public health strategy, and central government took a passive approach to the development of public health activities. Expenditure on health education was increased but interventionist measures were avoided. The government was reluctant to provide extra resources to encourage prevention, for example refusing to divert resources from high technology medicine.

■ Public health under the Conservatives

□ *Public health policies*

The Thatcher government gave added impetus to prevention, putting its faith in high-profile health education. It spent around £2 million on drug abuse campaigns in the early 1980s, a figure later exceeded by campaigns on heart disease and AIDS. Spending on mass media campaigns rose from £1.6 million to £11.4 million per annum between 1979 and 1988 (Whitehead, 1989), and this figure has since continued to grow. In 1995 the Department of Health spent £30 million on such campaigns.

During the 1980s high-level ministerial committees were established to discuss specific public health issues such as AIDS, and drug and alcohol abuse. This led to several policy initiatives. In the case of alcohol abuse, the rules governing alcohol advertising were tightened-up, further restrictions imposed on drinking and driving, and local inter-agency collaboration on alcohol problems encouraged (Lord President of the Council, 1991).

The Thatcher government actively supported clinical prevention by encouraging screening programmes for breast and cervical cancer. This included a national breast cancer screening programme, and a national call–recall appointment system to extend cervical cancer screening. By the mid-1990s the breast cancer programme was screening over 70 per cent of all women aged between 50 and 64 (the age group invited for screening at three-yearly intervals). The proportion of women in the 20 to 64 age group screened for cervical cancer also rose, to over 80 per cent by the mid-1990s.

The shake-up of primary care, in the form of the White Paper *Promoting Better Health,* further emphasised clinical prevention. This initiative, discussed in Chapter 9, introduced financial incentives for GPs achieving target rates for child immunisation and cervical cancer screening. GPs were also paid to undertake specific health promotion activities such as monitoring the health of their patients at certain intervals.

Despite the Thatcher government's encouragement of preventive medicine, critics attacked its policies on a number of grounds (Public Health Alliance, 1988). The main criticisms, which persisted under the Major government of the 1990s, were as follows.

☐ *Education and clinical prevention*

There were reservations about the emphasis on high-profile health education campaigns. There was particular criticism of the government's drug abuse campaign, which some believed was unhelpful because it reinforced the 'heroin addict' stereotype. Likewise, the government's hostility to low-profile community education campaigns was also criticised, and there was concern about GP-based health promotion. Subsequent evaluation of health promotion in general practice revealed that the benefits of such schemes were modest relative to the costs involved (see Chapter 9). The system of paying GPs for specific health promotion activities was later substantially reformed.

The emphasis on cancer screening was challenged in some quarters. On the one hand there was concern about the quality of services. In particular the failure of screening systems to detect cancers where one in five women screened will not have their cancers detected. On the other hand, in 95 per cent of cases where problems are found the abnormality will be non-cancerous. This creates unnecessary anguish, and in some cases unnecessary treatment as well. On top of this is concern about the quality of treatment services following diagnosis (House of Commons, 1995g). A further line of criticism is more fundamental. While recognising that breast and cervical cancer represent major threats to women's health, some argue that the potential benefits of such screening programmes are low in terms of numbers of lives saved compared with the resources invested (McCormick, 1989).

Government policy was further challenged on the grounds that it did not tackle the imbalance between prevention and treatment services. A report on coronary heart disease by the Public Accounts Committee of the House of Commons (House of Commons, 1989b) revealed that 50 times more was being spent on the treatment of this disease than on prevention. A subsequent report by the Audit Commission (1995f) showed that health authorities were still failing to give priority to the prevention of coronary heart disease. One of the reasons is that, until fairly recently, health authorities' efforts to improve public health have not been closely monitored and much has depended on local commitment to prevention initiatives.

The lack of priority given to public health was also revealed by examples of poor coordination within central government. Although, as mentioned earlier, special interdepartmental committees were established to tackle particular issues, this was not normal practice. Indeed on some issues departments were openly at loggerheads with each other, as revealed by a succession of food scandals, including the crises surrounding salmonella in eggs (Doig, 1990) and BSE (Lacey, 1994).

☐ *Individual responsibility*

The Thatcher and Major governments accepted that many health problems were associated with social habits such as drinking, smoking and poor diet, but took a rather narrow view of how these lifestyles developed, attributing them largely to ignorance. There were fears that this was tantamount to 'victim blaming'. An alternative view is that lifestyles, environment and social conditions interact in a complex manner. Policies which seek merely to inform and educate are likely to be ineffective if social conditions and the environment are not conducive to the development of responsible and healthy lifestyles (Jacobson, Smith and Whitehead 1991).

In order to prevent smoking-related diseases it may be necessary to regulate more effectively the marketing activities of the tobacco industry. Norway, for example, has operated a comprehensive Tobacco Act involving a total ban for nearly two decades on the advertising and promotion of tobacco products. For many years Britain avoided taking similar steps. However, a commitment to ban tobacco advertising and sponsorship was made by the Blair government in 1997, which promised tough action on smoking.

Intervention to protect public health was at odds with the Thatcher government's philosophy, and this was also true of the Major government. Even so, previous governments, both Conservative and Labour, demonstrated a reluctance to tackle industries whose products and practices are linked to public health problems, namely the alcohol, tobacco and food industries. It is easy to understand why. These industries are wealthy, they have considerable political leverage and can persuade governments not to intervene in their commercial affairs (Taylor, 1984).

☐ *Social and economic policy*

The social and economic policies of the Thatcher and Major governments were criticised for their impact upon public health. The policy of deregulation was blamed for a number of problems ranging from inadequate health and safety standards, to food scandals such as the BSE crisis (Gifford, 1996).

Another main feature of government policy in the 1980s and 1990s – privatisation – also had health implications. Most of the utility companies increased prices following privatisation, with consequences for the poor. Prices later fell but this was offset by the imposition of VAT on gas and electricity. The restructuring of public utilities following privatisation also had an impact on health. The newly-privatised companies sought to reduce costs by cutting jobs, leading to economic insecurity and unemployment –

both associated with ill-health. Finally, the utilities adopted a more commercial attitude towards customers and were more willing to disconnect services to those who failed to pay their bills. For those deprived of basic necessities such as heat, light and clean water the health consequences were obviously serious. The privatisation of the water authorities attracted most concern given the importance of water and sewerage services in the maintenance of public health (Barnardo's, 1993).

The key economic policy aims of the Thatcher and Major governments were to control inflation, cut public spending and taxation, and improve economic incentives to encourage enterprise and wealth creation. Other economic priorities of the postwar period, such as employment protection and income redistribution, were disregarded. Policies were introduced which led to greater inequality: reducing the burden of taxation for those on high incomes, reducing entitlement to welfare benefits, and the abandonment of low wage regulation.

As inquiries from the Joseph Rowntree Foundation (1995) and the Commission for Social Justice (1994) found economic inequality increased substantially in this period. In 1979 the richest fifth of the population received 36 per cent of the total household disposable income. By 1995 this share was 40 per cent. Meanwhile the share of the poorest fifth of the population fell over the same period from 9.4 per cent to 7.9 per cent. According to the Joseph Rowntree Foundation inquiry, income inequality grew rapidly between 1977 and 1990 reaching a level not seen in the UK since 1945. The bottom 10 per cent of the income distribution did not benefit from the general increase in incomes (a 36 per cent rise before deduction of housing costs) which occurred between 1979–92. The top tenth of the income distribution enjoyed more than a 60 per cent increase in income (after housing costs), while the income of the bottom tenth actually fell by 17 per cent. Poverty and deprivation also increased in the 1980s and early 1990s. In 1993, 25 per cent of households were living on below half the average income (after deduction of housing costs), compared with 9 per cent of households in 1979 (Department of Social Security, 1995).

According to some observers these changes reflected profound changes in the social and economic framework of society. Hutton (1996), for example, identified the emergence of the 40:30:30 society: 40 per cent with secure permanent jobs; 30 per cent having insecure or casual employment; the bottom 30 per cent being marginalised, unemployed or working for poverty wages. Similarly Galbraith (1992), in an American context, has written of a 'culture of contentment' where the experience of a contented majority contrasts sharply with that of a deprived underclass.

The health effects of social and economic inequality on this scale are serious. There has been a widening of health inequalities between the social classes since the late 1970s. Mortality rate differentials for men between social classes I and V have widened from a two-fold difference in the early 1970s, to almost a three-fold difference in the early 1990s (Drever, Whitehead and Roden, 1996). Other research reveals that the more unequal a society in terms of its income distribution, the greater the degree of health inequalities. Wilkinson (1992; 1996) found that income inequality was the key determinant of average life expectancy in developed countries. Although his findings have not gone unchallenged (Judge, 1995), other studies (Kennedy, Kawacki and Prothrow-Smith, 1996; Kaplan *et al.*, 1996) confirm a relationship between unequal income distribution and mortality. In addition, studies of particular localities in the UK have identified a relationship between widening income inequalities and growing health inequalities (Drever and Whitehead, 1995; Phillimore, Beattie and Townsend, 1994; McLoone and Boddy, 1994).

The Thatcher and Major governments denied that material inequalities directly caused ill-health. While accepting the existence of health inequalities, they pointed out that the variation between the health of different social classes could be explained in other ways. Indeed, it has been argued that the method of identifying social class – by occupation – artificially exaggerates inequalities in health (Illsley, 1986). Misrecording of occupations is also believed by some to contribute to the distortion of these figures. Mortality rates are calculated on the basis of the occupation of the deceased taken from the death certificate; previous occupations which might place people in a higher social category are not therefore taken into account.

Accurate measurement of health inequalities over a period of time is difficult, and reclassification of occupations adds to these difficulties. The changing size of the social classes themselves (between 1931 and 1981 social class V shrank by 55 per cent while social class I grew by 217 per cent) means that one is not comparing like with like. The widening gap between the social classes may reflect the growth in the middle classes and the shrinking working class. However, even when the changing size of classes is taken into account, health inequalities remain significant (Goldblatt, 1989; Fox, Goldblatt and Jones, 1990; Pamuk, 1985; Smith, Blane and Bartley, 1994).

Another potential explanation for health inequalities lies in social selection. According to this argument social class differences result from healthy people moving up the social ladder, and unhealthy people moving downwards (Stern, 1983). In other words healthy people are upwardly mobile, being better able to hold down jobs, own their own homes, and so on. There is, however, little evidence to support this theory (Blane, Smith and Bartley, 1993; Goldblatt, 1989; Fox, Goldblatt and Jones, 1990), though health status does influence the selection of occupation, a factor which should be noted when comparing mortality rates of workers in different jobs (Goldblatt, Fox and Leon, 1990).

A third alternative explanation focuses on the behaviour of individuals within the social classes. Manual classes, according to this explanation, adopt less healthy lifestyles. In particular, drinking, smoking and eating habits are held responsible for much of the burden of ill-health. While these factors may well be important, this behavioural explanation of health inequalities diverts attention from the social conditions within which individuals make choices. It is clear that individuals do not make choices within a social vacuum. Eating, smoking and drinking habits, for example, are shaped by class and income as well as personal preference.

Studies attributing health inequalities to material circumstances and social class structure were rejected, particularly by the Thatcher government. In 1980 the report of a DHSS Working Party (the Black report) was treated with contempt for putting this case forward (DHSS, 1980; Townsend, Davidson, Whitehead, 1992). In 1987 an updated version of the Black report received a similar response (Whitehead, 1987; Townsend, Davidson and Whitehead, 1992). This report confirmed that inequalities in health had persisted into the 1980s, and pointed out that the situation was deteriorating. Increasing homelessness (which, even according to official figures, almost doubled during the 1980s), greater income inequality, poverty and mass unemployment lay behind these trends. The report pointed out a particularly disturbing increase in child poverty and criticised the lack of a coordinated strategy to tackle the social roots of ill-health.

■ Towards a public health strategy?

During the latter part of the 1980s the Thatcher government came under increasing pressure to adopt a comprehensive health strategy. A number of factors were behind this: international developments, local initiatives, and a series of public health crises.

□ International developments

Increasingly the British government's approach seemed out of step with other countries. The UK was formally committed to the World Health Organisation's *Health For All* initiative, which set objectives to be achieved by the year 2000. These included greater equity in health, the development of healthy public policies, reducing accidents, and many others. In addition, other more specific targets were set by the World

Health Organisation for European countries (WHO, 1985). The revised targets are set out in Exhibit 12.1.

On top of this, the European Union began to take a growing interest in public health problems. It imposed a common set of health warnings on tobacco products in member countries – a move vigorously and unsuccessfully opposed by the UK. Following the Maastricht Treaty of 1992 the role of European institutions has extended further into the health sphere. For example, in 1995 the European Commission launched a five-year plan to promote public health, including a programme of cancer prevention, AIDS, communicable diseases, and drug addiction.

☐ *Local and regional developments*

For most of the 1980s the British government acknowledged international developments but failed to formulate its own national strategy. Many local authorities bypassed central government and established their own initiatives. Some built on the experience of the World Health Organisation's *Healthy Cities* initiative which began in 1986. This programme sought to establish comprehensive strategies aimed at improving the health of people within particular localities (Davies and Kelly, 1993), and it was targeted at cities with the worst health and social problems. The cities in the UK which participated in the programme were Liverpool, Belfast, Glasgow and the London Borough of Camden. But within the NHS such initiatives had a fairly low priority. Although most health authorities established local priorities in line with *Health for All*, only a minority allocated resources to implement local strategies.

Elsewhere in the UK attempts were made to develop clearer health strategies. In Wales, during the late 1980s, ten key problem areas including heart and circulatory disease, respiratory illness and unhealthy environments were identified. Resources were geared to tackling these specific problems with a view to increasing life expectancy and the quality of life (Health Promotion Authority for Wales, 1990). Meanwhile, in Northern Ireland a consultation document was published on the subject of health promotion (Northern Ireland Health Promotion Agency, 1990). In Scotland plans set attainment targets for improving health for the under-65s by the year 2000 (Scottish Office, 1991). This was followed by moves to implement a Scottish health strategy (Scottish Office, 1992).

☐ *Crises and scandals*

A series of public health crises added to the pressure for action. In the latter part of the 1980s public anxiety was raised by a series of potential threats to health: salmonella in eggs, BSE, AIDS and other infectious

---

Exhibit 12.1   World Health Organisation: Health for All by the Year 2000

Regional targets for Europe (base year 1980) as revised in 1991. Targets to be achieved by the Year 2000:

1. The differences in health status between countries and between groups within countries should be reduced by at least 25 per cent, by improving the level of health of disadvantaged nations and groups.
2. All people should have the opportunity to develop and use their health potential to live socially, economically and mentally fulfilling lives.
3. People with disabilities should be able to lead socially, economically and mentally fulfilling lives with the support of special arrangements that improve their relative physical, social and economic opportunities.
4. There should be a sustained and continuing reduction in morbidity and disability due to chronic disease in the Region.
5. There should be no indigenous cases of poliomyelitis, diphtheria, neonatal tetanus, measles, mumps and congenital rubella in the Region and there should be a sustained and continuing reduction in the incidence and adverse consequences of other communicable diseases, notably HIV infection.
6. Life expectancy at birth in the Region should be at least 75 years and there should be a sustained and continuing improvement in the health of all people aged 65 years and over.
7. The health of all children and young people should be improved, giving them the opportunity to grow and develop to their full physical, mental and social potential.
8. There should be a sustained and continuing improvement in the health of all women.
9. Mortality from diseases of the circulatory system should be reduced, in the case of people under 65 years by at least 15 per cent, and there should be progress in improving the quality of life of all people suffering from cardiovascular disease.
10. Mortality from cancer in people under 65 should be reduced by at least 15 per cent and the quality of life of all people with cancer should be significantly improved.
11. Injury, disability and death arising from accidents should be reduced by at least 25 per cent.
12. There should be a sustained and continuing reduction in the prevalence of mental disorders, an improvement in the quality of life of all people with such disorders and a reversal of the rising trends in suicide and attempted suicide.
13. All Member States should have developed, and be implementing, intersectoral policies for the promotion of healthy lifestyles, with systems ensuring public participation in policy-making and implementation.
14. All settings of social life and activity, such as the city, school, workplace, neighbourhood and home, should provide greater opportunities for promoting health.
15. Accessible and effective education and training in health promotion should be available in all Member States, in order to improve public and professional competence in promoting health and increasing health awareness in other sectors.
16. There should be continuous efforts in all Member States to actively promote and support healthy patterns of living through balanced nutrition, appropriate physical activity, healthy sexuality, good stress management, and other aspects of positive health behaviour.
17. The health-damaging consumption of dependence-producing substances such as alcohol, tobacco and psychoactive drugs should have been significantly reduced in all Member States.
18. All Member States should have developed, and be implementing, policies on the environment and health that ensure ecologically sustainable development, effective prevention and control of environmental health risk and equitable access to healthy environments.

$\longrightarrow$

Exhibit 12.1 continued

→

19. There should be effective management systems and resources in all Member States for putting policies on environment and health into practice.
20. All people should have access to adequate supplies of safe drinking water and the pollution of groundwater sources, rivers, lakes and seas should no longer pose a threat to health.
21. Air quality in all countries should be improved to a point where recognised air pollutants do not pose a threat to public health.
22. Health risks due to micro-organisms or their toxins, to chemicals and to radioactivity in food should have been significantly reduced in all Member States.
23. Public health risks caused by solid and hazardous wastes and soil pollution should be effectively controlled in all Member States.
24. Cities, towns and rural communities throughout the Region should offer physical and social environments supportive to the health of their inhabitants.
25. The health of workers in all Member States should be improved by making work environments more healthy, reducing work-related disease and injury, and promoting the well-being of people at work.
26. All Member States should have developed, and be implementing, policies that ensure universal access to health services of quality, based on primary care and supported by secondary and tertiary care.
27. Health service systems in all Member States should be managed cost-effectively, with resources being distributed according to need.
28. Primary health care in all Member States should meet the basic health needs of the population by providing a wide range of health promotive, curative, rehabilitative and supportive services and by actively supporting self-help activities of individuals, families and groups.
29. Hospitals in all Member States should be providing cost-effective secondary and tertiary care and contribute actively to improving health status and patient satisfaction.
30. People in all Member States needing long-term care and support should have access to appropriate services of a high quality
31. There should be structures and processes in all Member States to ensure continuous improvements in the quality of health care and appropriate development and use of health technologies.
32. Health research should strengthen the acquisition and application of knowledge in support of health for all development in all Member States.
33. All Member States should have developed, and be implementing, policies in line with the concepts and principles of the European health for all policy, balancing lifestyle, environment and health service concerns.
34. Management structures and processes should exist in all Member States to inspire, guide, and coordinate health development, in line with health for all principles.
35. Health information systems in all Member States should actively support the formulation, implementation, monitoring and evaluation of health for all policies.
36. Education and training of health and other personnel in all Member States should actively contribute to the achievement of health for all.
37. In all Member States a wide range of organisations and groups throughout the public, private and voluntary sectors should be actively contributing to the achievement of health for all.
38. All Member States should have mechanisms in place to strengthen ethical considerations in decisions relating to the health of individuals, groups and populations.

Source: World Health Organisation, Regional Office for Europe *Health for All Targets: The Health Policy for Europe* Updated Edition September 1991 (WHO, 1993) reproduced with permission.

diseases such as meningitis and Legionnaire's disease. Meanwhile, failures of public health planning at local level and a shortage of medical expertise in environmental health were exposed by public inquiries into two serious outbreaks of infectious disease. The food poisoning incident at Stanley Royd Hospital in Wakefield, which claimed 19 lives (Cmnd 9716, 1986), and the outbreak of Legionnaire's disease at Stafford General Hospital where 39 people died (Cmnd 9772, 1986).

□　*The emergence of a health strategy*

The public concern generated by these incidents led to the establishment of a further inquiry by the Chief Medical Officer (then Sir Donald Acheson) into the problems of the public health function in England. The Acheson report suggested a number of changes which provided the basis for a more focused approach to public health (Cm 289, 1988). These included: a public health monitoring unit within the Department of Health, clearer definition of health authorities' responsibility for the health of their populations, appointment of directors of public health within each health authority to monitor and produce annual reports on the health of the local population, and closer monitoring of health authorities' performance with regard to public health.

Nevertheless, the Thatcher government remained opposed to the idea of a national health strategy, and only after Thatcher's departure in 1990 did it seem possible that such a strategy might emerge. After months of speculation the Major government published a Green Paper (Cm 1523, 1991), followed by the *Health of the Nation* White Paper (Cm 1986, 1992) that set out a health strategy for England.

■　The health strategy for England

The stated goal of the strategy was to secure continuing improvement in the health of the population. First by adding years to life, which means increasing life expectancy and reducing premature death, second by adding life to years, that is increasing the quality of life and minimising illness. At the heart of the plan was the selection of key areas, based on several criteria: that the health problem in question must be a major cause of premature death or avoidable ill-health; it must be responsive to effective intervention; and be amenable to the setting of objectives, targets and monitoring.

The Green Paper had set out a number of possible key areas, including causes of substantial mortality such as coronary heart disease, stroke, cancers and accidents. Causes of substantial ill-health such as mental

health problems, diabetes and asthma were also included. So were f
contributing to both mortality and morbidity such as smoking, al
consumption and lack of exercise. Areas where there was considerable
scope for improving health were identified, including the health of the
elderly, pregnant women, infants and children, dental health, rehabilitation of the physically disabled, back pain, drug misuse, and the
environment. Finally, a number of other health problems were identified
where there was great potential for harm, such as HIV/AIDS, other
communicable diseases such as hospital-acquired infections, and food
safety.

The White Paper narrowed these possibilities down. Some were
discarded because the government argued that they were already
sufficiently well-developed, including childhood immunisation, maternal
and child health, and food safety. Others were not designated as key areas
because, the government claimed, further research was needed before
national targets could be set. These included rehabilitation, the health of
the elderly, asthma, back pain and drug misuse. Three other possibilities –
diabetes, hospital-acquired infections and breastfeeding – were acknowledged by government as areas where improvements should occur but
nevertheless did not qualify for key area status.

The remaining five priorities – cancer; heart disease and stroke; mental
illness; HIV/AIDS and sexual health; and accidents – were regarded as
suitable key areas. Two types of targets were identified for each category.
Main targets, setting out reductions in the incidence of illness and
mortality in various key areas; and risk factor targets, aimed at tackling
some of the causes of these illnesses. These are detailed in Exhibit 12.2.

☐ Implementing the strategy

Central government's main contribution was to coordinate the activities of
the various departments of state. It introduced guidance on policy
appraisal and health, with the expressed intention of assessing all policies
in terms of their consequences for health. A ministerial cabinet committee
(involving ministers drawn from eleven government departments) was
established to oversee the implementation of the strategy for England and
to coordinate UK-wide issues affecting health. A number of other
committees were set up to support the ministerial committee: the 'Wider
Health Working Group' (chaired by a Health Minister); the 'Health
Priorities Working Group' (chaired by the Government's Chief Medical
Officer); and the 'Working Group on Implementation in the NHS' (chaired
by the NHS Chief Executive). In addition the Chief Medical Officer
chaired an interdepartmental group on public health comprising officials
from departments with public health interests.

Exhibit 12.2 The Health of the Nation: main targets and risk factor targets

Main targets

Coronary heart disease and stroke

Targets
- To reduce death rates in the under 65 age group for both coronary heart disease (CHD) and stroke by 40 per cent by the year 2000 (from a 1990 baseline).
- To reduce death rate for CHD in people aged 65–74 by at least 30 per cent by the year 2000 (from a 1990 baseline).
- To reduce death rate for stroke in people aged 65–74 by at least 40 per cent by the year 2000 (1990 baseline).

Cancer

Targets
- To reduce the death rate from breast cancer in the screened population by at least 25 per cent by the year 2000 (1990 baseline).
- To reduce the incidence of invasive cervical cancer by at least 20 per cent by the year 2000 (1986 baseline).
- To reduce the death rate for lung cancer under the age of 75 by at least 30 per cent in men and by at least 15 per cent in women by 2010 (1990 baseline).
- To halt the year-on-year increase in skin cancer by 2005.

Mental health

Targets
- To improve significantly the health and social functioning of mentally-ill people.
- To reduce the overall suicide rate by at least 15 per cent by the year 2000 (1990 baseline).
- To reduce the suicide rate of severely mentally-ill people by at least 33 per cent by the year 2000 (1990 baseline).

HIV/AIDS and sexual health

Targets
- To reduce the incidence of gonorrhoea by at least 20 per cent by 1995 (1990 baseline) as an indicator of HIV/AIDS trends.
- To reduce by at least 50 per cent the rate of conceptions among the under-16s by the year 2000 (1989 Baseline).

Accidents

Targets
- To reduce the death rate for accidents among children aged under 15 by at least 33 per cent by 2005 (1990 baseline).
- To reduce the death rate for accidents among young people aged 15–24 by at least 25 per cent by 2005 (1990 baseline).
- To reduce the death rate for accidents among people aged 65 and over by at least 33 per cent by 2005 (1990 baseline).

$\longrightarrow$

Exhibit 12.2 continued

⟶

Risk factor targets

Diet and nutrition

Targets

- To reduce the proportion of men drinking more than 21 units of alcohol (roughly 10.5 pints of beer) per week, and the proportion of women drinking more than 14 units per week, by 30 per cent by 2005 (1990 baseline).
- To reduce the proportion of obese men and women in the 16–64 age group by 25 per cent and 33 per cent respectively by 2005 (baseline, 1986/7).
- To reduce the average percentage of food energy derived by the population from saturated fat by at least 35 per cent by 2005 (baseline, 1990).
- To reduce the average percentage of food energy derived from total fat by the population by at least 12 per cent by 2005 (baseline, 1990).

Smoking

Targets

- To reduce the proportion of men and women smoking cigarettes to no more than 20 per cent by the year 2000 – a reduction of around a third (baseline, 1990).
- To reduce the consumption of cigarettes by 40 per cent by the year 2000 (baseline, 1990).
- To reduce the prevalence of smoking among 11–15 year olds by at least 33 per cent by 1994 (baseline, 1988).
- To reduce smoking among women at the start of pregnancy by at least 33 per cent by the year 2000.

Blood pressure

Target

- To reduce mean systolic blood pressure in the adult population by at least 5mm Hg by 2005 (baseline to be established by a new national survey).

HIV/AIDS

Target

- To reduce the percentage of injecting drug misusers who report sharing injecting equipment in the previous 4 weeks from 20 per cent in 1990 to no more than 10 per cent by 1997 and no more than 5 per cent by the year 2000.

Note: In 1996 the Major government announced its intention to make the environment the sixth key area. Five topic areas were identified for the purpose of setting targets: outdoor air quality, indoor air quality, radon concentrations, lead concentrations in drinking water, and noise levels. The *Health of the Nation* strategy is likely to undergo further changes following the change of government in 1997; the Labour government signalled its commitment to alter the targets to reflect the impact of poverty, unemployment and poor housing on health.

Source: The Health of the Nation, Cm 1986, 1992.

The NHS was expected to operate within the framework of the national health strategy. Health authorities' role in monitoring the health of their populations, promoting health, and planning services in relation to needs was set out following the Acheson report. It was also thought that, in view of their commissioning role within the new internal market, health authorities would shift resources towards strategies that would maximise health, thereby re-emphasising the importance of health promotion and preventive medicine alongside care and treatment services.

Health authorities were expected to collaborate with other agencies in an attempt to tackle the main health problems identified by national strategy and local plans. Regional coordinators were subsequently appointed, to assist with the implementation process by ensuring the dissemination of good practice. The NHSE also established 'focus groups' for each of the key areas, to emphasise their importance within the NHS. In addition, collaboration between the NHS and other agencies was promoted by the formation of task forces, incorporating individuals from government, business, the NHS, and academia. Their function was to draw up coordinated programmes of action for specific areas of the strategy, to promote cooperation between the parties involved and to ensure effective implementation.

Collaboration was a central theme of the new strategy. Local authorities were identified as key collaborators given their responsibilities for environmental health. Other agencies such as the Health Education Authority, the voluntary sector, the media and employers were also identified, and were expected to cooperate and collaborate with government agencies.

The government promoted the formation of 'healthy alliances' to improve health in the key areas. In some localities alliances already existed to promote healthy eating, to combat smoking-related illness, and to prevent sexually transmitted diseases. Several settings were identified as possible arenas where healthy alliances could flourish: 'healthy cities', 'healthy schools', 'healthy hospitals', 'healthy homes', 'healthy work-places', 'healthy prisons' and 'healthy environments'.

Finally, a series of measures were announced in an effort to improve the information base for public health decision-making. These included more surveys of health and illness, a public health information strategy, and new research and development priorities to reflect the health strategy.

☐ *The impact of the health strategy and further developments*

Many were cynical about the impact of the new coordination arrangements within central government. Other government departments resisted efforts to align their policy objectives to those of the Health departments. There were renewed calls for a minister for public health to coordinate health aspects of policy-making, but the Major government resisted this. However, on taking office in 1997 the Blair government did create such a post.

Critics of the Major government's health strategy pointed out the inconsistencies between the health strategy and other reforms, in particular the internal market (Moran, 1989; Ewles, 1993), and the subsequent structural reorganisation of the mid-1990s. Although, as suggested earlier, purchasing authorities had a greater incentive to commission services more relevant to the promotion of public health, they did not necessarily do this. A key factor was the lack of new resources for public health initiatives which limited the ability of purchasers to move towards a prevention-orientated strategy.

The internal market undermined public health strategy in a number of ways. The fragmentation of the NHS into purchasers and providers made it difficult to take a broad overview of the population's health needs (Whitty and Pollock, 1992). This also added to the problems of collaboration between the NHS and other agencies (Nocon, 1993; Delaney, 1994). However, despite this some 'healthy alliances' flourished, encouraged to a limited extent by a national award scheme introduced in 1994 recognising good practice (Trevett, 1997).

The restructuring of the NHS that followed the introduction of the internal market had additional implications for public health. Regional directors of public health became civil servants, and some believed this would compromise their ability to speak out independently on public health matters (see Chadda, 1996). The reorganisation of public health functions following the demise of the RHAs was also viewed suspiciously. Many functions were devolved to the district health authority level, and there were fears that this would lead to further fragmentation of responsibility for public health.

Central government did respond by clarifying the responsibilities for public health at every level within the NHS (DoH, 1994h). Regional directors of public health were charged with ensuring collaboration between the health authorities within their region, and health authorities were expected to develop local health strategies and alliances necessary to implement these plans. In addition, health authority boards were required to include a director of public health as an executive member. In response to concerns about coordination, the Major government re-emphasised the role of the public health network – a system of national and local committees designed to improve the exchange of information between public health practitioners at all levels. It is too early to tell whether these efforts to improve collaboration have been successful or not.

The *Health of the Nation's* focus on specific health targets was also challenged. Some believed that an emphasis on targets downgraded health problems that were serious but which could not easily be quantified (Faculty of Public Health Medicine, 1991b). In addition the justification for many of the targets was based on inadequate scientific evidence (Akehurst, Godfrey and Robertson, 1991). Furthermore, the targets chosen reflected a medical rather than a social perspective, as the Radical Statistics Health Group (1991) observed. As a result the targets related more to the prevention of specific diseases rather than to the promotion of health of the community and of particularly vulnerable groups. It was also argued that some of the targets were not as tough as they appeared, and most would be achieved anyway if current trends continued (Mooney and Healey, 1991). This may partly explain why in many of the key areas, the targets have been achieved (DoH, 1995j); even so, the National Audit Office (1996c) discovered good progress in less than half of the 27 target areas. There are three areas where progress has been poor. Women's alcohol consumption, smoking among children, and obesity in both men and women. The proportion of women drinking above recommended sensible levels rose from 11 per cent to 13 per cent between 1990–94. Smoking among 11–15 year olds increased from 8 per cent to 12 per cent between 1988–94. Meanwhile the proportion of obese adult males of working age rose from 7 per cent in 1986 to 13 per cent by 1994. Over the same period, obesity among women rose from 12 per cent to 16 per cent.

These underperforming areas reveal the limits to which government was prepared to intervene to promote health in the period following the publication of the White Paper. The Major government, like its predecessor, resisted strong pressure to ban tobacco advertising. This was in spite of evidence that a ban could be effective in reducing smoking (DoH, 1992c; White *et al.*, 1996). It was also reluctant to take on the alcohol industry. In 1995 it reduced the 'safe drinking' limits for alcohol in spite of warnings from the majority of medical opinion, charities dealing with alcohol abuse and other organisations, including the World Health Organisation. In addition it refused to impose further restrictions on the sale of so-called 'alcopops', special designer drinks which, researchers have shown, appeal to children (Hughes *et al.*, 1997). However it did impose a higher level of duty on these products in the 1996 budget, bringing them into line with those levied on other alcoholic drinks. The Blair government subsequently introduced new proposals to tackle under-age drinking.

In addition the Major government was keen to avoid confrontation with the food industry which remained a powerful lobby group during the 1990s. The industry vigorously opposed some of the activities of government-sponsored bodies such as the Committee on the Medical Aspects of Food (COMA), the Health Education Authority, and the

Nutrition Task Force. Significantly the latter was abolished after unsuccessfully recommending a large-scale official campaign to promote healthy eating (DoH/NTF, 1996a). Its fate was perhaps sealed by the report of the project team (DoH/NTF, 1996b) which called for a strategy to improve nutrition for those on low incomes. Furthermore, in 1994 it was announced that the Health Education Authority, which has often upset vested interests in the past, would have its annual grant withdrawn and would instead compete for government contracts, further reducing its autonomy and independence. This followed earlier controversies which led to its reconstitution as a health authority rather than a semi-independent board during 1980s. Finally, COMA which comprises medical and scientific experts in the field of diet and health was vociferously attacked by the food industry for its recommendations to reduce consumption of products which have a high sugar and fat content (COMA, 1994; *Economist*, 1994).

In the 1980s and 1990s there has been a crisis in public confidence about the state's ability to safeguard public health, particularly where commercial interests are involved. This was clearly illustrated by the BSE crisis (Ford, 1996). In March 1996, after years of denials, the government finally recognised the possibility of a link between BSE in cattle and a similar disease – Creutzfeldt-Jakob disease (CJD) – in humans. The claims of those who warned of such a link in the mid-1980s had been ignored (Lacey, 1994), and in retrospect their views should have been taken more seriously by government. Instead it appears that the short-term interests of the farming, feed and food processing industries prevailed, though ultimately this cost them dear as the market for British beef collapsed amid consumer panic and a worldwide export ban imposed by the European Union.

Serious food poisoning outbreaks continued to undermine confidence in the public health system during the mid-1990s. In November 1996, for example, there was a major outbreak of *E-coli* food poisoning in Lanarkshire, Scotland which affected almost 500 people, 20 of whom later died. The inquiry into the incident called among other things for more research into the disease, better surveillance and reporting systems for food poisoning, improved coordination plans between health and local authorities, and tougher controls on premises handling meat products, including a licensing system for such establishments (Scottish Office, 1996b, 1997).

Although the *E-coli* inquiry related specifically to Scotland, it had a wider impact. The Major government reacted by proposing an independent food safety advisor, supported by a food safety council. Others, including the Labour Party, called for an independent food agency to ensure high standards of food quality. Following its election victory in

1997, Labour re-affirmed its commitment to the establishment of such an agency.

Further criticism was levelled at the Major government's failure to consider the role of inequality and social deprivation in ill-health. In the Appendix to its Green Paper the Major government admitted that the WHO's regional target of reducing health inequalities by at least 25 per cent by the year 2000 would probably not be achieved. The relationship between poverty and ill-health was not explicitly discussed in either the Green or White Paper. A section on the relationship between housing and ill-health, which allegedly appeared in an earlier draft, was omitted from the final published version of the Green Paper. In the White Paper healthy homes were identified as a 'setting' on which to focus, but no clear commitments made to improving poor housing conditions or reducing homelessness. The government merely stated that it would 'continue to pursue its policies to promote choice and quality in housing, having regard to health and other benefits' (Cm 1986, 1992, p. 28).

Following the publication of the White Paper, the Department of Health found it difficult to ignore the evidence regarding health inequalities and the public health aspects of poverty, deprivation and economic inequality (see Benzeval, Judge and Whitehead, 1995). Pressure came not only from the political left, but from within the NHS and particularly from health professionals (who were often reminded of the relationship between socio-economic conditions and health in everyday practice; see BMA, 1995b; Health Visitors' Association, 1996).

The Department responded by establishing a review of 'health variations' (rather than the more politically-charged term 'inequalities'). Although the review was undertaken by experts in the field, it was confined to what the NHS and the Department of Health could do about the problem. Its report accepted that 'an important way of achieving *Health of the Nation* targets is by improving the health of the least healthy groups to the levels attained by the most healthy groups' (DoH, 1995k, p. 74). However, its recommendations were rather weak, the main focus being placed on health authorities and commissioning groups at local level to identify and tackle variations and coordinate action.

On a more positive note, the Department and other research bodies began to invest in research into health variations (DoH, 1995k). In the longer run this is likely to reinforce calls for more comprehensive action to tackle health inequalities. The election of a Labour government in 1997 which stated a commitment to tackle the social and economic roots of ill-health added to this momentum. The Blair government launched a review of health inequalities and explored ways of amending the *Health of the Nation* targets so that they would reflect the impact of deprivation on health.

■ Conclusion

Many factors lay behind the revival of public health: growing media interest in environmental and public health issues; the Thatcher and Major governments' support for certain prevention policies; and pressures from within the NHS, from local authorities and from international agencies to adopt public health strategies.

Following its election in 1997 the Labour government stated its commitment to tackling the social and economic roots of illness, proposed a food standards agency and initiated plans for a ban on tobacco advertising and sponsorship.* It also introduced new plans to tackle under-age drinking and drug abuse. The new government created a minister for public health and explored ways of strengthening intersectoral collaboration within government and between local government and the NHS. It also examined the public health functions of the NHS and launched a review of the *Health of the Nation* targets. A Green Paper (*Our Healthier Nation*), outlining the Blair government's plans on public health, will be published in 1998.

Such developments will strengthen the public health approach. But the power of vested interests – commercial, professional and bureaucratic – should never be underestimated. Commercial interests have wealth and political influence to bring to bear. In addition, the dominant professional interests are closely tied to care and treatment services and are likely to oppose radical moves to shift resources towards prevention. Similarly, bureaucracies both within the NHS and in central government can be expected to resist initiatives which subvert their arenas of decision-making to a broader philosophy based on public health.

Note: The government granted a controversial exemption for Formula 1 racing, arguing that the sport could evade the sponsorship ban by moving to other locations. It then became known that prior to the General Election the Labour Party had accepted a large donation (subsequently returned) from the vice-president of the Formula 1 Association. Both parties involved denied that the donation was linked to influence over policy. Meanwhile the European Union was considering a directive banning tobacco advertising and sponsorship and it was believed that the UK's actions could prevent agreement on this issue. Eventually a compromise was reached when Formula 1 racing was given extra time to comply with the proposed directive.

■ *Chapter 13* ■

Conclusion

■ The challenges

As this book has shown, the British health care system continues to face a number of significant challenges. These include: demographic pressures; rising expectations; changing patterns of illness; premature mortality and preventable morbidity; mental illness; the persistence of variations in health status; economic constraints; and technological factors.

A number of important strategic, resource and accountability issues must be resolved if these health challenges are to be tackled effectively. First, it is vital that the health care system has a clear purpose. Its various parts must collaborate effectively to achieve stated objectives. Furthermore, as much illness is shaped by social, economic and environmental trends, a broad perspective incorporating these factors should be adopted when setting policy objectives in other sectors such as food, transport, housing, education, the environment and taxation.

Second, the availability and allocation of health care resources must be considered in the light of changing needs. In particular, the level of public funding for health care deserves closer scrutiny. It is important that a consensus be established regarding the appropriate mix of private, voluntary and public health care. In addition, given the scarcity of resources relative to need it is vital that funding, irrespective of source, is allocated efficiently, effectively and equitably.

Third, there is a need for greater accountability in health care. Improved financial accountability is, of course, an important goal. There must also be greater accountability and responsiveness to the users of health services, particularly as health and social care needs become more complex and as public expectations rise. In addition, the accountability of the NHS must be clarified both with regard to central government and to the communities it serves.

■ The ideas and the reforms

□ *Ideas*

As we noted in Chapter 5, almost all health care systems in the industrialised countries face similar challenges and have embarked upon a search for policy solutions. Specific proposals vary between countries but there are a number of common themes: a growing interest in managed competition between providers of health care; more emphasis on monitoring the effectiveness, cost and quality of health care; greater encouragement of primary care and care in community settings; and a sharper focus on public health strategies. These themes all featured in health care reforms undertaken in Britain in the 1980s and 1990s.

During the postwar period the problems facing the British health care system were countered mainly by reorganisation and restructuring. By and large such changes were intentionally cautious and incremental. New structures were either grafted on to existing ones, or bore strong similarities to those they replaced. New planning, management and resource allocation systems introduced in the 1970s had a more radical edge, but were implemented in an incremental fashion and in practice represented marginal rather than radical reform.

The Conservative government of Margaret Thatcher was more open to radical proposals. Its policies reflected many aspects of the economic critique of health care outlined in Chapter 3, viewing the NHS as an inefficient, public sector bureaucracy, largely unaccountable for the resources it consumed, and dominated by self-interested professionals. The Thatcher and Major governments favoured more evaluation and control of professional activity, placed greater emphasis on financial and managerial accountability, saw a greater role for markets and the private sector, and emphasised the role of the patient as a consumer of health care. Conservative administrations also drew on other critiques of health care and of orthodox medicine. The public health model was viewed sympathetically because it enabled greater emphasis upon individual responsibility for health, raising the possibility of saving resources through prevention. There was also an element of technological pessimism in the Conservatives' policies, again mainly on cost grounds.

Unwittingly perhaps, the antagonism of the Conservative governments (particularly the Thatcher government during the late 1980s) towards the medical profession had some affinity with the anti-medical thesis of Illich (1975). The feminist critique too had some influence on the context of debate. The Thatcher and Major governments responded with initiatives to make health services more responsive to women's needs, notably in the area of maternity services, and measures to improve the career prospects of female doctors.

Socialist ideas, in contrast, had little impact on policy during the 1980s and 1990s. This was reflected in the Conservative government's endorsement of market forces in health care, the refusal to admit that poor social and economic conditions were associated with ill-health, and the failure to accept that commercial interests had the capacity to undermine the nation's health.

☐ *Policies*

Nevertheless, as Wistow (1992) observed, the basic principles of the NHS survived. The Thatcher government learned at an early stage that NHS reform must be handled with care. Following the political uproar over allegations of health care privatisation in the early 1980s there was a return to a more cautious and pragmatic approach. Private health care and competitive tendering were encouraged and a more 'businesslike' management style was pursued within the NHS. But the implementation of reform was gradual, reflecting the political sensitivity of health care issues and the practical difficulties associated with change. Moreover, despite the rhetoric about devolving management responsibility, central government found itself taking an even closer interest in the detailed operation of health services. Meanwhile the Conservatives continued to spend large amounts of public money on health care, and were not afraid to boast about their commitment to the NHS in order to placate the electorate.

The prospects for radical change improved following the announcement of the NHS review in 1988. Although those on the political right were disappointed because a tax-funded system of health care was retained, the proposals set out in *Working for Patients* were nevertheless potentially far-reaching. However, the unpopularity of the reforms before the General Election of 1992 , combined with the practical problems of introducing the reforms quickly, meant that it was necessary to implement the changes in a gradual manner and a 'no surprises' approach prevailed.

Following Thatcher's departure, Conservative health policy continued to shift towards a more pragmatic approach. Some of the initiatives introduced by the Major government, notably market testing and the private finance initiative, were identified as ideological threats to the NHS. But they encountered a number of practical problems at the implementation stage and did not have as dramatic an impact as originally envisaged. Meanwhile, the Major government continued to regulate and intervene in the internal market until it looked less and less like the intellectual models devised in the late 1980s. Basic service standards in the form of *The Patient's Charter* were introduced and an overall health strategy was set out in the *Health of the Nation* document. The Major government reformed the internal market – reorganising the structure of the NHS, introducing new arrangements for planning and accountability, and embarking on a drive to reduce transactions and management costs.

The Conservatives' health policy addressed other concerns, such as the need to emphasise public health and to expand primary and community care. The tone of these policies reflected the government's pro-market principles, yet in practice there was a considerable degree of pragmatism and in some cases a departure from these principles. For example the Thatcher government's approach to community care produced a massive increase in public spending on residential care. It later accepted that local authorities should have the lead role in community care despite its hostility towards them. Radical proposals in primary care were toned down and amendments made to the controversial GP contract of 1990. The national health strategy adopted by the Major Government in 1992 can be seen as another change of direction, the Thatcher government having earlier rejected this approach.

■ A health care system for the 21st century?

After almost two decades of continuous reform, one might reasonably expect the health care system to be better equipped to deal with the challenges it faces. However, the sheer number and scope of the reforms, the absence of a proper evaluation programme, and shifts in government policy over time have made it extremely difficult to assess the impact of the changes (Ham, 1994; Powell, 1997).

Nevertheless, some developments have been viewed more positively than others. The Conservative governments placed a greater deal of emphasis on primary care, community care and public health. These reforms, though criticised on several grounds, at least focused attention on these neglected backwaters of health policy. Meanwhile the encouragement of the voluntary sector during this period was broadly welcomed in spite of warnings that it might displace statutory services.

The Conservatives' concern with management and efficiency in health care highlighted issues too long ignored. While the systems of management and cost-control introduced by the Thatcher and Major governments attracted criticism, with some justification, they nevertheless stimulated debate about important issues such as the measurement of costs, monitoring of service quality, effectiveness of interventions, assessment of needs, and the importance of setting clear objectives.

The management reforms and other policies such as the internal market provided to some extent a countervailing force to the medical profession. Given the various criticisms of the profession's dominance of health care (from across the political spectrum) this too may be seen in a positive light. Doctors (and other health professionals) should be accountable for their clinical actions and for the resources they use. They should also be sensitive to the needs of users. Although doctors remain powerful, the managerial reforms of the 1980s and 1990s have at the very least placed these issues on the agenda.

The division between purchasers (or in the current preferred terminology, commissioners) and providers of health care is credited by some with improving both health service planning and the use of resources. It is argued that commissioners can now focus more on identifying the health needs of the population and securing an appropriate package of clinically-effective services. Meanwhile providers can concentrate on managing their activities in such a way as to meet these needs. The value of this division of responsibilities is indicated by the fact that all the main political parties now endorse it in principle. However, the benefits of this division have not been fully realised in practice. Indeed, there is more than one model of the commissioner–provider division. The version introduced by the Conservatives was justly criticised for its high transaction costs and its negative impact on collaborative planning

☐ *Problems associated with the internal market reforms*

The Conservatives' internal market reforms were criticised on a number of grounds. Markets have a poor record in relation to health care, and internal markets have the potential to create similar problems of inequity. Without effective systems of regulation, 'high-risk' individuals – those who need health services the most – and users of 'unprofitable' services are likely to be marginalised. As a means of rationing scarce health care resources markets are a crude device. Because purchasing power does not necessarily correlate with need, services may be inappropriately and inefficiently allocated; greater variations in access and service quality are likely and there is some evidence to suggest this has happened.

Markets can frustrate planning and collaborative arrangements. Competitors have an incentive to avoid sharing information with each other, yet such communications are a necessary part of the health care planning process. The fragmentation of purchasers and providers compounds the difficulties of communication and collaboration. Following the creation of the NHS there was much evidence of these problems, particularly with relation to GP fundholders and trusts. Since then a new planning framework has sought to encourage greater collaboration at local level.

The introduction of the internal market incurred high administrative and regulatory costs. Some were associated with the establishment of the market, but others – such as the employment of staff to monitor and operate the market – were ongoing. The extra overhead and running costs incurred by the market offset to a considerable extent the efficiency gains claimed by its adherents.

□ *Public expenditure and efficiency*

Although public expenditure has risen, Britain continues to spend less on health care than comparable countries. As we saw in Chapter 7, there is evidence of underfunding both in relation to changing needs and the rising cost of health services. There is some scope for bridging this gap by improving efficiency. The Conservative governments of Thatcher and Major emphasised this approach as a means of securing extra resources for patient care. The Blair government has also stressed that additional resources must be generated internally by reorganisation and improvements in efficiency. However, there is a limit to the amount of money which can be produced by efficiency gains. Moreover, crude cost-cutting can cause inefficiency if it inhibits the development of services which in the long run may be more cost-effective.

In recent years there has been greater emphasis on explicit rationing of public sector resources, and this has been combined with a drive to encourage clinically-effective health care. It is of course important that health care resources be spent wisely on services where health gain can be maximised. However, the enthusiasm for new decision-making techniques in this field must not obscure the fact that there are important ethical and equity considerations to be taken into account. In addition some of the techniques promoted as aids to resource allocation and to decision-makers are rather insensitive to the needs of the individual patients.

□ *Private health care*

During the 1980s and 1990s government policy explicitly encouraged the private sector, both as a source of new finance and as an alternative mode of provision. As a result the private sector has grown rapidly, though the NHS remains the dominant funder and provider of health care in the UK.

There is still little consensus about the future of private health care. Supporters claim that it is a kind of safety valve for the NHS. It is seen by them as a model for the NHS in several respects, in particular with regard to the development of financial information systems and customer-responsiveness. Its opponents criticise the expansion of private health care for enabling widespread rationing by price for non-emergency treatments. In this way it is alleged that the private sector underpins a 'two-tier system', with different standards of care depending on ability to pay. The private sector is also seen as a drain on NHS resources by employing doctors and nurses trained at public expense. It is argued that the growth of the private sector has been unplanned, haphazard and is unrelated to health needs. In some areas, such as dentistry and longer term care critics argue that privatisation has occurred by default as a result of a deliberate attempt to curb public funding and provision.

The interdependence between private and public sectors must be addressed. The two can co-exist in their mutual interest. Joint working arrangements have expanded in recent years, and in view of the private finance initiative will increase further in the future. However, such arrangements must be monitored carefully to ensure that public funding of private care (as well as private funding of publicly-provided care) is appropriate, efficient and equitable. In addition, joint service developments must operate inside a broader framework of regulation and planning which ensures that the activities of the private sector are consistent with health care objectives, policies and standards.

Finally, it has been remarked with some irony that the commercialisation of the NHS in the 1990s has presented a serious challenge to the private sector. The internal market provided private hospitals with new and formidable competitors in the shape of NHS trusts. The private sector also began to face similar problems of competition in the social care sector, as noted in Chapter 10. Indeed private operators may well benefit from a more tightly regulated market in future if this allows protection from powerful public sector competitors. It is also possible that they may be persuaded to accept further restrictions on their own activities and participate more fully in planning and collaborative processes.

☐ *Management and accountability*

Turning now to the management reforms introduced by the Conservative governments during the 1980s and 1990s, despite the professed aims of these reforms central government continued to involve itself in operational matters. The formal separation of policy and management did not reduce ministerial intervention, nor did it entirely exempt ministers from responsibility when things went seriously wrong. However to some extent central government was able to distance itself from the problems faced by the NHS at local level, and from controversial decisions made by local managers, particularly with regard to rationing services.

At the same time local managers and professionals retained considerable influence over the implementation of policies and initiatives. They had considerable scope to develop their own local arrangements with regard to commissioning and needs-assessment in the context of performance targets set out by the centre. Nevertheless, the management structure of the NHS became more centralised and politicised during the 1980s and 1990s. As a result central government appeared to have far more scope to influence and manipulate the NHS for party political reasons than was previously the case.

The Conservatives' reforms added to confusion about the accountability and the responsibilities of the various tiers of the NHS. In 1996 a further re-organisation was undertaken: the regional health authorities were abolished, and mergers between local health authorities took place. It remains to be seen whether or not these changes have clarified the responsibilities of NHS bodies and enhanced their accountability.

There has been much concern about the public accountability of the NHS, particularly in the 1990s. In 1990, health authorities were reconstituted as management boards and were no longer obliged to contain local councillors. There was no requirement that their membership be constituted in such a way as to be representative of the local community. Not surprisingly, the under-representation of certain groups – younger people, women and ethnic groups – persisted. Others, such as political and business interests, were arguably over-represented. Another related issue was the lack of openness in the NHS. It was alleged that health authorities and other NHS bodies were reluctant to meet in public and were becoming more secretive.

In the 1990s, the Major government made a number of attempts to allay fears about public accountability and openness by changing appointments procedures, introducing codes of practice on accountability and openness, and urging NHS bodies to be more open with the public and with each other. However, these initiatives did little to arrest the growing culture of secrecy within the NHS which was reinforced by other factors. These included greater official secrecy as a result of the centralisation of the NHS management structure, while at the same time the advent of the internal market and joint ventures with the private sector led to an increasing emphasis on commercial secrecy.

Finally, under the Conservative government much effort went into the strengthening of financial accountability. Yet, paradoxically, this activity coincided with revelations about fraud and financial mismanagement. This of course may have reflected the greater effectiveness of audit procedures introduced during the 1980s and 1990s. On the other hand it could be argued that the commercialisation of the NHS, along with reforms and initiatives which reflected private sector ideals, created greater scope for actions regarded as inappropriate if not fraudulent within a public sector context.

☐ *The culture of the NHS*

The Thatcher and Major governments sought to change the culture of the NHS, to make it more businesslike. The Griffiths' management reforms and other NHS management initiatives sought to instil private sector management values into the service. Subsequently, the internal market introduced incentives that rewarded flexibility and entrepreneurial behaviour.

Did the culture of the NHS change as a result of these reforms? Cultural change is extremely difficult to measure, particularly in the short-term. However, one can make some observations. First, there is evidence of innovative activity, as exemplified by the diverse ways in which local NHS bodies responded to the new context. Positive changes in areas such as waiting times, diagnostic testing and hospital discharge appear to have resulted. However, the gains have not been uniform and may have been exaggerated by those with a stake in the success of such schemes.

NHS bodies have shown a greater readiness to engage in commercial enterprise and to adopt private sector management techniques. There is some evidence of a more entrepreneurial approach within health authorities and trusts (Ferlie, 1994), though some NHS organisations have been more resistant to change than others (Ranade, 1995b). Hence the variation in the adoption of market-testing, joint ventures and private finance schemes among health authorities and trusts (Decker, 1995).

There is little to suggest that the medical, nursing or other health professions shifted in their attitude to management or that they internalised entrepreneurial values to a significant degree with the possible exception of a minority of GPs (Harrison and Pollitt, 1994; Laughlin and Broadbent, 1994; Walby and Greenwell, 1994; Whynes, 1997). As noted in Chapter 6, the professions, particularly the medical profession, remain powerful and most managers realise that real and lasting change can only be brought about by persuasion. Doctors are still reluctant to undertake a management role, although GP fundholders again might be held up as a counter-example; yet even fundholders have expressed concern about their management workload. Moreover, the conversion of many GPs to fundholding perhaps had more to do with seizing an opportunity to redress the balance of power between themselves and hospital consultants than with cultural change.

☐ *Primary care, community care and public health*

The growing interest of policy-makers in community care, primary care and public health during the 1980s and 1990s was welcomed by most observers, though specific reforms attracted criticism. Changes in primary care were criticised for being too narrowly focused and too closely geared to the activities of the family practitioner professions (in particular GPs). The 'privatisation' of certain areas of primary care – such as NHS dentistry – and increased charges for optical and dental services were attacked for their impact on access to services. Furthermore, progress in the field of primary care was hampered by the deterioration in the relationship between the government and the family practitioner professions over new contracts.

The primary care reforms were poorly integrated with other key reforms in secondary care, community care and public health. Some reforms, notably GP fundholding, were at odds with the top-down managerial approach promoted within primary care and with efforts to promote coherent planning. Moreover, there was little attempt to blend in the primary care reforms with changes in community care in spite of the interdependence of the two sectors.

The often deplorable level of collaboration between the NHS and other agencies involved in community care has been well-documented. Critics of the Conservative government's community care policy highlighted the repeated delays which have prevented the kind of long-term planning urgently needed here. Both primary care and community care policies were criticised for encouraging commercial provision in areas where its contribution was at the very least unproven. There was particular criticism of the increasing reliance on informal carers in the absence of an adequate framework of support services.

The public health reforms introduced by the Conservatives, though seen by many as a step in the right direction, were regarded as fairly lightweight in a number of respects. The reluctance to tackle the social roots of ill-health and the failure to stand up to commercial interests was regarded as an indication of this weakness. Moreover, the setting of national health objectives, such as those listed in *The Health of the Nation* White Paper, did not sit easily with the fragmented, competitive market outlined in *Working for Patients*.

☐ *The impact on the public and patients*

The general public has always had a strong commitment to the NHS. Despite the well-publicised problems of the service during the 1980s and 1990s, the public retained its commitment to the fundamental principles of the NHS – a comprehensive service, available to all and free at the point of use (Jowell *et al.*, 1992; Bosanquet, 1994; Taylor-Gooby, 1995). But this was accompanied, paradoxically, by a greater willingness to use the private sector, a trend which threatened to undermine these principles.

The public also became more openly critical of the performance of the NHS, and this was reflected in the rising tide of complaints about the service. Attitude surveys detected increasing dissatisfaction with services provided. The British Social Attitudes survey calculated that the overall level of public dissatisfaction with the NHS increased from a quarter of the population to almost a half between 1983 and 1990, falling to 38 per cent by 1993 (Bosanquet, 1994). This survey also found high levels of dissatisfaction with particular services, such as outpatient and GP appointment systems, and long waiting lists.

While the public was prepared to be more openly critical of the NHS, it nevertheless reacted negatively to the Conservative government's reform programme, in particular the internal market. Between a half and three-quarters of the public were opposed to this policy at the time of its introduction. Opposition softened later, but many people continued to express concern about the changes. In 1994, the Conservatives were so concerned about the public reaction to its reforms that the deputy chairman of the Party, in an internal memorandum, called for 'zero media coverage' of the NHS in the run up to the next General Election. This came to naught. Health issues remain at the top of the political agenda, with a majority of people – over two thirds in most polls – naming health as one of the main issues facing the nation, and health services as the most important of the public services (Worcester, 1996; *The Times*, 1997).

Attitude surveys give an impression of the general public's view on health care, though as Judge and Solomon (1993) rightly warn they should be interpreted with caution. For example perceptions of change may relate more to media coverage than personal experience (see Karpf, 1988). Even when patients experience positive changes they may not attribute this to reform. Indeed, some of the changes in health care have arisen to some extent independently of the government's policies, such as many of the technological advances discussed in Chapter 3.

Yet the NHS reforms of the 1980s and 1990s undoubtedly had an impact on patient care over and above such changes in therapy. It is perhaps too early to make any final judgements on these reforms. Up to now the impact has been mixed: some patients have benefited from the shorter waiting times following the internal market, performance tables and *The Patient's Charter*, although as noted in Chapter 11 these statistics should be treated with caution.

Some patients seem to have benefited from the introduction of GP fundholding. They appear to have enjoyed quicker, more responsive service. It is difficult to escape the accusations of a two-tier service, notwithstanding arguments that the evidence is not conclusive or that the inequities identified are only short-term.

Something that patients will have noticed is the rising public relations profile of the NHS. Glossy brochures and leaflets abound. Marketing strategies and patients' charters may for a time convince patients and the wider public that all is well, but they won't in the long run obscure the perception of real service standards should these fail to match expectations. It is perhaps too early to tell whether or not services have actually become more responsive to users. There is little to suggest that patients have displayed consumerist values or that doctors are competing for patients in a way envisaged by the architects of the internal market reform. While there is evidence that many GP fundholders (and some non-fundholders) have sought to make services more responsive to the needs of patients, only a minority have so far actually made such changes.

The Major government emphasised the importance of the patient's perspective and listening to local opinion. *The Patient's Charter* and the *Local Voices* initiatives, discussed at length in Chapter 11, created a favourable environment in which some NHS organisations were able to experiment with various schemes to monitor local opinion and to involve patients. Although some of the initiatives were promising, it would be an exaggeration to say patients have been significantly empowered as a result. Furthermore, as mentioned earlier, other reforms inhibited a more open and consultative approach, thereby undermining public participation.

■ The future

In 1988 the Social Services Committee of the House of Commons commented that 'any new system of funding or delivering health care must be broadly agreed between the major parties. If it is not, it may not stand the test of time' (House of Commons, 1988c, p. ix). The ultimate test of any reform is its ability to withstand a change of government. The introduction of national health insurance in 1911 and the creation of the NHS in 1948 illustrate that it is possible to introduce durable reforms, even when opposition is strong at the time of their introduction.

During the 1980s, the health policies of the opposition parties differed considerably from those of the Conservative government. Both the Labour and Liberal Democrat parties argued strongly that the NHS was underfunded and called for a substantial increase in public spending on health. These parties disagreed with the Conservative government's management reforms and criticised specific policies in the field of community care, primary care and public health. However, the deepest divisions between the government and opposition parties were over privatisation and the internal market. Both opposition parties set out plans to abolish the internal market prior to the General Election in 1992 (Labour Party, 1992b; Liberal Democrats, 1992). Labour's policy was regarded as being particularly hostile to the involvement of private sector.

By the mid-1990s, however, Labour and the Liberal Democrats had come round to accept many of the changes introduced by the Conservatives. By the same token Conservative policies began to reflect some of the concerns raised by the opposition parties. Under the Major government the modification of the internal market arose from political criticism as well as practical difficulties of implementation. Moreover, policies such as *The Patient's Charter* and the *Health of the Nation* owed a significant debt to the opposition parties, which had earlier endorsed these ideas. In addition there were a number of issues on which all parties broadly agreed, such as the reform of complaints procedures and the promotion of clinical effectiveness.

The health policy documents issued by the opposition parties from 1992 onwards revealed their acceptance of key aspects of the Conservatives' reforms. The Liberal Democrats argued that 'those who propose the reversal of all the recent NHS reforms are living in the past' (Liberal Democrats, 1995, p. 8). A Labour Party document of the same year stated that 'it is clear that it is neither possible nor desirable to turn the clock back. Nor is there any appetite in the health service for huge upheaval. We do not intend to replace one dogmatic approach with another.'(Labour Party, 1995, p. 3)

Even where explicit commitments were made to reverse policies, such as Labour's pledge to abolish the internal market, closer inspection revealed much in common with the Conservatives' approach. Labour accepted the 'purchaser–provider split' and the need for explicit agreements on the quality and level of services provided. The party remained opposed to GP fundholding, though it later began to back-pedal on this too. There was also a softening of the stance on private sector involvement. Although the commitment to abolish certain tax reliefs on private health insurance remained, the Labour leadership began to support the use of private finance for NHS capital projects.

During the 1990s the opposition parties began to accept the importance of the issues identified by the Conservatives. Namely restraining public expenditure, improving 'value for money', encouraging voluntarism and self-help, exploring alternative sources of finance, the development of new managerialist techniques, and the extension of consumer choice. Operating within the constraints of this agenda the Liberal Democrat and Labour Party leaderships were reluctant to commit much in the way of additional public resources to health care. Both began to concede that there were limits to state care, accepting for example a larger role for the voluntary sector. Furthermore, they increasingly focused on the ways of improving efficiency, quality of service and consumer responsiveness, thereby accepting other key aspects of the Conservatives' reform agenda

How can the vitriolic debates over health care reform be squared with the gradual acceptance of important principles and assumptions under-lying the Conservatives policies? One explanation is that there has been a moving consensus (Rose and Davies, 1995) in health care. Despite the hostility between government and the opposition parties on health care issues, certain factors have led policies to converge in the longer term.

Governments, both in office and 'in waiting', are constrained by a range of factors which encourage policy convergence and continuity. Political limits are imposed by public opinion, the media and pressure groups, and can restrict the options available to the parties and influence decisions during the policy process. These political pressures were particularly evident at the implementation stage of health reform in the 1980s and 1990s. Such pressures had an impact on opposition parties too. During the early 1990s both the Labour Party (and the Liberal Democrats) consulted widely before publishing their definitive policy documents.

Their policies were shaped by two political perceptions. First, that many within the NHS opposed further radical reform. This pushed them in the direction of incremental, piecemeal reform rather than a 'big bang' approach. Secondly, there was an increasing awareness that some groups and individuals benefited from the reforms and might oppose future plans which threatened their gains. For example, Labour's plans on GP fundholding were heavily criticised by the National Association of Fundholding Practices, which warned that the abolition of the scheme could lead not only to protests from fundholding GPs and their patients, but to their exodus from the NHS.

Although the public had been hostile to many aspects of the Conservatives' reforms, it became obvious that public opinion could not necessarily be relied on to support a complete reversal of this programme. Indeed, as the reforms became entrenched significant elements of public opinion could conceivably be mobilised against such moves. For example by 1996 GP fundholding covered over half the population in England and Wales, and reversing this policy was therefore likely to be controversial, particularly as fundholders began to mobilise public support for the scheme. In the case of private health care similar considerations applied. Although only a minority of the population had private health insurance, and many of these used the NHS as well as the private sector, any future policy aimed at discouraging private care would be likely to offend a much larger proportion of the public than would have been the case in 1979.

Potential technical problems associated with future reform also shaped the policies of Labour and other opposition parties. As the new structures and processes introduced into the NHS by the Conservatives became entrenched, the costs of reversing the health reforms were increasingly perceived as prohibitive, both in terms of financial costs and opportunity costs (for example, legislative time involved in repealing the reforms and introducing an entirely new system). Moreover, it was conceded that, at least in the short-term, it would be practically impossible to reverse certain structural and procedural reforms, such as mergers, contracting processes and joint working arrangements between the NHS and the private sector.

Finally, significant shifts in the aims and values of the Labour Party reduced the prospects that the Conservatives' reforms would be overturned. The Labour leadership underwent a considerable shift in its stated values in the first half of the 1990s, accompanied by an influx of new members. Though these developments initially had little impact on health policy, some within Labour Party circles began to question some fundamental assumptions, such as whether collective provision was after all the best way of delivering efficient and equitable health care. In particular there emerged greater support for the non-state sector in the finance and provision of care, more emphasis on users, and broad support for the contract culture of welfare introduced by the Conservatives (see Abel-Smith and Glennerster, 1995; Jones, 1995; Mandelson and Liddle, 1996; Pollard, Liddle and Thompson, 1994).

□ New Labour: new NHS?

In the run-up to the 1997 General Election few observers believed that Labour would deviate significantly from the policies introduced by its predecessor. The size of Labour's election victory – giving it a majority of 179 seats – did however raise the possibility of a more radical approach. With such a majority the new government could quite easily force through the necessary legislation to reverse the Conservative reforms. There was anticipation that legislation would be introduced to replace GP fundholding by a locality commissioning system, as proposals along these lines had been announced prior to the election (Smith, 1996). But this was hardly a radical move since locality commissioning was already emerging as one of the more popular commissioning models (see Chapter 8). Moreover, closer scrutiny of Labour's pre-election plans suggested a lengthy period of grace before fundholding would cease in its present form, considerable local discretion in the adoption of local collaborative schemes, and the possibility of retaining practice-based budgets.

Initially at least, the Blair government appeared satisfied with some minor modifications of the existing system: encouraging longer-term contracts, greater collaboration, and simplified invoicing in an effort to reduce transaction costs. New measures were proposed to prevent unequal treatment of fundholder and non-fundholder's patients including common waiting lists. Regulations were announced to allow GP fundholder budgets to be re-examined when health authority budgets were under pressure, and to recoup windfall savings from fundholders. Applications to the GP fundholding scheme were deferred, but the scheme survived for the time being. Meanwhile, the government maintained it would pilot and evaluate various commissioning schemes before considering further structural changes, ironically using the previous government's NHS (Primary Care) Act of 1997 as a vehicle for this. It also announced the establishment of health action zones (HAZs) to pioneer new collaborative arrangements in public health and service provision at local level (see Exhibit 13.1).

The Blair government took care to diffuse expectations on NHS spending, despite inheriting plans that were below the level of any recent parliament. In its first budget, however, the Blair government shifted to some extent from its pre-election commitment to keep within existing spending plans. Further funding, subject to improvements in efficiency, was made available from contingency funds. Subsequently, a further amount was allocated in an effort to avert a funding crisis in the winter of 1997/8. At the same time a review of NHS finance was launched, and alternative funding schemes including earmarked taxes and new charges were not ruled out.

Labour's social policies and public health policies did seem to be geared more explicitly to tackling the social roots of ill-health than those of its predecessor. The Blair government signalled its commitment to alter *Health of the Nation* targets to reflect the contribution of socio-economic factors such as bad housing, unemployment and poverty. Economic policies were also aimed at tackling these problems. Yet the leadership showed little inclination to reverse significantly the economic inequalities generated in the previous two decades. Without such redistribution substantial reductions in inequality and levels of social deprivation seem unlikely to materialise in the short term.

The Labour government outlined its commitment to improve public health (see Exhibit 13.1), including the creation of a minister for public health and a promise of improved interdepartmental coordination on health matters. Plans to create an independent food standards agency were set in motion, and the new government also stated its intention to ban advertising and sponsorship by tobacco companies as well as tackle under-age drinking. These policies suggested that it would be less influenced than its predecessor by commercial interests in the food, tobacco and alcoholic drinks industries and other businesses having implications for health. However, in the light of the Blair government's handling of the tobacco sponsorship issue (see the note on p. 295) its determination to tackle the commercial roots of ill-health should not perhaps be taken at face value.

What does all this imply about the future direction of health policy? It seems that gradual change is the most likely outcome. Reform fatigue among those working in the health sector, emerging agreement between the parties on fundamental issues (in spite of the rhetoric which continues to characterise health debates), and continuing public support for the NHS, all point to this.

Exhibit 13.1   The Blair Government's health policies

Within the first six months of taking office, the Blair government announced a series of policy initiatives. Many of these were set out in its White Paper *The New NHS* in December 1997 (Cm 3807, 1997).

Health Care Resourcing

In its 1997 Budget, the Labour government found an extra £1.2 billion for the NHS for the following financial year (1998/9) resulting in a planned increase of 2.25 per cent over the estimated inflation rate. Meanwhile the new government launched a review of NHS funding which among other things considered alternative forms of finance such as earmarked taxes and user charges. Furthermore, National Lottery funding was permitted for certain health projects. The 1997 Budget also abolished tax relief on private health care and imposed insurance premium tax on some long term health care insurance products. The Private Finance Initiative was retained. New legislation was introduced to clarify the legality of PFI contracts. A review procedure was introduced to speed up and prioritise PFI projects. Also, pathology and radiology were excluded from the PFI programme. Meanwhile a review of market testing in the NHS was launched.

Health Authority Appointments and Openness

Under new arrangements local authorities and MPs were asked to nominate candidates for vacancies. Successful candidates would have to demonstrate a commitment to the NHS and live locally. Otherwise, the procedures for appointment remained much the same, with candidates having to conform to the rules drawn up in the light of the Nolan Committee recommendations (see Chapter 6). In a further move, the Department of Health proposed guidance forcing trusts to meet more often in public. Health ministers also declared their intention to outlaw 'gagging' clauses from NHS contracts.

Patient's Charter and Performance Indicators

Following the publication of the 1997 performance tables, the Blair government announced that it would be extending the process to include clinical indicators. 15 new clinical outcome indicators were proposed including: emergency readmissions to hospital within 28 days, deaths in hospital within 30 days of surgery, damage to organs following surgery, and adverse events related to the use of medicines. *The Patient's Charter* standards were reviewed with the intention of producing a new *NHS Charter* during 1998. Proposed changes included altering standards in Accident and Emergency, and stating patients' responsibilities more clearly.

Efficiency and Service Quality

Two new bodies have been proposed to improve the effectiveness and quality of services. A National Institute of Clinical Excellence and a Commission for Health Improvement (see Chapter 6). Trusts will be expected to monitor quality more closely and will be held accountable for shortcomings identified

Internal Market, Commissioning and Planning

It is intended that the fundholding scheme will be abolished by 1999. Contracts will be replaced by longer-term service level agreements. Primary Care Groups involving GPs and community nurses will commission services and in the longer term may acquire the responsibility of running local community health services.

→

Exhibit 13.1 *continued*

Health authorities are to have a stronger planning role, drawing up Health Improvement Programmes with trusts, GPs, local authorities and other interested parties. A statutory duty of cooperation will be placed on all those concerned.

Management Costs

The government signalled its intention to redeploy savings in management costs towards patient care, particularly to reduce waiting times for cancer services. Measures proposed to reduce costs included simplified invoicing, mergers of NHS trusts, and a reduction in the number of commissioning bodies.

Health Action Zones

The Labour government expressed interest in developing 'health action zones' as a means of improving planning and collaboration between different agencies at local level. Health action zones involve the development of local strategies on public health, community care and service reconfiguration by all the major service providers and funders of care – GPs, health authorities, community health and hospital trusts, as well as local authorities, the voluntary sector and local business.

Community Care and Primary Care

The Blair government established a Royal Commission on long-term care. For the moment it shelved the Major government's plans to encourage people to protect their assets through long-term care insurance. However, the previous government's support for a unified inspection process for nursing and residential care homes was endorsed. Health authorities and local authorities will in future be expected to collaborate more effectively on community care, drawing up joint investment plans for example. The Blair government maintained a commitment to primary care with the proposed creation of Primary Care Groups (see above).

London and Reconfiguration

Shortly after taking office, the Blair government initiated a further review of London's health and community care services. In the meantime certain hospital closures and mergers were put on hold. The government also explored new ways of encouraging the rationalisation of services throughout the NHS through mergers and integrated planning at local level (see 'health action zones' above).

Health of the Nation

Soon after it came to office the government created a new post of minister for public health. It also embarked on a review of public health. This involved an examination of how the *Health of the Nation* targets, introduced by its predecessor, could be altered. An inquiry into social deprivation, inequality and ill-health was also set in motion. The Blair government declared that its priorities would include tackling the social and economic roots of ill-health, the development of more specific targets to reduce deaths from heart disease and cancer, efforts to combat environmental pollution, policies to deal with ill-health and injury at work, the development of a healthy school philosophy, including nutritional standards for school meals, and a coordinated policy on illegal drug use. A Green Paper, outlining the Labour government's health strategy is expected in 1998. The government also announced its intention to ban tobacco advertising and sponsorship. Measures to discourage under-age drinking were also introduced during the summer of 1997.

Yet the policy process is rarely predictable, and much depends on the wider political environment within which government operates. In the case of the Blair Government, the size of its parliamentary majority gives it a great deal of scope for legislative action and it may sooner or later be tempted to be more ambitious about reform. It may also be pressured into new initiatives by those on the left of the party, who, though perhaps less numerous and vociferous than in the past, could undermine party discipline. At the time of writing this is already happening on other issues of welfare reform. Furthermore, despite the shifting values of the party leadership, the Blair government is likely to be more sympathetic to labour and trade union interests in the NHS than the Conservatives, and this too may generate new directions in policy. Finally, the media will no doubt continue to play a crucial role in the presentation of health policy issues and debates, forcing the government's hand. As former Labour health ministers will testify, the press and broadcasters have not in the past confined their criticism to the Conservatives' handling of the NHS (Castle, 1990). Indeed it may be increasingly difficult for the Blair government to pursue its chosen course in the face of continuing pressures on the NHS highlighted by the media.

Further Reading

☐ *Chapter 1*

Concepts of health are discussed further by Aggleton (1990). Sources on the health of the British population include the General Household Survey (OPCS, 1996) and progress reports on the *Health of the Nation* strategy (DoH, 1995j). The Office of Health Economics *Compendium* (1995) contains many useful statistics on health and health care. International comparisons of health can be found in WHO (1995). The threat of new infectious diseases is worryingly documented by Garrett (1995). The evidence regarding health inequalities is summarised in Townsend, Davidson and Whitehead (1992). Race and health issues are thoroughly explored in Ahmad (1993). Good sources on women's health include Miles (1991), Doyal (1995) and Foster (1995).

☐ *Chapter 2*

Inglis (1965) explores the history of medicine. Bynum (1994) focuses on the development of medical science in the nineteenth century. The history of the nursing profession is examined by Abel-Smith (1960). The role of the medical profession in relation to health, illness and health care is explored critically by Gould (1987), Inglis (1981), Illich (1975) and Kennedy (1981). The cultural aspects of medicine are examined by Payer (1989) and Helman (1990). Studies of alternative medicine include Saks (1995) and Sharma (1995). The restatement of the public health model by McKeown (1979) is still perhaps the best starting place for those interested in this field. The politics of the medical profession is examined by Watkins (1987). Moran and Wood (1992) provide a good analysis of the politics of medical regulation. The regulation of medical work is also examined by Allsop and Mulcahy (1996) and Stacey (1992). Histories of the BMA have been produced by Grey-Turner and Sutherland (1982) and Bartrip (1996).

The sociology of medicine is explored by Freidson (1988) and Turner (1987). Parry and Parry (1976) give an account of the rise of the medical profession. Lay beliefs about health are discussed by Calnan (1987) and Williams and Calnan (1996). Salvage (1985) and Davies (1995) examine the role and status of nursing. Deep-rooted inter-professional rivalries and political conflict between midwives and doctors are analysed by Donnison (1988).

☐ *Chapter 3*

The economic, moral and political dilemmas involved in the rationing of health care are analysed in Weale (1988). Honigsbaum (1992) examines the Oregon case. Klein, Day and Redmayne (1996) examine the management of scarcity in the NHS. The implications of high technology in medicine are discussed by Jennett (1986) and Stocking (1988). The Marxist perspective on health care is set out by

315

Doyal (1979). Broader socialist views on health are discussed in Carrier and Kendall (1990). Feminist perspectives are outlined by Doyal (1995), Wilkinson and Kitzinger (1994), and Foster (1995). Oakley (1980, 1984) analyses the particular case of women and childbirth.

☐ *Chapter 4*

A number of sources discuss the pre-NHS system of health care (Honigsbaum, 1979; Hodgkinson, 1967; Abel-Smith, 1964). The creation of the NHS is comprehensively analysed by Webster (1988) and Honigsbaum (1989). The history of the NHS and its problems since inception are covered by a number of books including Klein (1983, 1995), Haywood and Alaszewski (1980) and Webster (1988, 1996). Perhaps the best work on Thatcherism is Hugo Young's *One of Us* (1991). The impact of the Thatcher government on health policy is discussed by Wistow (1992) and Mohan (1995).

☐ *Chapter 5*

Field (1989) provides a useful overview of health care systems. A number of OECD publications (1994a, 1996) outline the problems facing health care systems in industrialised countries and show how different countries are responding. Health care reforms in a number of countries are discussed by Ham (1997). Navarro (1994) and Peters (1996) discuss the problems of reforming health care in the USA.

☐ *Chapter 6*

The impact of the Griffiths management reforms is assessed by Strong and Robinson (1990), Harrison *et al.* (1992) and Walby and Greenwell (1994). Harrison and Pollitt (1994), Laughlin and Broadbent (1994) and Marnoch (1996) further examine the organisational and managerial aspects of the NHS in the 1990s and the impact of reforms on the professions. Joss and Kogan (1995) analyse the management of quality in the NHS.

☐ *Chapter 7*

Appleby (1992) provides a comprehensive analysis of financial issues in the NHS. Public expenditure during the 1980s and early 1990s is examined by Bloor and Maynard (1993). Healthcare 2000 (1995) and Wordsworth, Donaldson and Scott (1996) examine the affordability of the NHS. Private health care is discussed by Higgins (1988), Calnan, Cant and Gabe (1993) and Yates (1995).

☐ *Chapter 8*

The politics behind the internal market reforms are discussed by Butler (1992) and Paton (1992). The implementation of planned markets in health care is explored in

Saltman and van Otter (1995). The impact of the internal market is examined by Le Grand and Robinson (1994) and by Powell (1997). GP fundholding is evaluated by the Audit Commission (1996b). Flynn *et al.* (1996) study the contracting process in the field of community health services.

☐ *Chapters 9 and 10*

The Audit Commission (1992a) provides a useful background to debates about the future of community health services. The volume edited by Griffin (1996) explores a number of key debates in primary care. The Institute for Public Policy Research (1995a) sets out options for future reform. Meads (1996) examines the practicalities of a primary care-led NHS. Means and Smith (1994) and Lewis and Glennerster (1996) analyse community care policy and practice. Wistow *et al.* (1994) and the Audit Commission (1996c) examine the impact of reform. Hancock and Jarvis (1995) study the long-term impact of being a carer. The Mental Health Foundation (1994) describe the reality of community care for mentally-ill people.

☐ *Chapter 11*

Williamson (1992) discusses the patient's perspective. Winkler (1987) outlines various models of consumer participation in health care. The Institute for Public Policy Research (1995b) examines the democratic deficit in health care.

☐ *Chapter 12*

The history of public health is discussed by Rosen (1993). Wohl (1984) explores Victorian public health. The revival of public health is discussed by Ashton and Seymour (1988). Specific issues are examined by the following authors: breast cancer screening (Hann, 1996); housing (Lowry, 1991); alcohol (British Paediatric Association and the Royal College of Physicians, 1995); inequalities (Benzeval, Judge and Whitehead, 1995; Wilkinson, 1996); tobacco control (Taylor, 1984), environment (Hall, 1990); and obesity (Office of Health Economics, 1994).

Bibliography

Aanchawan, T. (1996) 'Room at the Top', *Health Service Journal*, 7 March, 26–8.

Abbott, A. (1988) *The System of Professions: An Essay in the Division of Expert Labour* (Chicago, Chicago University Press).

Abel-Smith, B. (1960) *History of the Nursing Profession* (London, Heinemann).

Abel-Smith, B. (1964) *The Hospitals 1800–1948* (London, Heinemann).

Abel-Smith, B. (1994) *An Introduction to Health: Policy Planning and Financing* (London, Longman).

Abel-Smith, B. (1996) 'The Escalation of Health Care Costs: How Did We Get There', in OECD, *Health Care Reform: The Will To Change* (Paris, OECD), 17–30.

Abel-Smith, B. and Glennerster, H. (1995) 'Labour and the Tory Health Reforms', *Fabian Review*, 107 (3), 1–4.

Adams, B. (1991) 'Health Care Data Briefing: Unpaid Care', *Health Service Journal*, 7 February, 26.

Adams, C. (1995) 'OxDONS Syndrome: The Inevitable Disease of the NHS Reforms', *British Medical Journal*, 311, 1559–61.

Adams, J. (1995) 'With Complements', *Health Service Journal*, 1 June, 23.

Aggleton, P. (1990) *Health* (London, Routledge).

Ahmad, W. (ed.) (1993) *Race and Health in Contemporary Britain* (Buckingham, Open University Press).

Akehurst, R., Godfrey, J. and Robertson, E. (1991) *Health of the Nation: An Economic Perspective on Target Setting* (University of York, Centre for Health Economics).

Alaszewski, A. (1995) 'Restructuring Health and Welfare Professions in the United Kingdom: The Impact of Internal Markets on the Medical, Nursing and Social Work Professions', in Johnson, T., Larkin, G., Saks, M. (eds), *Health Professions and the State in Europe* (London, Routledge), 55–74.

Alchian, A. and Allen, W. (1974) *University Economics* (London, Prentice-Hall).

Alford, R. (1975) *Health Care Politics* (Chicago, Ill., University of Chicago Press).

Allen, I. (1994) *Doctors and their Careers: A New Generation* (London, Policy Studies Institute).

Allen, I., Bourke Dowling, S. and Williams, S. (1997) *A Leading Role for Midwives?* (London, Policy Studies Institute).

Allsop, J. and May, A. (1986) *The Emperor's New Clothes. Family Practitioner Committees in the 1980s* (London, King's Fund Institute).

Allsop, J. and Mulcahy, L. (1996) *Regulating Medical Work* (Buckingham, Open University Press).

Andrews, K., Murphy, L., Munday, R. and Littlewood, C. (1996) 'Misdiagnosis of the Vegatative State: Retrospective Study in a Rehabilitation Unit', *British Medical Journal*, 313, 13–16.

Andrews, L., Stocking, C., Krizeck, T., Gottlieb, L., Krizek, C., Vargish, T. and Seigler, M. (1997) 'An Alternative Strategy for Studying Adverse Events in Medical Care', *Lancet*, 349, 309–12.

Appleby, J. (1992) *Financing Health Care in the 1990s* (Buckingham, Open University Press).

Appleby, J. (1995) 'Managers in the Ascendancy', *Health Service Journal*, 21 September, 32–3.

Appleby, J. (1997) 'Promises, Promises', *Health Service Journal*, 8 May, 32–3.

Arblaster, L. and Hawtin, M. (1993) *Housing Health and Social Policy* (London, Socialist Health Association).

Armstrong, D. (1990) 'Medicine as a Profession: Times of Change', *British Medical Journal*, 301, 691–3.

Ashburner, L. and Cairncross, L. (1992) 'Just Trust Us', *Health Service Journal*, 14 May, 20–2.

Ashburner, L. and Cairncross, L. (1993) 'Membership of the "New Style", Health Authorities: Continuities or Change?', *Public Administration*, 71(3), 357–75.

Ashburner, L., Ferlie, E. and FitzGerald, L. (1994) 'Fast Forward', *Health Service Journal*, 6 January, 20–1.

Ashmore, M., Mulkay, M. and Pinch, T. (1989) *Health and Efficiency: A Sociology of Health Economics* (Buckingham, Open University Press).

Ashton, J. and Seymour, H. (1988) *The New Public Health* (Milton Keynes, Open University Press).

Association of Community Health Councils (1992) *A Health Standards Inspectorate* (London, Action for Victims of Medical Accidents).

Association of Community Health Councils (1993a) *The Internal Market and the NHS* (London, ACHCEW).

Association of Community Health Councils (1993b) *NHS Complaints Procedures* (London, ACHCEW).

Association of Community Health Councils (1994) *Access to Health Records Act 1990: The Concerns of CHCs* (London, ACHCEW).

Association of Metropolitan Authorities (1994) *The Future Role of Local Authorities in the Provision of Health Services* (London, Association of Metropolitan Authorities).

Audit Commission (1986) *Making a Reality of Community Care* (London, HMSO).

Audit Commission (1989) *Developing Community Care for Adults with a Mental Handicap* (London, HMSO).

Audit Commission (1990) *A Short Cut to Better Services: Day Surgery in England and Wales* (London, HMSO).

Audit Commission (1991a) *The Virtue of Patients: Making the Most of Ward Nursing Resources* (London, HMSO)

Audit Commission (1991b) *Report and Accounts* (London, HMSO).

Audit Commission (1992a) *Homeward Bound: A New Course for Community Health* (London, HMSO).

Audit Commission (1992b) *All in a Day's Work: An Audit of Day Surgery in England and Wales* (London, HMSO).

Audit Commission (1993a) *Their Health, Your Business: The Role of the District Health Authority* (London, HMSO).

Audit Commission (1993b) *Practices Make Perfect: The Role of the FHSA* (London, HMSO).

Audit Commission (1994a) *Annual Report and Accounts* (London, HMSO).

Audit Commission (1994b) *Protecting the Public Purse 2: Ensuring Probity in the NHS* (London, HMSO).

Audit Commission (1994c) *Taking Stock: Progress with Care in the Community* (London, HMSO).

Audit Commission (1994d) *Finding a Place: A Review of Mental Health Services for Adults* (London, HMSO).

Audit Commission (1995a) *Improving Your Image: How to Manage Radiology Services More Effectively* (London, HMSO).

Audit Commission (1995b) *Taken on Board: Corporate Governance in the NHS. Developing the Role of Non-executives* (London, HMSO).

Audit Commission (1995c) *The Doctor's Tale: The Work of Hospital Doctors in England and Wales* (London, HMSO).

Audit Commission (1995d) *A Price on Their Heads. Measuring Management Costs in NHS Trusts* (London, HMSO).

Audit Commission (1995e) *Briefing on GP Fundholding* (London, HMSO).

Audit Commission (1995f) *Commissioning Services for the Treatment and Prevention of Coronary Heart Disease* (London, HMSO).

Audit Commission (1996a) *The Doctor's Tale Continued – The Audit of Medical Staffing* (London, HMSO).

Audit Commission (1996b) *What the Doctor Ordered: A Study of GP Fundholders in England and Wales* (London, HMSO).

Audit Commission (1996c) *Balancing the Care Equation* (London, HMSO).

Audit Commission (1996d) *By Accident or Design: Improving Accident and Emergency Services in England and Wales* (London, HMSO).

Austoker, J. (1994) 'Diet and Cancer', *British Medical Journal*, 308, 1611–14.

Bach, S. (1994) 'Managing a Pluralist Health System: The Case of Health Care Reform in France', *International Journal of Health Studies*, 24 (4), 593–606.

Baggott, R. (1995) 'From Confrontation to Consultation? Pressure Group Relations From Thatcher to Major', *Parliamentary Affairs*, 48 (3), 484–502.

Bahl, V. (1993) 'Development of a Black and Ethnic Minority Health Policy at the Department of Health', in Hopkins, A. and Bahl, V. (eds), *Access to Health Care for People from Black and Ethnic Minorities* (London, Royal College of Physicians), 1–9.

Bailey, J., Black, M. and Wilkin, D. (1994) 'Specialist Outreach Clinics in General Practice', *British Medical Journal*, 308, 1083–6.

Bailey, S. and Bruce, A. (1994) 'Funding the NHS: The Continuing Search for Alternatives', *Journal of Social Policy*, 23 (4), 489–516.

Bakwin, H. (1945) 'Pseudoxia Pediatrica', *New England Journal of Medicine*, 232, 691–7.

Balarajan, R. (1989) 'Inequalities in Health within the Health Sector', *British Medical Journal*, 299, 822–5.

Balarajan, R. (1991) 'Ethnic Differences: Mortality from Ischaemic Heart Disease and Cerebrovascular Disease in England and Wales', *British Medical Journal*, 302, 560–4.

Balarajan, R. and Bulusu, L. (1990) 'Mortality Among Immigrants in England and Wales', in Britton, M. (ed.) *Mortality and Geography: A Review in the Mid-1980s DS9*, OPCS (London, HMSO), 103–21.

Balarajan, R. and Raleigh, V. (1993) *Ethnicity and Health: A Guide for the NHS* (London, Department of Health).

Baldwin, S. and Lunt, N. (1996) *Charging Ahead: Local Authority Charging Policies for Community Care* (Bristol, Policy Press).

Balogh, R. (1996) 'Exploring the Role of Localities in Health Commissioning: A Review of the Literature', *Social Policy and Administration*, 30 (2), 99–113.

Banta, H.D. (1993) 'Mimimally Invasive Surgery: Implications for Hospitals, Health Workers and Patients', *British Medical Journal*, 307, 1546–9.

Barnardo's (1993) *Liquid Gold* (Ilford, Barnardo's).

Barrow, S., Fisher, A., Seex, D. and Abdul, M. (1994) 'General Practitioner Attitudes to Day Surgery', *Journal of Public Health*, 16 (3), 318–20.

Bartlett, W. (1991) 'Quasi-Markets and Contracts: A Market and Hierarchies Perspective on NHS Reform', *Public Money and Management*, 11 (3), 53–62.

Bartley, M. and Owen, C. (1996) 'Relation between Socioeconomic Status, Employment and Health during Economic Change 1979–83', *British Medical Journal*, 313, 445–9.

Bartley, M., Montgomery, S., Cook, D. and Wadsworth, M. (1996) 'Health and Work Insecurity in Young Men', in Blane, D., Brunner, E. and Wilkinson, R. (eds), *Health and Social Organisation* (London, Routledge), 255–71.

Bartley, M., Popay, J. and Plewis, I. (1992) 'Domestic Conditions, Paid Employment and Women's Experience of Ill Health', *Sociology of Health and Illness*, 14 (3), 313–45.

Bartrip, P. (1996) *Themselves Writ Large: The BMA 1832–1966* (London, BMJ Publishing Group).

Baumol, W. (1995) *Health Care as a Handicraft Industry* (London, Office of Health Economics).

BBC (1994) 'The Greatest Nightmare', *Panorama*, 7 November.

Beardshaw, V. (1988) *Last on the List: Community Services for People with Physical Disabilities* (London, King's Fund Institute).

Beecham, L. (1994) 'Fundholders' Patients are Treated Quicker Says BMA', *British Medical Journal*, 308, 11.

Bennet, M., Smith, E. and Millard, P. (1995) *The Right Person? The Right Place? The Right Time?: An Audit of the Appropriateness of Nursing Home Placements Post Community Care Act*, Department of Geriatric Medicine (London, St George's Hospital Medical School).

Benster, R. (1994) 'Unfinished Business', *Health Service Journal*, 5 May, 27.

Benzeval, M., Judge, K. and New, B. (1991) 'Health and Health Care in London', *Public Money and Management*, 11 (1), 25–32.

Benzeval, M., Judge, K. and Whitehead, M. (eds) (1995) *Tackling Inequalities in Health: An Agenda for Action* (London, King's Fund).

Berwick, D. M., Enthoven, A. and Bunker, J. P. (1992) 'Quality Management in the NHS: The Doctors' Role', *British Medical Journal*, 304, 235–9.

Besley, T., Hall, J. and Preston, I. (1996) *Private Health Insurance and the State of the NHS* (London, Institute for Fiscal Studies).

Bethune, A. (1996) 'Economic Activity and Mortality of the 1981 Census Cohort in the OPCS Longitudinal Study', *Population Trends*, 83, 37–41.

Bevan, G., Holland, W., Maynard, A. and Mays, N. (1988) *Reforming UK Health Care to Improve Health: The Case for Research and Experiment* (University of York, Centre for Health Economics).

Bewley, C. and Glendinning, C. (1994) *Involving Disabled People in Community Care Planning* (York, Joseph Rowntree Foundation).

Birch, S. and Maynard, A. (1988) *Peformance Indicators* (Oxford, Policy Journals).

Bish, A., Armstrong, D., Jones, R. and Mitchell, P. (1996) 'Restricted Access', *Health Service Journal*, 7 November, 32–3.

Bjorkman, J. W. (1989) 'Politicising Medicine and Medicalising Politics: Physician Power in the United States', in Freddi, G. and Bjorkman, J. W., *Controlling Medical Professionals: The Comparative Politics of Health Governance* (London, Sage), 28–73.

Black, D. (1984) *An Anthology of False Antitheses* (London, Nuffield Provincial Hospitals Trust).

Black, D., Birchall, A. and Trimble, I. (1994) 'Non-fundholding in Nottingham: A Vision of the Future', *British Medical Journal*, 308, 930–2.

Black, N. (1996) 'Why We Need Observational Studies to Evaluate the Effectiveness of Healthcare', *British Medical Journal*, 312, 1215–18.

Black, N. and Thompson, E. (1993) 'Obstacles to Medical Audit: British Doctors Speak', *Social Science and Medicine*, 36 (7), 849–56.

Blackhurst, C. (1995) 'Finance Watchdog Prescribes Cure for Unhealthy NHS', *Independent*, 24 August, 10.

Blair, P., Fleming, P. and Bensley, D. (1996) 'Smoking and Sudden Infant Death Syndrome', *British Medical Journal*, 313, 195–8.

Blane, D., Smith, G. D. and Bartley, M. (1990) 'Social Class Differences in Years of Potential Life Lost: Size, Trends and Principal Causes', *British Medical Journal*, 301, 29–32.

Blane, D., Smith, G. D. and Bartley, M. (1993) 'Social Selection: What Does It Contribute to Social Class Differences in Health?', *Sociology of Health and Illness*, 15, 1–15.

Blaxter, M. (1990) *Health and Lifestyles* (London, Tavistock/Routledge).

Blom-Cooper, L. (1994) *Falling Shadow. One Patient's Mental Health Care 1978–93* (London, Duckworth).

Bloor, K. and Maynard, A. (1993) *Expenditure on the NHS During and After the Thatcher Years: Its Growth and Utilisation*. Centre for Health Economics (York, University of York).

BMA (British Medical Association) (1929) *A General Medical Service for the Nation* (London, BMA).

BMA (British Medical Association) (1942) *Draft Interim Report of the Medical Planning Commission* (London, BMA).

BMA (British Medical Association) (1962) *Report of the Medical Services Review Committee* (The Porritt Report) (London, BMA).

BMA (British Medical Association) (1986a) *Diet, Nutrition and Health* (London, BMA).

BMA (British Medical Association) (1986b) *Alternative Therapy* (London, British Medical Association).

BMA (British Medical Association) (1987) *Deprivation and Ill-Health* (London, BMA).

BMA (British Medical Association) (1993) *Complementary Medicine: New Approaches to Good Practice* (Oxford University Press).

BMA (British Medical Association) (1995a) *Survey on the Impact of the Implementation of the Community Care Reforms*. Health Policy and Economic Research Unit (London, BMA).

BMA (British Medical Association) (1995b) *Inequalities in Health*. Board of Science and Education Occasional Paper (London, BMA).

Bond, J., Cartlidge, A. M. and Gregson A. B. (1987) 'Inter-Professional Collaboration in Primary Care', *Journal of the Royal College of General Practitioners*, 37, 158–61.

Bone, M., Bebbington, A., Jagger, C., Morgan, K. and Nicholaas, G. (1995) *Health Expectancy and its Uses* (London, HMSO).

Bosanquet, N. (1975) *A New Deal for the Elderly* (London, Fabian Society).

Bosanquet, N. (1986) 'GPs as Firms: Creating an Internal Market for Primary Care', *Public Money and Management*, 6 (1), 53–62.

Bosanquet, N. (1994) 'Improving Health', in Jowell, R., Curtice, J., Brook, L. and Ahrendt, D. (eds) *British Social Attitudes: 11th Report* (Aldershot, Dartmouth).

Bowie, C., Richardson, A. and Sykes, W. (1995) 'Consulting the Public about Health Service Priorities', *British Medical Journal*, 311, 1155–58.

Bowling, A. (1996) 'Health Care Rationing: The Public's Debate', British Medical Journal, 312, 670–4.

Bowling, A., Jacobson, B. and Southgate, L. (1993) 'Health Service Priorities: Exploration in Consultation of the Public and Health Professionals on Priority Setting in an Inner London District', *Social Science and Medicine*, 37 (7), 851–7.

Bradlow, J. and Coulter, A. (1993) 'Effect of Fundholding and Indicative Prescribing on General Practitioner Prescribing Costs', *British Medical Journal*, 307, 1186–9.

Bradshaw, J. and Gibbs, I. (1988) *Public Support for Residential Care* (Aldershot, Avebury).

Brand, J. L. (1965) *Doctors and the State: The British Medical Profession and Government Action on Public Health: 1870–1912* (Baltimore Md., Johns Hopkins University Press).

Brazier, M., Lovecy, J., Moran, M. and Potton, M. (1993) 'Falling from a Tightrope? Doctors and Lawyers between the Market and State', *Political Studies*, 41 (2), 197–213.

Brewin, T. (1985) 'Orthodox and Alternative Medicine', *Scottish Medical Journal*, 30, 203–5.

British Association of Medical Managers, BMA, IHSM and RCN (1993) *Managing Clinical Services: A Consensus Statement of Principles for Effective Clinical Management* (London, IHSM).

British Association of Medical Managers (1996) *Putting Principles into Practice: The Involvement of Clinical Staff on the Management of NHS Trusts* (Manchester, BAMM).

British Cardiac Society (1987) *Report of the British Cardiac Society Working Group on Coronary Disease Prevention* (London, British Cardiac Society).

British Medical Journal (1994) 'The Rise of Stalinism in the NHS', *British Medical Journal*, 309, 17 December, 1640–5.

British Medical Journal (1996) 'Complementary Medicine is Booming Worldwide', *British Medical Journal*, 313, 20 July, 131–3.

British Paediatric Association (1993) *The Care of Critically Ill Children*. Report of a Multidisciplinary Working Party (London, BPA).

British Paediatric Association and the Royal College of Physicians (1995) *Alcohol and the Young* (London, The Royal College of Physicians).

Brittain, J. M. (1992) 'The Emerging Market for Information Professionals in the UK National Health Service', *International Journal of Information Management*, 12, 261–7.

Brittan, L. (1988) *A New Deal for Health Care* (London, Conservative Political Centre).

Brown, G. W. and Harris, T. (1982) 'Social Class and Affective Disorder', in Ihsan Al-Issa (ed.), *Culture and Psychopathology* (Baltimore Md., University Park Press).

Brown, M., Fallon, M., Favell, T., Forth, E., Hamilton, N., Heathcoat-Amory, D., Howarth, G., Jones, G., Leigh, E., Redwood, J., Stewart, A. and Twinn, I. (1988) *The NHS: A Suitable Case for Treatment* (London, Conservative Political Centre).

Bruce, A. and McConnell, A. (1995) 'Local Government and the NHS: Accountability in the Hollowed Out State', *Public Policy and Administration*, 10 (3), 15–28.

Bruster, S., Jarman, B., Bosanquet, N., Weston, D., Erens, R. and Delbanco, T. (1994) 'National Survey of Hospital Patients', *British Medical Journal*, 309, 1542–9.

Buchanan, D. (1996) *Representing Process: The Re-engineering Frame*, Occasional Paper 37 (Leicester, Leicester Business School).

Buck, N., Devlin, B. and Lunn, J. N. (1987) *Report of a Confidential Inquiry into Perioperative Deaths* (London, Nuffield Hospitals Provincial Trust).

Buckingham, R. A. and Buckingham, R. O. (1995) 'Robots in Operating Theatres', *British Medical Journal*, 311, 1479–82.

Bullock, S. (1994) *Women and Work* (London, Zed Press).

Bunker, J., Frazier., H. and Mostelle, F. (1994) 'Improving Health: Measuring Effects of Medical Care', *Milbank Quarterly*, 72 (2), 225–58.

Burke, C. and Goddard, A. (1990) 'Internal Markets: The Road to Inefficiency?', *Public Administration*, 68 (3), 389–96.

Butler, E. and Pirie, M. (1988) *The Health Alternatives* (London, Adam Smith Institute).

Butler, J. (1992) *Patients, Policies and Politics: Before and After 'Working for Patients'* (Buckingham, Open University Press).

Butler, P. (1995a) 'Hospital Closures Grind to a Halt in the Face of Opposition', *Health Service Journal*, 1 June, 5.

Butler, P. (1995b) 'Executive Orders Massive Increase in Market Testing', *Health Service Journal*, 11 May, 3.

Butler, P. (1995c) 'Trusts Aim to Streamline ECR System', *Health Service Journal*, 21 September, 6.

Bynum, W. (1994) *Science and the Practice of Medicine in the Nineteenth Century* (Cambridge University Press).

Byrne, P. S. and Long, B. E. (1976) *Doctors Talking to Patients* (London, HMSO).

Cadbury. A. (1992) *Report of the Committee on the Financial Aspects of Corporate Governance* (The Cadbury Report) (London, Gee and Co.).

Cairns, J. (1996) 'Measuring Health Outcomes', *British Medical Journal*, 313, 6.

Calnan, M. (1987) *Health and Illness* (London, Tavistock).

Calnan, M., Cant, S. and Gabe, J. (1993) *Going Private: Why People Pay for their Health Care* (Buckingham, Open University Press).

Cameron, H. M. and McCoogan, E. (1981) 'A Prospective Study of 1152 Hospital Autopsies', *Journal of Pathology*, 133, 273–85.

Campbell, E. J. M., Scadding, J. G. and Roberts, R. S. (1979) 'The Concept of Disease', *British Medical Journal*, 2, 757–62.

Camplin, E. A., Lunn, J. A. and Devlin, H. B. (1992) *The National Confidential Enquiry into Perioperative Deaths* (London, NCEPOD).

Camplin, E. A., Devlin, H. B., Hoile, R. and Lunn, J. A. (1995) *The National Confidential Enquiry into Perioperative Deaths 1992/3* (London, NCEPOD).

Cancer Research Campaign (1996) *Lung Cancer and Smoking. UK Factsheet* (London, CRC).

Cannon, G. (1987) *The Politics of Food* (London, Century Hutchinson).

Capewell, S. (1992) 'Clinical Directorates: A Panacea for Clinicians Involved in Management', *Health Bulletin*, 50 (6), 441–7.

Capewell, S. (1996) 'The Continuing Rise in Emergency Admissions', *British Medical Journal*, 312, 991–2.

Carers' National Association (1995) *Better Tomorrows?* (London, CNA).

Carr-Hill, R. (1991) 'Allocating Resources to Health Care: Is the Qaly a Technical Solution to a Political Problem?', *International Journal of Health Services*, 21 (2), 351–63.

Carr-Hill, R. and Morris, J. (1991) 'Current Practice in Obtaining the Q in Qalys: A Cautionary Note', *British Medical Journal*, 303, 699–701.

Carrier, J. and Kendall, I. (1990) *Socialism and the NHS* (Aldershot, Avebury).

Castle, B. (1990) *The Castle Diaries: 1974–6* (London, Macmillan).

Cd 4499 (1909) *Royal Commission on the Poor Laws and Relief of Distress*, Minority Report (London, HMSO).

Central Statistical Office (1992) *Social Trends 22* (London, HMSO).

Central Statistical Office (1995) *Social Trends 25* (London, HMSO).

Central Statistical Office (1996) *Social Trends 26* (London, HMSO).

Centre for Health Economics (1995) *A Stitch in Time: Minor Surgery in General Practice* (Centre for Health Economics, University of York).

Chadda, D. (1996) 'The Narked Civil Servants', *Health Service Journal*, 21 March, 11.

Chadwick, E. (1842) *Report on the Sanitary Condition of the Labouring Population of Great Britain* (London, Poor Law Commission).

Challis, L., Klein, R. and Webb, A. (1988) *Joint Approaches to Social Policy: Rationality and Practice* (Cambridge University Press).

Chamberlain, E. (1993) 'Sweet and Sour Charity', *Health Service Journal*, 30 September, 31.

Chaplin, N. W. (1982) *Getting it Right: The 1982 Reorganisation of the NHS* (London, Institute of Health Service Administrators).

Charlesworth, J., Clarke, J. and Cochrane, A. (1996) 'Tangled Webs? Managing Local Mixed Economies of Care', *Public Administration*, 74 (1), 67–88.

Charlton, J. (1996) 'Which Areas are the Healthiest?', *Population Trends*, 83, 17–24.

Chief Medical Officer (1996) *On the State of the Public Health 1995* (London, HMSO).

Clarke, A., McKee, J., Appleby, J. and Sheldon, T. (1993) 'Efficient Purchasing', *British Medical Journal*, 307, 1436–7.

Clinical Standards Advisory Group (1993) *Access to and Availability of Specialist Services* (London, HMSO).

Clinical Standards Advisory Group (1995) *Schizophrenia* (London, HMSO).

Cmd 693 (1920) *Interim Report on the Future Provision of Medical and Allied Services* (The Dawson Report) (London, HMSO).

Cmd 2596 (1926) *Report of the Royal Commission on National Health Insurance* (London, HMSO).

Cmd 6404 (1942) *Social Insurance and Allied Services* (The Beveridge Report) (London, HMSO).

Cmd 6502 (1944) *A National Health Service* (London, HMSO).

Cmd 9663 (1956) *Report of the Committee of Inquiry into the Cost of the National Health Service* (The Guillebaud Report) (London, HMSO).

Cmnd 1604 (1962) *A Hospital Plan for England and Wales* (London, HMSO).

Cmnd 1973 (1963) *Health and Welfare: The Development of Community Care. Plans for the Health and Welfare Services of the Local Authorities in England and Wales* (London, HMSO).

Cmnd 4683 (1971) *Better Services for the Mentally Handicapped* (London, HMSO).

Cmnd 5055 (1972) *National Health Service Reorganisation: England* (London, HMSO).
Cmnd 6018 (1975) *Report of the Committee of Inquiry into the Regulation of the Medical Profession* (London, HMSO).
Cmnd 6233 (1975) *Better Services for the Mentally Ill* (London, HMSO).
Cmnd 7047 (1977) *Prevention and Health* (London, HMSO).
Cmnd 7615 (1979) *Report of the Royal Commission on the NHS* (The Merrison Commission) (London, HMSO).
Cmnd 8173 (1981) *Growing Older* (London, HMSO).
Cmnd 9716 (1986) *Report of the Committee of Inquiry into an Outbreak of Food Poisoning at Stanley Royd Hospital* (London, HMSO).
Cmnd 9771 (1986) *Primary Health Care: An Agenda for Discussion* (London, HMSO).
Cmnd 9772 (1986) *First Report of the Committee of Inquiry into the Outbreak of Legionnaire's Disease in Stafford, April 1985* (London, HMSO).
Cm 249 (1987) *Promoting Better Health* (London, HMSO).
Cm 289 (1988) *Public Health in England*, Report of the Acheson Committee of inquiry into the Future Development of the Public Health Function (London, HMSO).
Cm 555 (1989) *Working for Patients* (London, HMSO).
Cm 849 (1989) *Caring for People* (London, HMSO).
Cm 1343 (1990) *The Government's Plans for the Future of Community Care* (London, HMSO).
Cm 1370 (1991) *Competing for Quality* (London, HMSO).
Cm 1523 (1991) *The Health of the Nation: A Consultative Document for Health in England* (London, HMSO).
Cm 1599 (1992) *The Citizen's Charter* (London, HMSO).
Cm 1986 (1992) *The Health of the Nation: A Strategy for Health in England* (London, HMSO).
Cm 2625 (1994) *Improving NHS Dentistry* (London, Department of Health).
Cm 2850 (1995) *Report of the Committee on Standards in Public Life* (The Nolan Report) (London, HMSO).
Cm 3242 (1996) *A New Partnership for Old Age* (London, HMSO).
Cm 3390 (1996) *Choice and Opportunity. Primary Care: The Future* (London, HMSO).
Cm 3555 (1997) *Developing Partnerships in Mental Health* (London, HMSO).
Cm 3807 (1997) *The New NHS: Modern, Dependable* (London, The Stationery Office).
Coburn, D. (1992) 'Freidson Then and Now. An Internalists' Critique of Freidson's Past and Present Views of the Medical Profession', *International Journal of Health Services*, 25 (3), 497–512.
Cochrane, A. L. (1971) *Effectiveness and Efficiency: Random Reflections on Health Services* (London, Nuffield Provincial Hospital Trust).
Cochrane, M., Ham, C., Heginbotham, C. and Smith, R. (1992) 'Rationing: At the Cutting Edge', *British Medical Journal*, 303, 1039–42.
Cochrane, R. and Bal, S. (1989) 'Mental Hospital Admission Rates of Immigrants to England: A Comparison of 1971 and 1981', *Social Psychiatry and Psychiatric Epidemiology*, 24, 2–11.
Cohen, D. (1994) 'Marginal Analysis in Practice: An Alternative to Needs Assessment for Contracting Health Care', *British Medical Journal*, 309, 781–5.
Cohen, G., Forbes, J. and Garraway, M. (1996) 'Can Different Patient Satisfaction

Survey Methods Generate Consistent Results?: Comparison of Three Surveys', *British Medical Journal*, 313, 841–4.

Coid, J. (1984) 'How Many Psychiatric Patients in Prison?', *British Journal of Psychiatry*, 145, 78–86.

Collier, J. (1989) *The Health Conspiracy* (London, Century Hutchinson).

Collins, E. and Klein, R. (1988) 'Equity and the NHS: Self-Reported Mobility, Access and Primary Care', *British Medical Journal*, 282, 1111–5.

COMA (Committee on Medical Aspects of Food Policy) (1994) *Nutritional Aspects of Cardiovascular Disease* (London, HMSO)

COMEAP (Committee on the Medical Effects of Air Pollutants) (1995) *Asthma and Outdoor Air Pollution* (London, HMSO).

Commission for Social Justice (1994) *Social Justice: Strategies for National Renewal* (London, Verso).

Consumers' Association (1992) 'Is it Worth Going Private?', *Which?*, August, 426–9.

Cope, R. (1989) 'The Compulsory Detention of Afro-Caribbeans Under the Mental Health Act', *New Community*, 15 (3), 343–56.

Coulter, A. and Mays, N. (1997) 'Deregulating Primary Care', *British Medical Journal*, 314, 510–3.

Council for Science and Society (1982) *Expensive Medical Technologies: Report of a Working Party* (London, Council for Science and Society).

Crail, M. (1995) 'Most Trust Managers Claim NHS Secrecy has Increased', *Health Service Journal*, 2 February, 5.

Cross, M. (1996) 'Developing Read Codes Cost £3.7m', *Health Service Journal*, 2 May, 4.

Crossman, R. (1977) *The Diaries of a Cabinet Minister Volume Three, Secretary of State for Social Services 1968–70* (London, Hamilton Cape).

Culyer, A. (1991) 'The Promise of a Reformed NHS: An Economist's Angle', *British Medical Journal*, 302, 1253–6.

Culyer, A. J., Brazier, J. E. and O'Donnell, O. (1988) *Organising Health Service Provision. Drawing on Experience* (London, Institute for Health Service Management).

Cutler, T. and Waine, B. (1994) *Managing the Welfare State* (London, Berg).

Dally, A. (1991) *Women Under the Knife* (London, Hutchinson).

Davies, B. (1994) 'Maintaining the Pressure in Community Care Reform', Social Policy and Administration, 28 (3), 197–205.

Davies, B., Bebbington, A. and Charnley, H. (1990) *Resources, Needs and Outcomes in Community-Based Care* (Aldershot, Avebury).

Davies, J. and Kelly, M. (1993) *Healthy Cities: Policy and Practice* (London, Routledge).

Davies, C. (1995) *Gender and the Professional Predicament in Nursing* (Buckingham, Open University Press).

Dawson, D. (1995) *Regulating Competition in the NHS*. Centre for Health Economics (University of York).

Day, P. and Klein, R. (1987) *Accountabilities: Five Public Services* (London, Tavistock).

Day, P. and Klein, R. (1990) *Inspecting the Inspectorates* (York, Joseph Rowntree Memorial Trust).

Day, P. and Klein, R. (1991) 'Variations in Budgets of Fundholding Practices', *British Medical Journal*, 303, 168–70.

Deakin, N. (1991) 'Government and the Voluntary Sector in the 1990s', *Policy Studies*, 12 (3), 11–21.

Decker, D. (1995) 'Market Testing: Does it Bring Home the Bacon?', *Health Service Journal*, 19 January, 26–8.

Delamothe, T. (1991) 'Social Inequalities in Health', *British Medical Journal*, 303, 1046–50.

Delaney, F. (1994) 'Making Connections: Research into Intersectoral Collaborations', *Health Education Journal*, 53, 474–85.

Demming, W. (1982) *Quality, Productivity, and Competitive Position* (Cambridge, Mass., Massachusetts Insttiute of Technology).

Department of Social Security (1995) *Households Below Average Income: A Statistical Analysis 1979–1992/3* (London, HMSO).

DHSS (Department of Health and Social Security) (1970) *National Health Service. The Future Structure of the National Health Service in England* (London, HMSO).

DHSS (Department of Health and Social Security) (1971) *National Health Service Reorganisation: A Consultative Document* (London, DHSS).

DHSS (Department of Health and Social Security) (1976a) *Priorities for Health and Personal Social Services in England: A Consultative Document* (London, HMSO).

DHSS (Department of Health and Social Security) (1976b) *Report of the Regional Chairmen's Enquiry into the Working of the DHSS, in Relation to Regional Health Authorities* (London, DHSS).

DHSS (Department of Health and Social Security) (1976c) *Prevention and Health: Everybody's Business* (London, HMSO).

DHSS (Department of Health and Social Security) (1977) *The Way Forward* (London, HMSO).

DHSS (Department of Health and Social Security) (1979) *Patients First* (London, HMSO).

DHSS (Department of Health and Social Security) (1980) *Report of the Working Group on Inequalities in Health* (The Black Report) (London, DHSS).

DHSS (Department of Health and Social Security) (1981a) *Care in Action* (London, HMSO).

DHSS (Department of Health and Social Security) (1981b) *The Primary Care Team: Report of a Joint Working* Group (The Harding Report) (London, HMSO).

DHSS (Department of Health and Social Security) (1981c) *Community Care* (London, DHSS).

DHSS (Department of Health and Social Security) (1981d) *Report of a Study on Community Care* (London, DHSS).

DHSS (Department of Health and Social Security) (1982) *The NHS Planning System* (London, DHSS).

DHSS (Department of Health and Social Security) (1983) *NHS Management Inquiry* (The Griffiths Management Report) (London, DHSS).

DHSS (Department of Health and Social Security) (1986a) *NHS Management Board. A National Strategic Framework for Information Management in the Hospital and Community Services* (London, DHSS).

DHSS (Department of Health and Social Security) (1986b) *Neighbourhood Nursing: A Focus for Care. Report of the Community Nursing Review* (The Cumberlege Report) (London, HMSO).

DHSS (Department of Health and Social Security) (1987) *Achieving a Balance: A Plan for Action* (London, DHSS).

DHSS (Department of Health and Social Security) (1988) *Community Care: Agenda for Action* (The Griffiths Community Care Report) (London, HMSO).

DHSS (Department of Health and Social Security) and Welsh Office (1973) *Report of the Committee on Hospital Complaints Procedures* (The Davies Report) (London, HMSO).

Dicker, A. and Armstrong, D. (1995) 'Patients' Views of Priority Setting in Health Care: An Interview Survey in One Practice', *British Medical Journal*, 311, 1137–9.

Dix, A. (1996) 'Tender Mercies', *Health Service Journal*, 23 May, 20–1.

Dixon, J. (1994) 'Can There Be Fair Fundholding for Fundholding Practices?', *British Medical Journal*, 308, 772–5.

Dixon, J., Dinwoodie, M., Hodson, D., Dodd, S., Poltorak, T., Garrett, C., Rice, P., Doncaster, I. and Williams, M. (1994) 'Distribution of NHS Funds Between Fundholding and Non-fundholding Practices' *British Medical Journal*, 309, 30–4.

DoH (Department of Health) (1990a) *Developing Districts* (London, HMSO).

DoH (Department of Health) (1990b) *Contracts for Health Services: Operating Contracts* (London, HMSO).

DoH (Department of Health) (1990c) *NHS Trusts: A Working Guide* (London, HMSO).

DoH (Department of Health) (1991) *The Patients', Charter* (London, HMSO).

DoH (Department of Health) (1992a) *Women and Alcohol* (London, DoH).

DoH (Department of Health) (1992b) *Health and Social Service Statistics 1991* (London, HMSO).

DoH (Department of Health) (1992c) *Effect of Tobacco Advertisements on Tobacco Consumption. A Discussion Document Reviewing the Evidence* (London, DoH, Economics and Operational Research Division).

DoH (Department of Health) (1993a) *Hospital Doctors. Training for the Future* (The Calman Report) (London, DoH).

DoH (Department of Health) (1993b) *Changing Childbirth* (London, DoH).

DoH (Department of Health) (1993c) *Making London Better* (London, DoH).

DoH (Department of Health) (1994a) *Supporting Research and Development in the NHS* (The Culyer Report) (London, HMSO).

DoH (Department of Health) (1994b) *The Review of the Wider Department of Health* (The Banks Report) (London, DoH).

DoH (Department of Health) (1994c) *Functions and Responsibilities in the New NHS* (London, DoH).

DoH (Department of Health) (1994d) *NHS Hospital and Community Health Services. Non-medical Staff in England 1989–93* (London, DoH).

DoH (Department of Health) (1994e) *The Operation of the Internal Market: Local Freedoms, National Responsibilities*, HSG 94/55 (London, DoH).

DoH (Department of Health) (1994f) *Being Heard: Report of a Review Committee on NHS Complaints Procedures* (The Wilson Committee) (London, DoH).

DoH (Department of Health) (1994g) *The Patient's Charter and Maternity Services* (London, DoH).

DoH (Department of Health) (1994h) *Public Health in England: Roles and Responsibilities of the Department of Health and the NHS* (London, DoH).

DoH (Department of Health) (1995a) *Confidential Enquiry into Stillbirth and Death in Infancy. Part I* (London, HMSO).

DoH (Department of Health) (1995b) *NHS Hospital and Community Health Services Non-medical Staff 1989–94* (London, DoH).

DoH (Department of Health) (1995c) *The NHS Performance Guide 1994–5* (London, Central Office of Information).

DoH (Department of Health) (1995d) *An Accountability Framework for GP Fundholding* (London, DoH).

DoH (Department of Health) (1995e) *A Policy Framework for the Commissioning of Cancer Services* (London, DoH).

DoH (Department of Health) (1995f) *NHS Responsibilities for Meeting Continuing Health Care Needs,* HSG (95) 8 (London, DoH).

DoH (Department of Health) (1995g) *Building Bridges* (London, DoH).

DoH (Department of Health) (1995h) *Acting on Complaints* (London, DoH).

DoH (Department of Health) (1995i) *Obesity. Reversing the Increasing Problem of Obesity in England* (London, DoH).

DoH (Department of Health) (1995j) *Fit for the Future: A Second Progress Report on The Health of the Nation* (London, DoH).

DoH (Department of Health) (1995k) *Variations in Health: What Can the Department of Health and the NHS Do?* (London, DoH).

DoH (Department of Health) (1996a) *Priorities and Planning Guidance for the NHS 1997/8* (London, DoH).

DoH (Department of Health) (1996b) *NHS Performance Guide 1995–6* (London, DoH).

DoH (Department of Health) (1996c) *Primary Care: The Future* (London, DoH).

DoH (Department of Health) (1996d) *The Spectrum of Care* (London, DoH).

DoH (Department of Health) (1996e) *Complaints. Listening. . . Acting. . . Improving. Guidance on NHS Complaints Procedure* (London, DoH).

DoH (Department of Health) (1996f) *The Patient's Charter and You* (London, DoH).

DoH (Department of Health) (1996g) *The Patient's Charter and Services for Young People* (London, DoH).

DoH (Department of Health) (1997a) *Mental Health Services* (London, DoH).

DoH (Department of Health((1997b) *NHS Performance Guide 1996–7* (London DoH).

DoH and NTF (Department of Health and Nutrition Task Force) (1996a) *Eat Well II* (London, DoH).

DoH and NTF (Department of Health and Nutrition Task Force) (1996b) Low Income Project Team (1996b) *Low Income, Food, Nutrition and Health: Strategies for Improvement* (London, DoH).

DoH and DOE (Department of Health and Department of the Environment) (1994) *A Framework for Local Community Care Charters in England* (London, DoH).

DoH and OPCS (Department of Health and Office of Population Censuses and Surveys) (1995) *Health Survey for England, 1993* (London, HMSO).

Doig, A. (1990) 'Routine Crisis and Muddle: Mishandling the Egg Crisis', *Teaching Public Administration,* 10 (1), 15–26.

Doll, R. and Peto, R. (1981) 'The Causes of Cancer', *Journal of the National Cancer Institute,* 66, 1191–1308.

Donaldson, L. (1994) 'Doctors with Problems in the NHS Workforce', *British Medical Journal,* 308, 1277–82.

Donnison, J. (1988) *Midwives and Medical Men: A History of Interprofessional Rivalries and Women's Rights* (London, Heinemann).

Doyal, L. (1979) *The Political Economy of Health* (London, Pluto).

Doyal, L. (1995) *What Makes Women Sick?* (London, Macmillan).

Drever, F. and Whitehead, M. (1995) 'Mortality in Regions and Local Authority

Districts in the 1990s: Exploring the Relationship with Deprivation', *Population Trends*, 82, 19–27.

Drever, F., Whitehead, M. and Roden, M. (1996) 'Current Patterns and Trends in Male Mortality by Social Class (based on occupation)', *Population Trends*, 86, 15–21.

Drucker, P. (1954) *The Practice of Management* (New York, Harper Row).

Dugdill, L. and Springett, J. (1994) 'Evaluation of Work Based Health Promotion: A Review', *Health Education Journal*, 53, 337–47.

Dunnell, K. (1995) 'Population Review (2): Are We Healthier?', *Population Trends*, 82, 12–18.

Dunnigan, M. G. (1993) 'The Problem with Cholesterol', *British Medical Journal*, 306, 1355–6.

Eastman, N. (1995) 'Anti-therapautic Mental Health Law', *British Medical Journal*, 301, 1081–2.

Eckstein, H. (1960) *Pressure Group Politics: The Case of the BMA* (London, George Allen & Unwin).

Economist (1994) 'The Battle of the Bulge', 20 August, 21–2.

Edwards, G. (ed.) (1994) *Alcohol Policy and the Public Good* (Oxford University Press).

Edwards, N. (1996) 'Lore Unto Themselves', *Health Service Journal*, 12 September, 26–7.

Edwards, N. and Raftery, J. (1995) 'Bedtime Stories', *Health Service Journal*, 2 March, 26–7.

Elcock, H. and Haywood, S. (1980) 'The Centre Cannot Hold', *Public Administration Bulletin*, 36, 53–62.

Elliott, P. *et al.* (1996) 'Intersalt Revisited: Further Analyses of 24 Hour Sodium Excretion and Blood Pressure Within and Across Populations', *British Medical Journal*, 312, 1249–53.

Ellis, K. (1993) *Squaring the Circle: User and Carer Participation in Needs Assessment* (York, Joseph Rowntree Foundation).

Ellwood, S. (1995) 'NHS Costing for Contracting Rules', *Public Money and Management*, 15 (2), 41–7.

Elston, M. (1991) 'The Politics of Professional Power: Medicine in a Changing Health Service', in Gabe, J., Calnan, M. and Bury, M., *The Sociology of the Health Service* (London, Routledge), 58–88.

Engel, G. (1977) 'The Need for a New Medical Model: A Challenge for Biomedicine', *Science*, 196, 129–36.

Enthoven, A. C. (1985) *Reflections on the Management of the National Health Service* (London, Nuffield Provincial Hospitals Trust).

EOC (Equal Opportunities Commission) (1991) *Equality Management: Women's Employment in the NHS* (London, EOC).

Ermisch, J. (1990) *Fewer Babies, Longer Lives* (York, Joseph Rowntree Foundation).

Etzioni, A. (1993) *The Spirit of Community* (USA, Crown).

Ewles, L. (1993) 'Hope Against Hype', *Health Service Journal*, 26 August, 30–1.

Faculty of Public Health Medicine (1991a) *Alcohol and the Public Health* (London, Macmillan).

Faculty of Public Health Medicine (1991b) *UK Levels of Health* (London, Faculty of Public Health Medicine).

Family Heart Study Group (1994) 'Randomised Controlled Trial Evaluating Cardiovascular Screening and Intervention in General Practice', *British Medical Journal*, 308, 313–20.

Farnham, D. and Horton, S. (1993) *Managing the New Public Services* (London, Macmillan).

Ferlie, E. (1994) 'The Creation and Evolution of Quasi-Markets in the Public Sector: Early Evidence From the National Health Service', *Policy and Politics*, 22 (2), 105–122.

Ferlie, E., Ashburner, L. and FitzGerald. L. (1993) 'Movers and Shakers', *Health Service Journal*, 18 November, 24–6.

Ferlie, E., FitzGerald, L. and Ashburner, L. (1996) 'Corporate Governance in the post–1990 NHS: The Role of the Board', *Public Money and Management*, 16 (2), 15–21.

Ferrie, J., Shipley, M., Marmot, M., Stansfield, S. and Smith, G. D. (1995) 'Health Effects of Anticipation of Job Change and Non Employment: Longitudinal Data From the Whitehall II Study', *British Medical Journal*, 311, 1264–9.

Field, F. (1988) 'Thoughts on Reforming the Health Service', *Catholic Herald*, 12 February.

Field, K., Thorogood, M., Silagy, C., Normand, C., O'Neill, C. and Muir, J. (1995) 'Strategies for Reducing Coronary Risk Factors in Primary Care: Which is the Most Cost-Effective?', *British Medical Journal*, 310, 1109–12.

Field, M. G. (ed.) (1989) *Success and Crisis in National Health Systems* (London, Routledge).

Fitzherbert, L. (1992) *Charity and NHS Reform* (London, Directory of Social Change).

Fitzherbert, L. and Giles, S. (1990) *Charity and The National Health: A Report on the Extent and Potential of Charitable Funds within the NHS* (London, The Directory of Social Change).

Fitzhugh, W. (1995) *The Fitzhugh Directory: Independent Health Care in Long Term Care 1995/6* (London, Health Care Information Services).

Fitzpatrick, R. (1984) 'Lay Concepts of Illness', in R. Fitzpatrick *et al.*, *The Experience of Illness* (London, Tavistock).

Flanagan, H. (1989) 'Effective or Efficient Management of Health Care?', *Health Services Management,* December 1989, 266–69.

Flynn, R. (1992) *Structures of Control in Health Management* (London, Routledge).

Flynn, R., Williams, G. and Pickard, S. (1996) *Markets and Networks: Contracting in Community Health Services* (Buckingham, Open University Press).

Ford, B. (1996) *BSE: The Facts* (London, Corgi).

Foster, P. (1995) *Women and the Health Care Industry: An Unhealthy Relationship* (Buckingham, Open University Press).

Foucault, M. (1973) *The Birth of the Clinic* (London, Tavistock).

Foucault, M. (1979) 'On Governmentality', *Ideology and Consciousness*, 6, 5–22.

Fowler, N. (1991) *Ministers Decide: A Personal Memoir of the Thatcher Years* (London, Chapman).

Fox, A. and Shewry, M. (1988) 'New Longitudinal Insights into Relationships Between Unemployment and Mortality', *Stress Medicine*, 4, 11–19.

Fox, J. (ed.) (1989) *Health Inequalities in European Countries* (Aldershot, Gower).

Fox, J., Goldblatt, P. and Jones, D. (1990) 'Social Class Mortality Differentials: Artefact, Selection, or Life Circumstances?', in Goldblatt, P. (ed.), *Longitudinal Study: Mortality and Social Organisation 1971–81*, OPCS LS 6 (London, HMSO), 100–8.

Frankel, S. and West, R. (eds) (1993) *Rationing and Rationality in the National Health Service: The Persistence of Waiting Lists* (London, Macmillan).

Freddi, G. and Bjorkman, J. (1989) *Controlling Medical Professionals: The Comparative Politics of Health Governance* (London, Sage).

Freemantle, N. (1992) 'Spot the Flaw', *Health Service Journal*, 9 July, 122–3.

Freidson, E. (1988) *Profession of Medicine* (London, University of Chicago Press).

Fuchs, V. (1974) *Who Shall Live?* (New York, Basic Books).

Fulder, S. (1992) 'Alternative Therapists in Britain', in Saks, M. P. (ed.), *Alternative Medicine in Britain* (Oxford, Clarendon), 166–82.

Gaines, A. (1979) 'Definitions and Diagnoses: Cultural Implications of Psychiatric Help Seeking and Psychiatrists', Definitions of the Situation in Psychiatric Emergencies', *Culture, Medicine and Psychiatry*, 3 (4), 381–428.

Galbraith, J. K. (1992) *The Culture of Contentment* (London, Sinclair-Stevenson).

Gamble, A. (1994) *The Free Economy and the Strong State. The Politics of Thatcherism*, 2nd edition (London, Macmillan).

Garrett, L. (1995) *The Coming Plague: Newly Emerging Diseases in a World Out of Balance* (Harmondsworth, Penguin).

Garrow, J. (1991) 'The Importance of Obesity', *British Medical Journal*, 303, 704–6.

George, S. (1976) *How the Other Half Dies: The Real Reasons for World Hunger* (Harmondsworth, Penguin).

Giddings, P. (1993) 'Complaints, Remedies and the Health Service Commissioner', *Public Administration*, 71 (3) 377–94.

Gifford, C. (1996) *Deregulation, Disasters and BSE* (Nottingham, European Labour Forum).

Ginzberg, E. (1990) *The Medical Triangle: Physicians, Politicians and the Public* (Cambridge, Mass., Harvard University Press).

Gladstone, D. (1992) *Opening up the Medical Monopoly: Consumer Choice Versus Professional Power* (London, Adam Smith Institute).

Glennerster, H., Matsaganis, M. and Owens, P. (1994) *Implementing GP Fundholding: Wild Card or Winning Hand?* (Buckingham, Open University Press).

Godt, P. (1987) 'Confederation, Consent and Corporation: State Strategies and the Medical Profession in France, Great Britain and West Germany', *Journal of Health Politics, Policy and Law*, 12 (3), 459–80.

Goffman, E. (1968) *Stigma: Notes on the Management of Spoiled Identity* (Harmondsworth, Penguin).

Goldacre, M. and Harris R. (1980) 'Mortality, Morbidity, Resource Allocation and Planning: A Consideration of Disease Classification', *British Medical Journal*, 281, 1515–19.

Goldblatt, P. (1989) 'Mortality by Social Class 1971–85', *Population Trends* (London, HMSO).

Goldblatt, P., Fox, J. and Leon, D. (1990) 'Mortality of Employed Men and Women', in Goldblatt, P. (ed.), *Longitudinal Study: Mortality and Social Organisation, 1971–81*, OPCS LS 6 (London, HMSO), 67–80.

Goldsmith, M. and Willetts, D. (1988) *Managed Health Care Organisations: A New System for a Better Health Service* (London, Centre for Policy Studies).

Goldstein, H. and Spiegelhalter, D. (1996) 'League Tables and their Limitations: Statistical Issues in Comparisons of Institutional Performance', *Journal of the Royal Statistical Society*, 159 (3), 385–443.

Gould, D. (1987) *The Medical Mafia* (London, Sphere).

Graffy, J. and Williams, J. (1994) 'Purchasing for All: An Alternative to Fundholding', *British Medical Journal*, 308, 391–4.

Graham, H. (1984) *Women, Health and the Family* (Brighton, Wheatsheaf).

Graham, H. (1993) *Hardship and Health in Women's Lives* (Brighton, Harvester Wheatsheaf).

Gray, D., Hampson, J., Bernstein, S., Kosekoff, J. and Brook, R. (1990) 'Clinical Practice: The Appropriateness of Performing Coronary Artery Bypass Grafts', *Lancet, 335,* 1317–20.

Green, D. G. (1986) 'Joint Finance: An Analysis of the Reasons for its Limited Success', *Policy and Politics,* 14 (2), 209–20.

Green, D. G. (1988) *Everyone a Private Patient* (London, Institute for Economic Affairs).

Green, D. G., Neuberger, J., Lord Young and Burstall, M. (1990) *The NHS Reforms: What Happened to Consumer Choice?* (London, Institute for Economic Affairs).

Green, D. S. (1987) *The New Right: The Counter Revolution in Political, Economic and Social Thought* (Brighton, Wheatsheaf).

Green, H. (1988) *General Household Survey 1985: Series GHS15A – Informal Carers* (London, HMSO).

Grey-Turner, E. and Sutherland, F. M. (1982) *History of the BMA Part 2, 1932–81* (London, BMA).

Griffin, J. (ed.) (1996) *The Future of Primary Care* (London, Office of Health Economics).

Griffiths, D. (1971) 'Inequalities and Management in the NHS', *The Hospital,* July 1971, 229–33.

Griggs, E. (1991) 'The Politics of Health Care Reform in Britain', *Political Quarterly,* 62 (4), 419–30.

Grol, R. (1990) 'National Standard Setting for Quality of Care in General Practice: Attitudes of GPs and a Response to a Set of Standards', *British Journal of General Practice,* 40, 361–4.

Groves, T. (1990) 'The Future of Community Care', *British Medical Journal,* 300, 923–4.

Guardian (1992) 'Carers Made Ill by Strains of Duties', 22 May, 4.

Hacking, J. (1995) 'For Richer, For Poorer', *Health Service Journal,* 24 July, 22–4.

Hacking, J. (1996) 'Weight Watchers', *Health Service Journal,* 2 May, 28–9.

Hadley, R. and Clough, R. (1996) *Care in Chaos: Frustration and Challenge in Community Care* (London, Cassell).

Hadley, R. and Forster, D. (1993) *Doctors as Managers: Experiences From the Front Line* (London, Longman).

Hadley, T. and Goldman, H. (1995) 'Effect of Recent Health and Social Service Policy Reforms on Britain's Mental Health System', *British Medical Journal,* 311, 1556–8.

Hall, R. H. (1990) *Health and the Global Environment* (Oxford, Polity).

Ham, C. (1986) *Managing Health Services: Health Authority Members in Search of a Role* (University of Bristol, School for Advanced Urban Studies).

Ham, C. (1994) 'Where Now for the NHS Reforms?', *British Medical Journal,* 309, 351–2.

Ham, C. (ed.) (1997) *Healthcare Reform: Learning from International Experience* (Buckingham, Open University Press).

Ham, C. and Matthews, T. (1991) *Purchasing with Authority: The New Role of DHAs* (London, King's Fund College Paper).

Hambleton, R. (1983) 'Health Planning – A Second Chance', *Policy and Politics,* 11 (2), 198–201.

Hancock, C. (1993) 'Time to Ask a Leading Question', *Health Service Journal*, 29 June, 21.

Hancock, C. (1995) 'Nurses Right to be On Board', *Health Service Journal*, 3 May, 23.

Hancock, G. and Carim, E. (1987) *AIDS: The Deadly Epidemic* (London, Gollancz).

Hancock, R. and Jarvis, C (1995) *The Long Term Effects of Being a Carer* (London, HMSO).

Hann, A. (1996) *The Politics of Breast Cancer Screening* (Aldershot, Avebury).

Hansard (1992) House Of Commons Official Report, volume 214, 23 November, 497–8.

Hansard (1993) House Of Commons Official Report, volume 217, 26 January, *864*.

Hansard (1994) House Of Commons Official Report, volume 239, 17 March, *833*.

Harding, S. (1995) 'Social Class Differences in Mortality of Men: Recent Evidence from the OPCS Longitudinal Study', *Population Trends*, 80, 31–7.

Harrison, G. and Bartlett, P. (1994) 'Supervision Registers for Mentally Ill People', *British Medical Journal*, 309, 551–2.

Harrison, S. (1988) 'The Workforce and the New Managerialism', in R. Maxwell (ed.), *Reshaping the NHS* (Oxford, Policy Journals), 141–52.

Harrison, S and Pollitt, C. (1994) *Controlling Health Professionals* (Buckingham, Open University Press).

Harrison, S. and Schulz, R. I. (1989) *Clinical Autonomy in the UK and the US: Contrasts and Convergence*, in Freddie, G. and Bjorkman, J. W. (eds), *Controlling Medical Professionals* (London, Sage), 198–209.

Harrison, S., Hunter, D. J., Marnoch, G. and Pollitt, C. (1992) *Just Managing: Power and Culture in the National Health Service* (London, Macmillan).

Hart, M. (1996) 'Incorporating Outpatient Perceptions into Definitions of Quality', *Journal of Advanced Nursing*, 24, 1234–40.

Harvard Medical Practice Study (1990) *Patients, Doctors and Lawyers: Medical Injury Malpractice and Patient Compensation in New York* (Boston, Harvard Medical Practice Study).

Hashemi, K. and Merlin, M. (1987) 'Are Routine Bacteriological Cultures Necessary in an Accident and Emergency Department?', *British Medical Journal*, 294, 1462–3.

Hawley, K. and Hudson, B. (1996) *Community Care and the Prospects for Service Development* (London, King's Fund).

Hayward, S. and Fee, E. (1992) 'More in Sorrow than in Anger: The British Nurses' Strike of 1988', *International Journal of Health Services*, 22 (3), 397–416.

Haywood, S. (1990) 'Efficiency and the NHS', *Public Money and Management*, 10 (2), 51–4.

Haywood, S. and Alaszewski, A. (1980) *Crisis in the Health Service* (London, Croom Helm).

Health Advisory Service (1987) *Annual Report* (Sutton, HAS).

Healthcare 2000 (1995) *UK Health and Healthcare Services: Challenges and Policy Options* (London, Healthcare 2000).

Health Care Information Services (1995) *The Fitzhugh Directory of Independent Health Care Financial Information* 10th edition 1995/6 (London, HCIS).

Health Care Parliamentary Monitor (1995a), 13 November, 8.

Health Care Parliamentary Monitor (1995b), 23 January, 19.

Health Care Parliamentary Monitor (1995c), 20 March, 14.

Health Promotion Authority for Wales (1990) *Health for All in Wales: Health Promotion Challenges for the 1990s* (Cardiff, HPAFW).

Health Rights (1995), Summer, 5.

Health and Safety Executive (1990) *Surveillance of People Exposed to Health Risks at Work* (London, HMSO).

Health and Safety Executive (1994) *The Cost to the British Economy of Work Accidents and Work-related Ill-Health* (London, HSE).

Health Service Commissioner (1994) (HCP 197) 2nd Report 1993/4, *Failure to Provide Long Term Care for a Brain Damaged Patient* (London, HMSO).

Health Service Commissioner (1996a) (HC 87) 2nd Report 1996/7, *Selected Investigations Completed April to September* (London, HMSO).

Health Service Commissioner (1996b) (HCP 62) 1st Report 1996/7, *Selected Investigations. Access to Official Information in the NHS* (London, HMSO).

Health Service Commissioner (1996c) (HCP 380) 4th Report 1995/6, *Report of the Health Service Commissioner: Investigations of Complaints about Continuing NHS Inpatient Care* (London, HMSO).

Health Service Commissioner (1996d) (HCP 504) 5th Report 1995/6, *Report of the Health Service Commissioner: Investigations of Complaints about Long Term NHS Inpatient Care* (London, HMSO).

Health Service Journal (1995) 'Manager Doctor Relations are Fine', 2 March, 8.

Health Services Management Unit (1996a) *The Future Healthcare Workforce* (Manchester, HSMU).

Health Services Management Unit (1996b) *The Evaluation of the NHS Resource Management Programme in England* (Manchester, HSMU).

Health Visitors Association (1996) *Health Visitors Association Centenary Survey. Return of Diseases and Social Conditions of the Nineteenth Century* (London, HVA).

Hellander, I., Moloo, J., Himmelstein, D., Woolhandler, S. and Wolfe, S. (1995) 'The Growing Epidemic of Uninsurance: New Data on the Health Insurance Coverage of Americans', *International Journal of Health Services*, 25 (3), 377–92.

Helman, C. (1990) *Culture, Health and Illness*, 2nd edn (London, Wright).

Hennessy, P. (1988) *Whitehall* (London, Secker & Warburg).

Henwood, M. (1992) *Through a Glass Darkly: Community Care and Elderly People* (London, King's Fund Institute).

Henwood, M. (1995) *Making a Difference?: Implementation of the Community Care Reforms Two Years On* (London, King's Fund).

Henwood, M. and Wistow, G. (1995) 'The Tasks in Hand', *Health Service Journal*, 13 April, 24–5.

Henwood, M., Wistow, G. and Robinson, J. (1996) 'Halfway There?: Policy, Politics and Outcomes in Community Care', *Social Policy and Administration*, 30 (1), 39–53.

Herzlich, C. and Pierret, J. (1985) 'The Social Construction of the Patient: Patients and Illnesses in Other Ages', *Social Science and Medicine*, 25, 1019–32.

Hibbard, J. and Weekes, E. (1987) 'Consumerism in Health Care: Prevalence and Predictors', *Medical Care*, 25 (11), 1019–32.

Hicks, D. (1976) *Primary Health Care: A Review* (London, HMSO).

Higgins, J. (1988) *The Business of Medicine: Private Health Care in Britain* (London, Macmillan).

Higgins, J. (1989) 'Defining Community Care: Realities and Myths', *Social Policy and Administration*, 23 (1), 3–16.

Hoare, J. (1992) *Tidal Wave: New Technology, Medicine and the NHS* (London, King's Fund).

Hodgkinson, R. (1967) *The Origins of the NHS: The Medical Services of the New Poor Law* (London, Wellcome Foundation).

Hoffenberg, R. (1987) *Clinical Freedom* (London, Nuffield Hospital Provincial Trust).

Hogg, C. (1986) *Community Health Councils: A Review of Their Role and Structure* (London, ACHCEW).

Home Office (1995) *Statistics of Drug Addicts Notified to the Home Office*, UK 1994. Home Office Bulletin 95/17 (London, Home Office).

Honigsbaum, F. (1979) *The Division in British Medicine* (London, Kogan Page).

Honigsbaum, F. (1989) *Health, Happiness and Security: The Creation of the NHS* (London, Routledge and Chapman & Hall).

Honigsbaum, F. (1990) 'The Evolution of the NHS', *British Medical Journal*, 301, 694–9.

Honigsbaum, F. (1992) *Who Shall Live? Who Shall Die?*, Oregon's Health Financing Proposals (London, King's Fund College Papers).

Hopkins, A. and Bahl, V. (eds) (1993) *Access to Health Care for People from Black and Ethnic Minorities* (London, The Royal College of Physicians).

Horrobin, D. (1977) *Medical Hubris: A Reply to Illich* (London, Churchill Livingstone).

House of Commons (1985) (HC 13) *2nd Report 1985/6. Community Care with Special Reference to Adult Mentally Ill and Mentally Handicapped People*, Social Services Committee (London, HMSO).

House of Commons (1986) (HC 387) *4th Report 1985/6. Public Expenditure in the Social Services*, Social Services Committee (London, HMSO).

House of Commons (1988a) (HC 494) *8th Report 1987/8. Civil Service Reform: The Next Steps.* Treasury and Civil Committee (London, HMSO).

House of Commons (1988b) (HC 300) *26th Report 1987/8. Community Care Developments*, Public Accounts Committee (London, HMSO).

House of Commons (1988c) (HC 613) *5th Report 1987/8. The Future of the NHS*, Social Services Committee (London, HMSO).

House of Commons (1989a) (HC 108) *1st Report 1988/9. Salmonella in Eggs*, Select Committee on Agriculture (London, HMSO).

House of Commons (1989b) (HC 249) *26th Report 1988/9. Coronary Heart Disease*, Public Accounts Committee (London, HMSO).

House of Commons (1989c) (HC 214.III) *8th Report 1988/9. Resourcing the NHS: The Government's Plans for the Future of the NHS*, Social Services Committee (London, HMSO).

House of Commons (1990a) (HC 163) *28th Report 1989/90. The NHS and the Independent Hospitals*, Public Accounts Committee (London, HMSO).

House of Commons (1990b) (HC 410) *5th Report 1989/90. Community Care: Carers*, Social Services Committee (London, HMSO).

House of Commons (1990c) (HC 444) *6th Report 1989/90. Choice for Service Users*, Social Services Committee (London, HMSO).

House of Commons (1990d) (HC 580) *8th Report 1989/90. Community Care: Planning and Co-operation*, Social Services Committee (London, HMSO).

House of Commons (1990e) (HC 558) *9th Report 1989/90. Community Care: Quality*, Social Services Committee (London, HMSO).

House of Commons (1990f) (HC 664) *11th Report 1989/90. Community Care: Services for People with Mental Handicap and People with Mental Illness*, Social Services Committee (London, HMSO).

House of Commons (1991a) (HC 429) *1st Report 1990/1. Public Expenditure on Health Services. Waiting Lists,* Health Committee (London, HMSO).

House of Commons (1991b) (HC390) *6th Report 1990/1. Elective Surgery,* Welsh Affairs Committee (London, HMSO).

House of Commons (1992) (HC 29) *2nd Report 1991/2. Maternity Services,* Health Committee (London, HMSO).

House of Commons (1993a) (HCP 275) *26th Report 1992/3. The Chelsea and Westminster Hospital,* Public Accounts Committee (London, HMSO).

House of Commons (1993b) (HC 485) *57th Report 1992/3. West Midlands Regional Health Authority: Regionally Managed Services Organisation,* Public Accounts Committee (London, HMSO).

House of Commons (1993c) (HC 658) *63rd Report 1992/3, Wessex Regional Health Authority Regional Information Systems Plan,* Public Accounts Committee (London, HMSO).

House of Commons (1993d) (HC 309) *3rd Report 1992/3. Community Care: Funding from April 1993,* Health Committee (London, HMSO).

House of Commons (1994) (HC102) *1st Report 1993/4. Better Off in the Community. The Care of People who are Seriously Mentally Ill,* Health Committee (London, HMSO).

House of Commons (1995a) (HCP 264) *27th Report 1994/5. GP Fundholding in England,* Public Accounts Committee (London, HMSO).

House of Commons (1995b) (HC 134) *1st Report 1994/5. Priority Setting in the NHS,* Health Committee (London, HMSO).

House of Commons (1995c) (HC 32) *2nd Report 1995/6. Health Care International (Scotland) Ltd,* Public Accounts Committee (London, HMSO).

House of Commons (1995d) (HC19) *1st Report 1995/6. NHS Responsibilities for Meeting Continuing Healthcare Needs* (London, HMSO).

House of Commons (1995e) (HC 20) *2nd Report 1994/5. London Ambulance Service,* Health Committee (London, HMSO).

House of Commons (1995f) (HC 448) *42nd Report 1995/6. NHS Outpatient Services in England and Wales,* Public Accounts Committee (London, HMSO).

House of Commons (1995g) (HC 324) *3rd Report 1994/5. Breast Cancer Services,* Health Committee (London, HMSO).

House of Commons (1996a) (HC 59) *3rd Report 1995/6. Long Term Care. Future Provision and Funding,* Health Committee (London, HMSO).

House of Commons (1996b) (HC 304) *31st Report 1995/6. Clinical Audit in England,* Public Accounts Committee (London, HMSO).

House of Commons (1996c) (HC 39) *3rd Report 1995/6. Report of the Health Service Ombudsman for 1994/5,* Select Committee on the Parliamentary Commissioner for Administration (London, HMSO).

House of Commons (1996d) (HC 146) *6th Report 1995/6. The Private Finance Initiative,* Public Accounts Committee (London, HMSO).

House of Commons (1996e) (HC 477) *2nd Report 1995/6. Allocation of Resources of Health Authorities,* Health Committee (London, HMSO).

Howie, J., Heaney, D. and Maxwell, M (1995) *General Practice Fundholding Shadow Project and Evaluation* (Edinburgh, University of Edinburgh).

Hoyes, L., Lart, R., Means, R. and Taylor, M. (1994) *Community Care in Transition* (York, Joseph Rowntree Foundation).

Hudson, B. (1992) 'Quasi-Markets in Health and Social Care in Britain. Can The Public Sector Respond?', *Policy and Politics,* 20 (2), 131–42.

Hudson, B. (1995) 'Joint Commissioning: Organisational Revolution or Misplaced Enthusiasm?', *Policy and Politics*, 23 (3), 233–49.

Hughes, K, MacKintosh, A. M., Hasting, G., Wheeler, C., Watson, J. and Inglis., J. (1997) 'Young People, Alcohol, and Designer Drinks. Quantitative and Qualitative Study', *British Medical Journal*, 314, 414–18.

Hunt, P. (1995) 'Accountability in the National Health Service', *Parliamentary Affairs*, 48 (2), 297–305.

Hunter, D. (1993) 'Protect and Survive', *Health Service Journal*, 18 November, 21.

Hunter, D. J. and Webster, C. (1992) 'Here We Go Again', *Health Services Journal*, 5 March, 26–7.

Hunter, H. (1995) 'CHCs Challenge Attempt to Undermine Autonomy', *Health Service Journal*, 14 July, 8.

Huntington, J. (1993) 'From FPC to FHSA To. . . Health Commission?', *British Medical Journal*, 306, 33–6.

Hutton, W. (1996) *The State We're In* (London, Vintage).

Iliffe, S. (1988) *Strong Medicine: Health Service Politics for the 21st Century* (London, Lawrence & Wishart).

Illich, I. (1975) *Limits to Medicine* (Harmondsworth, Penguin).

Illsley, R. (1986) 'Occupational Class Selection and the Production of Inequalities in Health', *Quarterly Journal of Social Affairs*, 2 (2), 151–65.

Imperial Cancer Research Fund Oxcheck Study Group (1995) 'Effectiveness of Health Checks Conducted by Nurses in Primary Care', *British Medical Journal*, 310, 1099–1104.

Independent Scientific Committee on Smoking and Health (1988) *4th Report* (London, HMSO).

Independent (1995) 'NHS Dentists Drop', 12 May, 10.

Inglis, B. (1965) *A History of Medicine* (London, Weidenfeld & Nicolson).

Inglis, B. (1981) *The Diseases of Civilisation* (London, Hodder & Stoughton).

Insight Management Consulting (1996) *Resourcing and Performance Management in Community Health Councils* (London, Department of Health).

Institute of Health Service Management (IHSM) (1993) *Future Health Care Options* (London, IHSM).

Institute of Health Service Management (IHSM) (1995) *Current Issues in Acute Care: Reconfiguring Acute Services II* (London, IHSM).

Institute for Public Policy Research (1995a) *Primary Health Care: A Prognosis* (London, IPPR).

Institute for Public Policy Research (1995b) *Voices Off: Tackling the Democratic Deficit in Health* (London, IPPR).

Institute for Public Policy Research (1996) *Paying for Long Term Care* (London, IPPR).

Jackman, J. (1995) 'Filling In', *Health Service Journal*, 31 August, 24–5.

Jacobs, D., Blackburn, H., Higgins, M., Reed, D., Iso, H. and McMillan, G. (1992) 'Report of the Conference on Low Blood Cholesterol: Mortality Associations', *Circulation*, 86, 1046–60.

Jacobson, B., Smith, A. and Whitehead, M. (1991) *The Nation's Health: A Strategy for the 1990s*, 2nd edn (London, King's Fund Centre).

Jamdagni, L. (1996) *Purchasing for Black Populations* (London, King's Fund).

James, A. (1994) *Managing to Care: Public Services and the Market* (London, Longman).

Jarman, B. (1993) 'Is London Overbedded?', *British Medical Journal*, 306, 979–82.

Jarvis, C., Hancock, Askham, J. and Tinker, A. (1996) *Getting Around After 60: A Profile of Britain's Older Population* (London, HMSO).

Jenkins, J. (1985) *Caring for Women's Health* (London, Search Press).

Jenkins, P. (1987) *Mrs Thatcher's Revolution: The Ending of the Socialist Era* (London, Jonathan Cape).

Jenkins, R. (1993) 'Defining the Problem. Stress, Depression and Anxiety: Causes, Prevalence and Consequences', in Jenkins, R. and Warman, D. (eds), *Promoting Mental Health Policies in the Workplace* (London, HMSO).

Jennett, B. (1986) *High Technology Medicine* (Oxford University Press).

Johnson, M. (1993) 'Equal Opportunities in Service Delivery. Response to a Changing Population?', in Ahmad, W. (ed.) (1993) *Race and Health in Contemporary Britain* (Buckingham, Open University Press), 183–200.

Johnson, N. (1989) 'The Privatisation of Welfare', *Social Policy and Administration*, 23 (2), 17–30.

Johnson, P., Conrad, C. and Thomson, D. (1989) *Workers versus Pensioners* (London, Centre for Economic Policy Research).

Johnson, T. (1972) *Professions and Power* (London, Macmillan).

Johnson, T. (1995) 'Governmentality and the Institutionalisation of Expertise', in Johnson, T., Larkin, G. and Saks, M. (eds), *Health Professsions and the State in Europe* (London, Routledge), 7–24.

Joint NHS Privatisation Unit (1990) *The Privatisation Experience* (London, JNHSPU).

Jones, A. and Duncan, A. (1995) *Hypothecated Health Taxes: An Evaluation of Recent Proposals* (London, Office of Health Economics).

Jones, B. (1994) 'Nursing, Obstetrics and Gynaecology', in Burrows, M., Dyson, R., Jackson, P. and Saxton, H. (eds), *Management for Hospital Doctors* (Oxford, Butterworth-Heinemann).

Jones, I. and Higgs, P. (1990) 'Putting People before Logic', *Health Service Journal*, 31 May, 814–5.

Jones, K. (1995) *Accountability Not Ownership: Labour and the NHS* (London, Fabian Society).

Jönsson, B. (1990) 'What can Americans Learn from Europeans?', in OECD, *Health Care Systems in Transition* (Paris, OECD).

Joseph Rowntree Foundation (1995) *Income and Wealth* (York, Joseph Rowntree Foundation).

Joseph Rowntree Foundation (1996) *Inquiry into Meeting the Cost of Continuing Care* (York, York Publishing Services).

Joss, R. and Kogan, M. (1995) *Advancing Total Quality: Total Quality Management in the National Health Service* (Buckingham, Open University Press).

Jowell, R., Witherspoon, F. and Brook, L. (1989) *British Social Attitudes Survey* (London, Social and Community Planning Research).

Jowell, R., Brooke, L., Prior, G. and Taylor, B. (1992) *British Social Attitudes: The 9th Report*, 1992/3 edn, Social and Community Planning Research (Aldershot, Dartmouth).

Judge, K. (1995) 'Income Distribution and Life Expectancy: A Critical Appraisal', *British Medical Journal*, 311, 1282–5.

Judge, K. and Solomon, M. (1993) 'Public Opinion and the NHS: Patterns and Perspectives in Consumer Satisfaction', *Journal of Social Policy*, 22 (3), 299–327.

Kammerling, R. and Kinnear, A. (1996) 'The Extent of the Two Tier Service for Fundholders', *British Medical Journal*, 312, 1399–1401.

Kaplan, G., Pamuk, E., Lynch, J., Cohen, R. and Balfour, J. (1996) 'Inequality in Income and Mortality in the United States', *British Medical Journal*, 312, 999–1003.

Karpf, A. (1988) *Doctoring the Media: The Reporting of Health and Medicine* (London, Routledge).

Kavanagh, D. (1990) *Thatcherism and British Politics* (Oxford University Press).

Kelleher, D. (1994) 'Self-Help Groups and their Relationship with Medicine', in Gabe, J., Kelleher, D. and Williams, G. (eds), *Challenging Medicine* (London, Routledge), 104–17.

Kendrick, K., Weir, P. and Rosser, E. (1995) *Innovations in Nursing Practice* (London, Edward Arnold).

Kennedy, I. (1981) *The Unmasking of Medicine* (London, Allen & Unwin).

Kennedy, B., Kawacki, I. and Prothrow-Smith, D. (1996) 'Income Distribution and Mortality: Cross Sectional Ecological Study of the Robin Hood Index in the United States', *British Medical Journal*, 312, 1004–7.

Kerr, A and Radford, M. (1994) 'TUPE or not TUPE: Competitive Tendering and the Transfer Laws', *Public Money and Management*, 14 (4), 37–45.

Key, T., Thorogood, M., Appleby, P. and Burr, M. (1996) 'Dietary Habits and Mortality in 11000 Vegetarians and Health Conscious People: Results of a 17 Year Follow-up', *British Medical Journal*, 313, 775–9.

King, D. S. (1987) *The New Right: Politics Markets and Citizenship* (London, Macmillan).

King's Fund (1992) *London Health Care 2010* (London, King's Fund).

King's Fund (1995) *London Monitor No.2: Focusing on London's Health Services* (London, King's Fund).

Kirkness, B. (1996) *Putting Patients First. The Emerging Role of Patients in the Provision of Healthcare* (London, Association of British Pharmaceutical Industry).

Klein, R. (1977) 'The Health Commissioner: No Cause for Complaint', *British Medical Journal*, 22 January, 248–9.

Klein, R. (1980) 'Between Nihilism and Utopia in Health Care', Lecture, Yale University, New Haven (Unpublished).

Klein, R. (1983) *The Politics of the National Health Service*, 1st edn (London, Longman).

Klein, R. (1989) 'The Role of Health Economics', *British Medical Journal*, 299, 275–6.

Klein, R. (1990a) 'The State and the Profession: The Politics of the Double Bed', *British Medical Journal*, 301, 700–2.

Klein, R. (1990b) 'What Future for the Department of Health?', *British Medical Journal*, 301, 481–4.

Klein, R. (1994) 'Lessons from the Financial Scandals in Wessex and the West Midlands', *British Medical Journal*, 308, 22 January, 215–16.

Klein, R. (1995) *The New Politics of the NHS* (London, Longman).

Klein, R. and Lewis, J. (1976) *The Politics of Consumer Representation* (London, Centre for Studies in Social Policy).

Klein, R. and Day, P. (1992) 'Constitutional and Distributional Conflict in British Medical Politics: The Case of General Practice 1911–1991', *Political Studies*, 40 (3), 462–78.

Klein, R., Day, P. and Redmayne, S. (1996) *Managing Scarcity. Priority–Setting and Rationing in the NHS* (Buckingham, Open University Press).

Kleinman, A. (1978) 'Concepts and a Model for the Comparison of Medical Systems as Cultural Systems', *Social Science and Medicine*, 12 (2B), 85–93.

Krause, R. (1981) *The Restless Tide: The Persistent Challenge of the Microbial World* (Washington DC, National Foundation for Infectious Diseases).

Labour Party (1992a) *No Previous Experience Required: A Survey of 3rd Wave Trusts* (London, Labour Party).

Labour Party (1992b) *Your Good Health* (London, Labour Party).

Labour Party (1995) *Renewing the NHS* (London, Labour Party).

Labour Research Department (1994) 'The NHS: Unelected Tory Quangos', *Labour Research*, December.

Lacey, R. (1994) *Mad Cow Disease* (St Helier, Cypsela Publications).

Laidlaw, D., Bloom, P., Hughes, A., Sparrow, J. and Marmion, V. (1994) 'The Sight Test Fee: Effect on Ophthalmology Referrals and Rate of Glaucoma Detection', *British Medical Journal*, 309, 634–6.

Laing, W. (1995) *Care of Elderly People. Market Survey* (London, Laing & Buisson).

Laing, W. (1996) *Laing's Review of Private Health Care 1996* (London, Laing & Buisson).

Langan, M. (1990) 'Community Care in the 1990s. The Community Care White Paper "Caring for People" ', *Critical Social Policy*, 29, 58–71.

Langham, S. and Black, N. (1995) 'The Evolution of a Public Sector Market for Cardiac Services in the UK 1991–4', *Public Money and Management*, 15 (3), July–September, 31–8.

Larkin, G. (1983) *Occupational Monopoly and Modern Medicine* (London, Tavistock).

Larson, M. (1977) *The Rise of Professionalism* (Berkeley, University of California Press).

Laughlin, R. and Broadbent, J. (1994) 'The Managerial Reform of Health and Education in the UK: Value for Money or a Devaluing Process', *Political Quarterly*, 65 (2), 152–67.

Law, M., Thompson, S. and Wald, N. (1994) 'Assessing Possible Hazards of Reducing Serum Cholesterol', *British Medical Journal*, 308, 373–9.

Law, M., Wald, N., Wu, T., Hackshaw, A. and Bailey, A. (1994) 'Systematic Underestimation of Association Between Serum Cholesterol Concentrations and Ischaemic Heart Disease in Observational Studies', *British Medical Journal*, 308, 363–6.

Lawrence, M. (ed.) (1987) *Fed Up and Hungry: Women, Oppression and Food* (London, Womens', Press).

Lawrence, M. and Williams, T. (1996) 'Managed Care and Disease Management in the NHS', *British Medical Journal*, 313, 125–6.

Lawson, N. (1992) *The View from Number 11. Memoirs of a Tory Radical* (London, Bantam Press).

Leadbeater, M. (1996) 'Why Essex Kept Together', *Care Plan*, 3 (2), 9–10.

Leadbeater, P. (1990) *Partners in Health: The NHS and the Independent Sector* (Birmingham, National Association of Health Authorities and Trusts).

Leavey, R., Wilkin, D. and Metcalfe, D. (1989) 'Consumerism and General Practice', *British Medical Journal*, 298, 737–9.

Leese, B. (1996) 'Dr Livingstone I Presume?', *Health Service Journal*, 5 December, 24–6.

Leese, B. and Bosanquet, N. (1995a) 'Change in General Practice and its Effects on Service Provision in Areas with Different Socioeconomic Characteristics', *British Medical Journal*, 311, 546–7.

Leese, B. and Bosanquet, N. (1995b) 'Family Doctors and Change in Practice Strategy Since 1986', *British Medical Journal*, 310, 705–8.

Leeson, J. and Gray, J. (1978) *Women and Medicine* (London, Tavistock).

Le Grand, J. (1978) 'The Distribution of Public Expenditure and the Case of Health Care', *Economica*, 45, 125–42.

Le Grand, J. (1994) 'Internal Market Rules OK', *British Medical Journal*, 309, 1596.

Le Grand, J. and Bartlett, W. (1993) *Quasi-Markets and Social Policy* (London, Macmillan).

Leichter, H. M. (1979) *A Comparative Approach to Policy Analysis: Health Care Policy in Four Nations* (London, Cambridge University Press).

Leonard, O., Allsop, J., Taket, A. and Wiles, R. (1997) *'User Involvement in Two Primary Health Care Projects in London'*, Social Science Research Paper 5 (London, South Bank University).

Levick, P. (1992) 'The Janus Face of Community Care Legislation: An Opportunity for Radical Possibilities', *Critical Social Policy*, 34, 75–92.

Lewis, J. (1987) *What Price Community Medicine?* (Brighton, Wheatsheaf).

Lewis, J. and Glennerster, H. (1996) *Implementing the New Community Care* (Buckingham, Open University Press).

Lewis, J., Bernstock, P., Bovell, V. and Wookey, F. (1996) 'The Purchaser–provider Split in Social Care: Is it Working?', *Social Policy and Administration*, 30 (1), 1–19.

Ley, P. (1982) 'Satisfaction, Compliance and Communication', *British Journal of Clinical Psychology*, 21, 241–54.

Liberal Democrats (1992) *Restoring the Nation's Health*, Federal Paper Number 5 (London, Liberal Democrats).

Liberal Democrats (1995) *Building on the Best of the NHS* (London, Liberal Democrats).

Light, D. (1991) 'Professionalism as Countervailing Power', *Journal of Health Politics, Policy and Law*, 16, 499–506.

Limb, M. (1995) 'Banham Delivers Scathing Attack on NHS Governance', *Health Service Journal*, 30 November, 6.

Lock, S. (1986) 'Self Help Groups: The Fourth Estate in Medicine', *British Medical Journal*, 293, 159–60.

Loewy, E. H. (1980) 'Cost Should Not Be A Factor In Medical Care', *New England Journal of Medicine*, 302, 697.

Lord President of the Council (1991) *Action Against Alcohol Misuse* (London, HMSO).

Loveridge, R. and Starkey, K. (1992) *Continuity and Crisis in the NHS* (Buckingham, Open University Press).

Lowry, S. (1988) 'Focus on Performance Indicators', *British Medical Journal*, 296, 992–4.

Lowry, S. (1991) *Housing and Health* (London, British Medical Journal Publications).

Lowy, A., Brazier, J., Fall, M., Thomas, K., Jones, N. and Williams, B. (1993) 'Minor Surgery by General Practitioners Under the 1990 Contract: Effect on Hospital Workload', *British Medical Journal*, 307, 413–17.

Lupton, D., Donaldson, C. and Lloyd, P. (1991) 'Caveat Emptor or Blissful Ignorance: Patients and the Consumerist Ethos', *Social Science and Medicine*, 33, 559–68.

Maddock, S. (1995) 'Is Macho Management Back?', *Health Service Journal*, 23 February, 26–7.

Mahon, A., Wilkin, D. and Whitehouse, C. (1994) 'Choice of Hospital for Elective Surgery Referral: GPs' and Patients' Views', in Robinson, R. and Le Grand, J. (1994) *Evaluating the NHS Reforms* (Newbury, Policy Journals), 108–29.

Majeed, A., Troy., G., Nicholl, J., Smythe, A., Reed, M., Stoddart *et al.* (1996) 'Randomised, Prospective Single Blind Comparison of Laparoscopic versus Small Incision Cholecystectomy', *Lancet*, 347, 989–94.

Mandelson, P. and Liddle, R. (1996) *The Blair Revolution: Can New Labour Deliver?* (London, Faber & Faber).

Mann, J. (ed.) (1993) *Aids in the World: A Global Report* (Cambridge University Press, Harvard).

Manton, K. Stalland, E. and Corder, L. (1995) 'Changes in Morbidity and Chronic Disability in the US Elderly Population. Evidence from 1982, 1984 and 1989 National Long Term Care Survey', *Journal of Gerontology*, 50B, S104–204.

Marinker, M. (ed.) (1990) *Medical Audit and General Practice* (London, British Medical Journal).

Marks, D. (1995) 'Balancing Act', *Health Service Journal*, 13 April, 26–7.

Marks, L. (1988) *Promoting Better Health: An Analysis of the Government's Programme for Improving Primary Care,* Briefing Paper no. 7 (London, King's Fund Institute).

Marmot, M. G., Davey-Smith, G., Stansfield, S., Patel, C., North, F., Head, J., White, I., Brunner, E. and Feeney, A. (1991) 'Health inequalities among British Civil Servants: the Whitehall II Study', *Lancet*, 337, 1387–93.

Marmot, M. and McDowall, M. (1986) 'Mortality Decline and Widening Social Inequalities', *Lancet*, 2, 274–76.

Marmot, M. and Shipley, M (1996) 'Do Socioeconomic Differences in Mortality Persist After Retirement? 25 Year Follow Up of Civil Servants from the First Whitehall Study', *British Medical Journal*, 313, 1177–80.

Marnoch, G. (1996) *Doctors and Management in the NHS* (Buckingham, Open University Press).

Marsh, D. and Rhodes, R. (1992) *Implementing Thatcherite Policies* (Buckingham, Open University Press).

Martin, C. (1992) 'Attached, Detached or New Recruits?', *British Medical Journal*, 305, 348–50.

Martin, J. (1984) *Hospitals in Trouble* (Oxford, Blackwell).

Mather, H. and Elkeles, R. (1995) 'Attitudes of Consultant Physicians to the Calman Proposals: A Questionnaire Survey', *British Medical Journal*, 311, 1060–2.

Mays, N. and Bevan, G. (1987) *Resource Allocation in the Health Service* (London, Bedford Square Press).

McCormick, A., Fleming, D. and Charlton, J. (1995) *Morbidity Statistics from General Practice, 4th National Study 1991/2* (London, HMSO).

McCormick, S. S. (1989) 'Cervical Smears: A Questionable Practice?', *The Lancet*, 2, 207.

McIver, S. (1991) *An Introduction to Obtaining the Views of Users of Health Services* (London, King's Fund Centre).

McKeown, T. (1979) *The Role of Medicine: Dream, Mirage or Nemesis?* (Oxford, Blackwell).

McKinlay, J. (1979) 'Epidemiological and Political Developments of Social Policies Regarding the Public Health', *Social Science and Medicine,* 13A, 541–8.

McKinlay, J. (ed.) (1988) 'The Changing Character of the Medical Profession', *Milbank Quarterly* 66, Supplement 2.

McLachlan, G. (1990) *What Price Quality? The NHS in Review* (London, Nuffield Provincial Hospitals Trust).

McLoone, P and Boddy, F. (1994) 'Deprivation and Mortality in Scotland: 1981–91', *British Medical Journal*, 309, 1465–70.

McPherson, K., Strong, P. M. and Epstein, A. (1981) 'Regional Variations in the Use of Common Surgical Procedures: Within and Between England and Wales, Canada and the USA', *Social Science and Medicine*, 15A, 273–88.

Meade, T., Dyer, S., Browne, W. and Frank, A. (1995) 'Randomised Comparison of Chiropractic and Hospital Outpatient Management for Low Back Pain: Results From Extended Follow Up', *British Medical Journal*, 311, 349–51.

Meads, G. (1996) *A Primary Care Led NHS: Putting it into Practice* (London, Churchill Livingstone).

Means, R and Smith, R. (1994) *Community Care: Policy and Practice* (London, Macmillan).

Mechanic, D. (1961) 'The Concept of Illness Behaviour', *Journal of Chronic Diseases*, 15, 189–94.

Mechanic, D. (1991) 'Sources of Countervailing Power in Medicine', *Journal of Health Policy, Politics and Law* 16, 485–98.

Meltzer, H., Gill, B., Petticrew, M. and Hinds, K. (1995) *The Prevalence of Psychiatric Morbidity Among Adults Living in Private Households* (London, HMSO).

Mental Health Act Commission (1995) *Sixth Biennial Report 1993–5* (London, HMSO).

Mental Health Foundation (1994) *Report on Community Care* (London, Mental Health Foundation).

Mercer, J. and Talbot, I. C. (1985) 'Clinical Diagnosis: A Post Mortem Assessment of Accuracy in the 1980s', *Post Graduate Medical Journal*, 61, 713–16.

Micozzi, M. (1995) *Fundamentals of Complementary and Alternative Medicine* (London, Churchill Livingstone).

Mihill, C. (1996) 'GPs Pay the Price for Wrong Medicine', *Guardian*, 4 June, 7.

Miles, A. (1991) *Women, Health and Medicine* (Buckingham, Open University Press).

Millar, B. (1995) 'Time Machine', *Health Service Journal*, 20 April, 11.

Miller, P and Plant, M. (1996) 'Drinking, Smoking and Illicit Drug Use Among 15–16 Year Olds in the United Kingdom', *British Medical Journal*, 313, 394–7.

Mills, A and Zwi, A. (1995) *Health Policies in Developing Countries* (Chichester, John Wiley).

Millstone, E. (1986) *Food Additives* (Harmondsworth, Penguin).

Milne, R. (1987) 'Competitive Tendering in the NHS: An Economic Analysis of the Early Implementation of HC (83)18', *Public Administration*, 65 (2), 145–60.

Ministry of Health (1954) *Report of the Committee on Economic and Financial Problems of Old Age* (The Phillips Report) (London, HMSO).

Ministry of Health (1959) *Report of the Committee on Maternity Services* (The Cranbrook Report) (London, HMSO).

Ministry of Health (1963) *The Field of Work of the Family Doctor* (The Gillie Report) (London, HMSO).

Ministry of Health (1968) *The National Health Service. The Administrative Structure of the Medical and Related Services in England and Wales* (London, HMSO).

Mohan, J. (1995) *A National Health Service?* (Basingstoke, Macmillan).

Monopolies and Mergers Commission (1993) *Private Medical Services: A Report on Agreements and Practices Relating to Charges for the Supply of Private Medical Services by NHS Consultants* (London, HMSO).

Montgomery, H., Hunter, S., Morris, S., Naunton-Morgan, R. and Marshall, R. (1994) 'Interpretation of Electrocardiograms by Doctors', *British Medical Journal*, 309, 1551–2.

Moon, G. and Lupton, C. (1995) 'Within Acceptable Limits: Health Care Provider Perspectives on Community Health Councils in the Reformed British National Health Service', *Policy and Politics*, 23 (4), 335–46.

Mooney, G. H. and Healey, A. (1991) 'Strategy full of good intentions', *British Medical Journal*, 303, 1119–20.

Moore, W (1995) 'Is Doctors' Power Shrinking?', *Health Service Journal*, 9 November, 24–7.

Moran, G. (1989) 'Public Health at Risk', *Health Service Journal*, 1 June, 668–9.

Moran, M. (1991) *Welfare State, Health Care State*, Paper given at the Political Studies Annual Conference, Lancaster.

Moran, M. (1994) 'Reshaping the Health Care State', *Government and Opposition*, 29 (1), 48–63.

Moran, M. and Wood, B. (1992) *States, Regulation and the Medical Profession* (Buckingham, Open University Press).

Morris, J. K., Cook, D. and Shaper, A. (1994) 'Loss of Employment and Mortality', *British Medical Journal*, 308, 1135–9.

Morris, J. N. (1980) 'Are Health Services Important to People's Health?', *British Medical Journal*, 280, 167–8.

Morse, S. (ed.) (1993) *Emerging Viruses* (Oxford University Press).

Moser, K., Goldblatt, P., Fox., J. and Jones, D. (1990) 'Unemployment and Mortality', in Goldblatt, P. (ed.), *Longitudinal Study: Mortality and Social Organisation 1971–81*, OPCS LS 6 (London, HMSO), 81–97.

Mullen, P. (1995) 'The Provision of Specialist Services Under Contracting', *Public Money and Management*, 15 (3), 23–30.

Mulube, M. (1996) 'Myths Dispelled About Chronic Fatigue Syndrome', *British Medical Journal*, 313, 839.

NAHA and NCVO (National Association of Health Authorities and National Council for Voluntary Organisations) (1987) *Partnerships for Health* (Birmingham, NAHA).

NAHAT (National Association of Health Authorities and Trusts) (1990) *Healthcare Economic Review* (Birmingham, NAHAT).

NAHAT (National Association of Health Authorities and Trusts) (1995) *Testing the Market*, Research Paper 18 (Birmingham, NAHAT).

NAHAT (National Association of Health Authorities and Trusts) (1996) *The Update. What Makes NHS Boards Effective?* (Birmingham, NAHAT).

Nairne, P. (1984) 'Parliamentary Control and Accountability', in R. Maxwell and R. Weaver (eds), *Public Participation in Health* (London, King Edward's Hospital Fund for London), 33–51.

NAO (National Audit Office) (1987) (HC 108) *Community Care Developments 1987/88* (London, HMSO).

NAO (National Audit Office) (1988) (HC 498) *Management of Family Practitioner Services* (London, HMSO).

NAO (National Audit Office) (1989a) (HC 106) *The NHS and the Independent Hospitals* (London, HMSO).

NAO (National Audit Office) (1989b) (HC 566) *Financial Management in the NHS* (London, HMSO).

NAO (National Audit Office) (1993) (HC 605) *Income Generation in the NHS* (London, HMSO).

NAO (National Audit Office) (1995a) (HC 359) *NHS Outpatient Services in England and Wales* (London, HMSO).

NAO (National Audit Office) (1995b) (HC 261) *Contracting for Acute Health Care in England* (London, HMSO).

NAO (National Audit Office (1996a) (HC 332) *The NHS Executive: The Hospital Information Support Systems Initiative* (London, HMSO).

NAO (National Audit Office) (1996b) (HC 280) *Inquiry Commissioned by the NHS Chief Executive into Matters Concerning the former Yorkshire Regional Health Authority* (London, HMSO).

NAO (National Audit Office) (1996c) (HC 656) *Health of the Nation: A Progress Report* (London, HMSO).

Nath, U. (1986) *Smoking: Third World Alert* (Oxford, University Press).

National Consumer Council (1992) *Quality Standards in the NHS. The Consumer Focus* (London, NCC).

National Consumer Council (1995) *Charging Consumers for Social Services: Local Authority Policy and Practice* (London, NCC).

National Economic Research Associates (1995) *Healthcare Report: Are Pay Beds Profitable?* (Eastleigh, Norwich Union).

National Institute for Social Work (1988) *Residential Care: A Positive Choice Report of the Independent Review of Residential Care* (The Wagner Report) (London, HMSO).

Navarro, V. (1978) *Class Struggle, the State and Medicine* (Oxford, Martin Robertson).

Navarro, V. (1994) *The Politics of Health Policy: The US Reforms 1980–94* (Massachusetts, Blackwell).

Newbrander, W. and Parker, D. (1992) 'The Public and Private Sectors in Health and Economic Issues', *International Journal of Health Planning and Management,* 7, 37–49.

Newton, J., Henderson, J. and Goldacre, M. (1995) 'Waiting List Dynamics and the Impact of Earmarked Funding', *British Medical Journal,* 311, 783–5.

NHSE (NHS Executive) (1994a) *Code of Conduct and Accountability* EL (94) 40 (Leeds, NHSE).

NHSE (NHS Executive) (1994b) *NHS Responsibilities for Meeting Long Term Health Care Needs* HSG (94) (Leeds, NHSE).

NHSE (NHS Executive) (1995a) *Code of Practice on Openness in the NHS* (Leeds, NHSE).

NHSE (NHS Executive) (1995b) *Priorities and Planning Guidance for the NHS 1996/7* (Leeds, NHSE).

NHSE (NHS Executive) (1995c) *Patients Not Paper. Report of the Efficiency Scrutiny into Bureaucracy in General Practice* (Leeds, NHSE).

NHSE (NHS Executive) (1996a) *Promoting Clinical Effectiveness* (Leeds, NHSE).

NHSE (NHS Executive) (1996b) *Seeing the Wood, Sparing the Trees* (Leeds, NHSE).

NHSE/SSI (NHSE and Social Services Inspectorate) (1995) *Community Care Monitoring Report 1994* (London, DoH).

NHSME (NHS Management Executive) (1992) *Local Voices* (London, Department of Health).

NHS Trust Federation (1995) *Behind Closed Doors: Boardroom Practice in NHS Trusts* (London, NHS Trust Federation).

Nicholl, J. P., Beeby, N R. and Williams B. T. (1989a) 'Comparison of the Activity at Short Stay Independent Hospitals in England and Wales, 1981 and 1986', *British Medical Journal,* 298, 239–42.

Nicholl, J. P., Beeby, N. R. and Williams B. T. (1989b) 'Role of the Private Sector in Elective Surgery in England and Wales', *British Medical Journal, 298*, 243–7.

Nikolaides, K., Barnett, A. H., Spiliopoulos, A. J. and Watkins, P. J. (1981) 'West Indian Diabetic Population of a Large Inner City Diabetic Clinic', *British Medical Journal, 283*, 1374.

Nocon, A. (1993) 'Made in Heaven', *Health Service Journal,* 2 December, 24–6.

Nocon, A. (1994) *Collaboration in Community Care in the 1990s* (Sunderland, Business Education Publishers).

Normand, C. (1991) 'Economics, Health and the Economics of Health', *British Medical Journal, 303*, 1572–7.

North, N. (1995) 'Alford Revisited: The Professional Monopolisers, Corporate Rationalisers, Community and Markets', *Policy and Politics,* 23 (2), 115–25.

Northern Ireland Health Promotion Agency (1990) *Health Promotion in Northern Ireland. A Discussion Paper* (Belfast, NIHPA).

North West London Mental Health Trust (1994) *The Report of the Independent Panel of Inquiry Examining the Case of Michael Buchanan* (London, NW London Mental Health Trust).

Oakley, A. (1980) *Women Confined* (Oxford, Martin Robertson).

Oakley, A. (1984) *The Captured Womb: A History of the Medical Care of Pregnant Women* (Oxford, Blackwell).

O'Connor, J. (1973) *The Fiscal Crisis of the State* (New York, St Martin's Press).

O'Donnell, O., Propper, C. and Upward, R. (1991) *An Empirical Study of Equity in the Finance and Delivery of Health Care in Britain,* Discussion Paper No. 85 (Centre for Health Economics, University of York).

OECD (Organisation for Economic Co-operation and Development) (1990) *Health Care Systems in Transition: The Search for Efficiency* (Paris, OECD).

OECD (Organisation for Economic Co-operation and Development) (1993) *Health Systems: Facts and Trends 1960–1991* (Paris, OECD).

OECD (Organisation for Economic Co-operation and Development) (1994a) *Health Care Reform: A Review of Seventeen OECD Countries* (Paris, OECD).

OECD (Organisation for Economic Co-operation and Development) (1994b) *Economic Surveys 1993–4: United Kingdom* (Paris, OECD).

OECD (Organisation for Economic Co-operation and Development) (1996) *Health Care Reform: The Will To Change* (Paris, OECD).

Offe, C. (1984) *The Contradictions of the Welfare State* (London, Hutchinson).

Office of Fair Trading (1996) *Health Insurance* (London, OFT).

Office of Health Economics (1984) *Compendium of Health Statistics* (London, Office of Health Economics).

Office of Health Economics (1994) *Obesity* (London, OHE).

Office of Health Economics (1995) *Compendium of Health Statistics* (London, OHE).

OPCS (Office of Population Censuses and Surveys) (1988) *OPCS Surveys of Disability in Great Britain: The Prevalence of Disability Among Adults* (London, HMSO).

OPCS (Office of Population Censuses and Surveys) (1992) *Mortality Statistics: Perinatal and Infant Mortality: Sociological and Biological Factors England and Wales 1990* (London, HMSO).

OPCS (Office of Population Censuses and Surveys) (1995) *General Household Survey 1993* (London, HMSO).

OPCS (Office of Population Censuses and Surveys) (1996) *Living in Britain: Results From the General Household Survey 1994* (London, HMSO).

Orchard, C. (1993) 'Strained Legacy', *Health Service Journal*, 2 December, 27.

Ottewill, R. and Wall, A. (1990) *The Growth and Development of the Community Health Services* (Sunderland, Business Education Publishers).

Owen, D. (1988) *Our NHS* (London, Pan).

Owens, P. and Glennerster, H. (1990) *Nursing in Conflict* (London, Macmillan).

Packwood, T., Keen, J. and Buxton, M. (1991) *Hospitals in Transition. The Resource Management Experiment* (Buckingham, Open University Press).

Packwood, T., Kerrison, S. and Buxton, M. (1994) 'The Implementation of Medical Audit', *Social Policy and Administration*, 28 (4), 299–315.

Pamuk, E. R. (1985) 'Social Class Inequality in Mortality from 1971–72 in England and Wales', *Population Studies*, 39, 17–31.

Parker, H., Measham, F. and Aldridge, J. (1995) *Drugs Futures: Changing Patterns of Drug Use Among English Youth* (London, Institute for Drug Dependency).

Parliamentary Office of Science and Technology (1994) *Breathing in Our Cities* (London, HMSO).

Parry, N. and Parry, J. (1976) *The Rise of the Medical Profession* (London, Croom Helm).

Parsons, T. (1951) *The Social System* (New York, Free Press of Glencoe).

Paton, C. (1992) *Competition and Planning in the NHS. The Danger of Unplanned Markets* (London, Chapman & Hall).

Paton, C. (1993) 'Devolution and Centralism in the National Health Service', *Social Policy and Administration*, 27 (2), 83–108.

Paton, C. (1995a) 'Contriving Competition', *Health Service Journal*, 30 March, 30–1.

Paton, C. (1995b) 'Present Dangers and Future Threats: Some Perverse Incentives in the NHS Reforms', *British Medical Journal*, 310, 1245–8.

Payer, L. (1989) *Medicine and Culture* (London, Gollancz).

Payne, S. (1991) *Women, Health and Poverty: An Introduction* (Brighton, Harvester Wheatsheaf).

Peck, E. (1995) 'The Performance of an NHS Trust Board: Actors Accounts, Minutes and Observation', *British Journal of Management*, 6, 135–56.

Pereira, J. (1993) 'What Does Equity in Health Mean?', *Journal of Social Policy*, 22 (1), 19–48.

Perkin, H. (1989) *The Rise of Professional Society* (London, Routledge).

Perrin, J. (1988) *Resource Management in the NHS* (London, Chapman & Hall).

Petchey, R. (1987) 'Health Maintenance Organisations: Just What the Doctor Ordered?', *Journal of Social Policy*, 16 (4), 489–507.

Petchey, R. (1993) 'NHS Internal Market 1991–2: Towards a Balance Sheet', *British Medical Journal*, 306, 699–701.

Peters, B. G. (1996) 'Is it the Institutions? Explaining the Failure of Health Care Reform in the United States', *Public Policy and Administration*, 11 (1), 8–15.

Peters, T. and Waterman, R. (1982) *In Search of Excellence* (New York, Harper & Row).

Pettigrew, A., Ferlie, E., FitzGerald, L. and Wensley, R. (1991) *Research in Action: Authorities in the NHS* (University of Warwick, Centre for Corporate Strategy and Change).

Phillimore, P., Beattie, A. and Townsend, P. (1994) 'Widening Inequality of Health in Northern England', *British Medical Journal*, 308, 1125–8.

Phillips, A. and Rakusen, J. (1989) *The New 'Our Bodies Ourselves'* (Harmondsworth, Penguin).

Phillips, D. R. (1990) *Health and Healthcare in the Third World* (London, Longman).

Phillips, G. (1996) 'A Worrying Statistic?', *British Medical Journal*, 312, 1586.

Pickard, S., Williams, G. and Flynn, R. (1995) 'Local Voices in an Internal Market: The Case of Community Health Services', *Social Policy and Administration*, 29 (2), 135–49.

Political and Economic Planning (1937) *Report on the British Health Services* (London, Political and Economic Planning).

Pollard, S., Liddle, T. and Thompson, B. (1994) *Towards a More Co-operative Society: Ideas on the Future of the British Labour Movement and Independent Health Care* (London, Independent Health Care Association).

Pollitt, C. (1985) 'Measuring Performance: A New System for the NHS', *Policy and Politics*, 13 (1), 1–15.

Pollitt, C. (1993a) *Managerialism and the Public Services: The Anglo American Experience*, 2nd edn (Oxford, Blackwell).

Pollitt, C. (1993b) 'The Struggle for Quality: The Case of the NHS', *Policy and Politics*, 21 (3), 161–70.

Pollock, A. (1992) 'Local Voices', *British Medical Journal*, 305, 535–6.

Pollock, A. and Whitty, P. (1990) 'Crisis in our Hospital Kitchens: Ancillary Staffing during an Outbreak of Food Poisoning in a Long-stay Hospital', *British Medical Journal*, 300, 383–5.

Popay, J. and Williams, G. (1994) 'Local Voices in the National Health Service: Needs, Effectiveness and Sufficiency', in Oakley, A. and Williams, A. (eds), *The Politics of the Welfare State* (London, UCL Press), 75–97.

Powell, M. (1990) 'Need and Provision in the NHS: An Inverse Care Law?', *Policy and Politics*, 18, 31–8.

Powell, M. (1992) 'A Tale of Two Cities: a Critical Evaluation of the Geographical Provision of Health Care Before the NHS', *Public Administration*, 70 (1), 67–80.

Powell, M. (1997) *Evaluating the National Health Service* (Buckingham, Open University Press).

Power, C. (1994) 'Health and Social Inequality in Europe', *British Medical Journal* 308, 1153–6.

Powles, J. (1973) 'On the Limitations of Modern Medicine', *Science, Medicine and Man*, 1, 1–30.

Poxton, R. (1994) *Joint Commissioning: The Story So Far*, Briefings nos 1 and 2 (London, King's Fund).

Price, D. (1996) 'Lessons for Health Care Rationing from the Case of Child B', *British Medical Journal*, 312, 167–9

Pritchard, C. (1992) 'What Can We Afford for the NHS?', *Social Policy and Administration*, 26 (1), 40–54.

Pritchard, P. (1978) *Manual of Primary Care: Its Nature and Organisation* (Oxford University Press).

Pritchard, P. (ed.) (1981) *Patient Participation in General Practice* (London, Royal College of General Practitioners).

Public Health Alliance (1988) *Beyond Acheson* (Birmingham, PHA).

Pyper, R. (ed. (1996) *Aspects of Accountability in the British System of Government* (Eastham, Tudor).

Radical Statistics Health Group (1977) *RAWP Deals: A Critique of 'Sharing Resources for Health in England'* (London, Radical Statistics Health Group).

Radical Statistics Health Group (1991) 'Let Them Eat Soap', *Health Service Journal*, 14 November, 25–7.

Radical Statistics Health Group (1995) 'NHS "Indicators of Success": What Do They Tell Us?', *British Medical Journal*, 310, 1045–50.

Ranade, W. (1995a) 'The Theory and Practice of Managed Competition in the National Health Service', *Public Administration*, 73 (2), 241–262.

Ranade, W. (1995b) 'US Health Care Reform: The Strategy that Failed', *Public Money and Management*, 15 (3), 9–16.

Rea, D. (1995) 'Unhealthy Competition: The Making of a Market for Mental Health', *Policy and Politics*, 23 (2), 141–55.

Read, S. and Graves, K. (1994) *Reduction of Junior Doctors' Hours in Trent Region: The Nursing Contribution* Sheffield Centre for Health and Related Research (Sheffield, Trent Regional Health Authority).

Redmayne, S. (1996) *Small Steps: Big Goals* (Birmingham, NAHAT).

Redwood, J. (1988) *In Sickness and in Health: Management Change in the NHS* (London, Centre for Policy Studies).

Regan, D. E. and Stewart, J. (1982) 'An Essay in the Government of Health: The Case for Local Authority Control', *Social Policy and Administration*, 16 (1), 19–42.

Reiser, J. (1978) *Medicine and the Reign of Technology* (Cambridge University Press).

Relman, A. (1980) 'The New Medical-Industrial Complex', *New England Journal of Medicine*, 303 (17), 963–70.

Richman, J. (1987) *Medicine and Health* (London, Longman).

Riddell, P. (1991) *The Thatcher Era and its Legacy* (Oxford, Blackwell).

Riley, C., Warner, M., Pullen, A. and Semple Piggott, C. (1995) *Releasing Resources to Achieve Health Gain* (London, Radcliffe Medical Press).

Rimm, E., Klatsky, A., Grobee, D. and Stampfer, M. (1996) 'Review of Moderate Alcohol Consumption and Reduced Risk of Coronary Heart Disease: Is the Effect due to Beer, Wine or Spirits?', *British Medical Journal*, 312, 731–6.

Ritchie, J., Dick, D. and Lingham, R. (1994) *The Report of the Inquiry into the Care and Treatment of Christopher Clunis* (London, HMSO).

Robb, B. (1967) *Sans Everything* (London, Nelson).

Roberts, H. (ed.) (1992) *Women's Health Matters* (London, Routledge).

Roberts, J. (1994) 'Health Reform is Dead: Long Live Health Reform', *British Medical Journal*, 309, 630.

Robins, A. and Wittenburg, R. (1993) *The Health of Elderly People – An Epidemiological Overview* (London, HMSO).

Robinson, D. (1971) *The Process of Becoming Ill* (London, Routledge).

Robinson, J. (1992) 'Introduction: Beginning the Study of Nursing Policy', in Robinson, J., Gray, A. and Elkan, R. (eds), *Policy Issues in Nursing* (Milton Keynes, Open University Press), 1–8.

Robinson, R. and Le Grand, J. (1994) *Evaluating the NHS Reforms* (Newbury, Policy Journals).

Rose, R. and Davies, P. (1995) *Inheritance in Public Policy: Change Without Choice in Britain* (New Haven, Yale University Press).

Rosen, H. (1993) *A History of Public Health*, expanded edition (New York, Johns Hopkins).

Rosser, R. and Watts, V. (1972) 'The Measurement of Hospital Output', *International Journal of Epidemiology*, 1, 361–8.

Rosser, R. and Kind, P. (1978) 'A Scale of Valuations of States of Illness: Is There A Social Consensus?', *International Journal of Epidemiology*, 7, 347–58.

Royal College of General Practitioners (1986) *Alcohol: A Balanced View*, Reports from General Practice (London, RCGP).

Royal College of Nursing (1990) *Memorandum to the House of Commons Social Services Committee 5th Report 1989/90. Community Care: Carers* (London, RCN).

Royal College of Physicians (1981) *Medical Aspects of Dietary Fibre* (London, Pitman).

Royal College of Physicians (1983a) 'Obesity', *Journal of the Royal College of Physicians,* 17, 5–64.

Royal College of Physicians (1983b) *Health or Smoking?* (London, Pitman).

Royal College of Physicians (1994) *Ensuring Equity and Quality of Care for Elderly People* (London, RCP).

Royal College of Physicians (1995) *Setting Priorities for the NHS: A Framework for Decision-making* (London, RCP).

Royal College of Physicians (1996) *Future Patterns of Care by General and Specialist Physicians* (London, Royal College of Physicians).

Royal College of Psychiatrists (1994) *Monitoring Inner London Mental Illness Services* (London, Royal College of Psychiatrists).

Royal College of Psychiatrists (1995) *Report of the Confidential Inquiry into Homicides and Suicides by Mentally Ill People* (London, Royal College of Psychiatrists).

Royal College of Radiologists (1992) 'Influence of the Royal College of Radiologists' Guidelines on Hospital Practice: A Multicentre Study', *British Medical Journal,* 304, 740–3.

Royal College of Surgeons (1994*) College Survey of Surgical Activity in the National Health Service* (London, RCS).

Sagan, L. A. (1987) *The Health of Nations* (New York, Basic Books).

Saks, M. P. (ed.) (1992) *Alternative Medicine in Britain* (Oxford, Clarendon).

Saks, M. P. (1995) *Professions and the Public Interest: Medical Power, Altruism and Alternative Medicine* (London, Routledge).

Salisbury, C. (1989) 'How Do People Choose Their Doctor?', *British Medical Association,* 299, 608–10.

Salmon, J. W. (1995) 'A Perspective on the Corporate Transformation of Health Care', *International Journal of Health Studies,* 25 (1), 11–42.

Salter, B. (1994) 'The Politics of Community Care: Social Rights and Welfare Limits', *Policy and Politics,* 22 (2), 119–31.

Salter, B. (1995) 'The Private Sector and the NHS: Redefining the Welfare State', *Policy and Politics,* 23 (1), 17–30.

Salter, B. (1996) 'Medicine and the State: Redefining the Concordat', *Public Policy and Administration* 10 (3), 60–87.

Salter, B. and Salter, C. (1993) 'Theatre of the Absurd', *Health Service Journal,* 11 November, 30–1.

Saltman, R. and von Otter, C. (eds) (1995) *Implementing Planned Markets in Health Care* (Buckingham, Open University Press).

Salvage, J. (1985) *The Politics of Nursing* (Oxford, Heinemann).

Salvage, J. (1992) 'The New Nursing', in Robinson, J., Gray, A. and Elkan, R., *Policy Issues in Nursing* (Milton Keynes, Open University Press), 9–23.

Salvage, J. and Wright, S. (1995) *Nursing Development Units: A Force for Change* (London, Scutari).

Sandler, G. (1979) 'Cost of Unnecessary Tests', *British Medical Journal,* 2, 21.

Sashidaran, S. and Francis, E. (1993) 'Epidemiology, Ethnicity and Schizophrenia', in Ahmad, W. (ed.) (1993) *Race and Health in Contemporary Britain* (Buckingham, Open University Press), 96–113.

Savage, R. and Armstrong, D. (1990) 'Effect of a GP's Consulting Style on Patients' Satisfaction: A Controlled Study', *British Medical Journal*, 301, 968–70.

Schieber, G. and Poullier, J. (1992) 'International Health Spending', *Health Affairs*, 10 (1), 106–16.

Schober, J. (1995) 'Nursing: Current Issues and the Patient's Perspective', in Schober, J. and Hinchcliffe, S., *Towards Advanced Nursing Practice* (London, Arnold), 94–108.

Scitovsky, A. (1988) 'Medical Care in the Last 12 Months of Life: The Relation Between Age, Functional Status, and Medical Care Expenditure', *The Milbank Quarterly*, 66 (4), 640–60.

Scope (1995) *Disabled in Britain: Behind Closed Doors – The Carer's Experience* (London, Scope).

Scottish Council for Independent Care (1995) *Closing the Door on the Private Sector* (Crieff, SCIC).

Scottish Office (1991) *Health Education in Scotland* (Edinburgh, HMSO).

Scottish Office (1992) *Scotland's Health: A Challenge For Us All* (London, HMSO).

Scottish Office (1995) *Clinical Outcome Indicators* (Edinburgh, Scottish Office).

Scottish Office (1996a) *Clinical Outcome Indicators* (Edinburgh, Scottish Office).

Scottish Office (1996b) Health Department *Interim Report and Recommendations of the Pennington Group* (Edinburgh, Scottish Office).

Scottish Office (1997) *The Pennington Group Report* (Edinburgh, The Stationery Office).

Scull, A. T. (1979) *Museums of Madness: The Social Organisation of Insanity in Nineteenth Century England* (London, Allen Lane).

Sculpher, M. (1993) *A Snip at the Price?* Health Economics Research Group (Uxbridge, Brunel University).

Sen, A. (1981) *Poverty and Famines: An Essay on Entitlement and Deprivation* (Oxford University Press).

Shackley, P. and Ryan, M. (1994) 'What is the Role of the Consumer in Health Care?', *Journal of Social Policy*, 23 (4), 517–41.

Shapiro, J. (1994) *Shared Purchasing and Collaborative Commissioning within the NHS* (Birmingham, NAHAT).

Sharma, U. (1995) *Complementary Medicine Today: Practitioners and Patients*, revised edn (London, Routledge).

Sheldon, T., Smith., P., Borwitz, M., Martin., S. and Carr-Hill, R. (1994) 'Attempt at Deriving a Formula for Setting General Practitioner Fundholder Budgets', *British Medical Journal*, 309, 1059–84.

Shepperd, S. and Iliffe, S. (1996) 'Hospital at Home', *British Medical Journal*, 312, 923–4.

Skinner, P. W., Riley, D. and Thomas, E. M. (1988) 'The Use and Abuse of Performance Indicators', *British Medical Journal*, 292, 1256–9.

Smaje, C. (1995) *Health, Race and Ethnicity: Making Sense of the Evidence* (London, King's Fund).

Smith, A. (1987) 'Qualms about QALYs', *The Lancet*, 1, 1134–6.

Smith, C. (1996) *A Health Service for a New Century: Labour's Proposals to End the Internal Market in the NHS*, speech made on 3 December.

Smith, F. B. (1979) *The People's Health* (London, Croom Helm).

Smith, G. D., Bartley, M. and Blane, D. (1990) 'The Black Report on Socioeconomic Inequalities in Health: 10 Years On', *British Medical Journal*, 301, 373–7.

Smith, G. D., Blane, D. and Bartley, M. (1994) 'Explanations for Socio-economic Differentials in Mortality', *European Journal of Public Health*, 4, 131–44.

Smith, R. (1987) *Unemployment and Health* (Oxford University Press).

Snashall, D. (1996) 'Hazards of Work', *British Medical Journal*, 313, 161–3.

Social Services Inspectorate (1995) *Social Services Departments and the Care Programme Approach* (London, Department of Health).

Social Services Inspectorate (1996) *Caring for People at Home: Part II. Report of a Second Inspection of Arrangements for Assessment and Delivery of Home Care Services* (London, Department of Health).

Spenceley, C., Craig, N., Denham, K. and Van Zwanenberg, T. (1994) 'NHS Funds for Fundholders and Non-fundholders', *British Medical Journal*, 309, 956.

Spencer, N. (1996) *Poverty and Child Health* (London, Radcliffe).

Spurgeon, P. (1993) 'Resource Management: A Fundamental Change in Managing Health Services', in Spurgeon, P., *The New Face of the NHS* (London, Longman), 96–101.

Stacey, M. (1992) *Regulating British Medicine: The General Medical Council* (Chichester, John Wiley).

Starr, P. and Immergut, E. (1987) 'Health Care and the Boundaries of Politics', in Maier, C. S. (ed.) *Changing Boundaries of the Political* (Cambridge University Press), 221–54.

Steele, K. (1992) 'Patients as Experts: Appraisal of Health Services', *Public Money and Management*, 12 (4), 31–8.

Stern, J. (1983) 'Social Mobility and the Interpretation of Social Class Mortality Differentials', *Journal of Social Policy*, 12 (1), 27–49.

Stern, R., Martin, V. and Cray, S. (1995) *Developing the Role and Purpose of NHS Boards Part One: Where Are We Now?* (Southborough, Salomons Centre).

Stewart, J., Kendall, E. and Coote, A. (1996) *Citizens' Juries* (London, Institute for Public Policy Research).

Stewart-Brown, S., Surender, R., Bradlow, J., Coulter, A. and Doll, H. (1995) 'The Effects of Fundholding in General Practice on Prescribing Habits Three Years After Introduction of the Scheme', *British Medical Journal*,311, 1543–7.

Stocking, B. (1988) *Expensive Medical Technologies* (Oxford University Press).

Stowe, K. (1989) *On Caring for the National Health* (London, Nuffield Provincial Hospitals Trust).

Strong, P. and Robinson, J. (1990) *The NHS: Under New Management* (Buckingham, Open University Press).

Szasz, T. S. and Hollender, M. H. (1956) 'A Contribution to the Philosophy of Medicine: The Basic Models of the Doctor–Patient Relationship', *American Medical Association, Archives of Internal Medicine*, 97, 585–92.

Szreter, S. (1988) 'The Importance of Social Intervention in Britain's Mortality Decline c1850–1914', *Social History of Medicine*, 1 (1), 1–38.

Taylor, D. (1988) 'Primary Care Services', in Maxwell, R. (ed.), *Reshaping the National Health Service* (Oxford, Policy Journals), 2–47.

Taylor, P. (1984) *The Smoke Ring: Tobacco, Money and Multi-National Politics* (London, Bodley Head).

Taylor-Gooby, D. (1995) 'Comfortable, Marginal and Excluded', in Jowell, R., Curtice, J., Park, A., Brook, L. and Ahrendt, D. (eds), *British Social Attitudes; The 12th Report 1995/6*, Social and Community Planning Research (Aldershot, Dartmouth), 1–17.

Taylor-Gooby, D. (1996) 'The Future of Health Care in Six European Countries: The Views of Policy Elites', *International Journal of Health Services*, 26 (2), 203–19.

Temple, J. and Wilson, J. (1988) 'Self-help Groups: A Useful Addition to Professional Care', *Geriatric Medicine*, 18 (3), 17–18.

Thane, P. (1987) 'The Growing Burden of an Ageing Population', *Journal of Public Policy*, 7 (4), 373–87.

Thatcher, M. (1982) Speech to Conservative Party Conference, Brighton, 8 October.

Thatcher, M. (1993) *The Downing Street Years* (London, Harper Collins).

The Times (1997) 'The Key Issues: Which Party is Best', report of a MORI poll, 28 February, 10.

Thomas, K., Fall., M., Parry., G. and Nicholl, J. (1995) *National Survey of Access to Complementary Health Care via General Practice*. Sheffield Centre for Health and Related Research (Sheffield, University of Sheffield).

Thomas, K., Nicholl, J. and Coleman, P. (1995) 'Assessing the Outcome of Making it Easier for Patients to Change General Practitioner: Practice Characteristics Associated with Patient Movements', *British Journal of General Practice*, 45, 581–6.

Thomas, R. (1994) 'Has HISS Run Out of Steam?', *Health Service Journal*, 28 July, 24–5.

Thompson, J. (1984) 'Compliance', in R. Fitzpatrick *et al.* (1984), *The Experience of Illness* (London, Tavistock).

Thwaites, B. (1988) *The Grand Dilemmas of a National Health Service* (Leeds, Nuffield Institute).

Timmins, N. (1988) *Cash, Crisis and Cure: The Independent Guide to the NHS Debate* (Oxford, Alden Press).

Timmins, N. (1995) *The Five Giants: A Biography of the Welfare State* (London, Harper Collins).

Tomlinson, B. (1992) *Report of the Inquiry into London's Health Service* (London, HMSO).

Townsend, P., Davidson, N. and Whitehead, M. (1992) *Inequalities in Health*, revised edition (Harmondsworth, Penguin).

Travers, A. (1996) 'Carers', *British Medical Journal*, 313, 482–6.

Trevett, N. (1997) 'Injecting New Life into the Wirral', *Healthlines*, 39, 20–1

Tuckett, D., Bolton, M., Olson, C. and Williams, A. (1985) *Meetings Between Experts: An Approach to Sharing Ideas in Medical Consultation* (London, Tavistock).

Tudor-Hart, J. (1971) 'The Inverse Care Law', *Lancet*, 27 February, 405–12.

Tudor-Hart, J. (1981) 'A New Kind of Doctor', *Journal of the Royal Society of Medicine*, 74, 871–83.

Tudor-Hart, J. (1994) *Feasible Socialism. The National Health Service: Past Present and Future* (London, Socialist Health Association).

Turnbull, D., Holmes, A., Shields, N., Cheyne, H., Twaddle, S., Harper Gilmour, W., McGinley, M., Reid, M., Johnstone, I., Geer, I., McIlwaine, G. and Burnett Lunan, C. (1996) 'Randomised Controlled Trial of Efficacy of Midwife Managed Care', *Lancet*, 348, 213–8.

Turner, B. (1987) *Medical Power and Social Knowledge* (London, Sage).

Twaddle, A. C. (1974) 'The Concept of Health Status', *Social Science and Medicine*, 8 (1), 29–38.

UKCC (UK Central Council for Nursing, Midwifery and Health Visiting) (1992a) *The Code of Professional Conduct for Nurses, Midwives and Health Visitors* (London, UKCC).

UKCC (UK Central Council on Nursing, Midwifery and Health Visiting) (1992b) *The Scope of Professional Practice* (London, UKCC).

UKCC (UK Central Council on Nursing, Midwifery and Health Visiting) (1996) *Guidelines for Professional Practice* (London, UKCC).

Vayda, E., Mindell, W. R. and Rutkow, I. M. (1982) 'A Decade of Surgery in Canada, England and Wales and the US', *Archives of Surgery*, 117, 846–53.

Walby, S. and Greenwell, J. (1994) *Medicine and Nursing: Professions in a Changing Health Service* (London, Sage).

Wall, A. (1996) 'Mine, Yours or Theirs?: Accountability in the New NHS', *Policy and Politics*, 24 (1), 1996.

Waller, D., Agass, M., Mant, D., Coulter, A., Fuller, A. and Jones, L. (1990) 'Health Checks in General Practice: Another Example of Inverse Care?', *British Medical Journal*, 300, 1115–8.

Warr, P. and Parry, G. (1982) 'Paid Employment and Women's Psychological Well Being', *Psychological Bulletin*, 91, 498–516.

Waterhouse, R. (1994a) 'Government Admits Flaw in Community Care Policy', *Independent*, 30 September, 10.

Waterhouse, R. (1994b) 'Unit With A Mission to be Honest', *Independent*, 20 December, 4.

Watkins, S. (1987) *Medicine and Labour. The Politics of a Profession* (London, Lawrence & Wishart).

Watterson, A. (1994) 'Threats to Health and Safety in the Workplace in Britain', *British Medical Journal*, 308, 1115–16.

Weale, A. (ed.) (1988) *Cost and Choice in Health Care* (London, King Edward's Hospital Fund for London).

Webb, N. (1994) *GP Fundholding: Market Effects and Allocation Issues* (London, Healthcare Financial Management Association).

Webster, C. (1988) *Health Services Since the War, Volume I: Problems of Health Care. The National Health Service before 1957* (London, HMSO).

Webster, C. (1996) *Government and Health Care, Volume 2: The National Health Service 1958–79* (London, HMSO).

Weller, M. (1989) 'Psychosis and Destitution at Christmas 1985–88', *The Lancet*, 2, 509–1.

White, D., Kelly, S., Huang, W and Charlton, A. (1996) 'Cigarette Advertising and the Onset of Smoking in Children: Questionnaire Survey', *British Medical Journal*, 313, 843–6.

White, D., Leach, K. and Christensen, L. (1996) 'Self-fulfilling Prophecies', *Health Service Journal*, 23 May, 31.

White, T. (1993) *Management for Clinicians* (London, Edward Arnold).

Whitehead, M. (1987) *The Health Divide* (London, Health Education Council).

Whitehead, M. (1989) *Swimming Upstream: Trends and Prospects in Health Education*, Research Report No. 5 (London, King's Fund).

Whitehead, M. (1994) 'Who Cares About Equity in the NHS?', *British Medical Journal*, 308, 1284–7.

Whitehouse, G. (1995) 'Use of Diagnostic Imaging Resources', in Riley, C., Warner, M., Pullen, A. and Semple Piggot, C. (1995) *Releasing Resources for Health Gain* (London, Radcliffe Medical).

Whitney, R. (1988) *National Health Crisis: A Modern Solution* (London, Shepherd-Walwyn).

Whitty. P. and Pollock, A. (1992) 'Public Health Heresy: A Challenge to the Purchasing Orthodoxy', *British Medical Journal*, 304, 1039–41.

WHO (World Health Organisation) (1946) *Constitution: Basic Documents* (Geneva, WHO).

WHO (World Health Organisation) (1978) *Alma Ata 1977: Primary Health Care* (Geneva, WHO/UNICEF).

WHO (World Health Organisation) (1985) *Targets for Health for All: Targets in Support of the European Regional Strategy for Health for All* (Copenhagen, WHO Regional Office for Europe).

WHO (World Health Organisation) (1986) *Health and the Environment* (Geneva, WHO).

WHO (World Health Organisation) (1988) *Healthy Nutrition. Preventing Nutrition-Related Disease in Europe* (Copenhagen, WHO).

WHO (World Health Organisation) (1993) *Health For All Targets: The Health Policy For Europe*, updated edition 1991 (Copenhagen, WHO Regional Office for Europe).

WHO (World Health Organisation) (1995) *The World Health Report: Bridging the Gaps* (Geneva, WHO).

WHO (World Health Organisation) (1996) *World Health Statistics Annual 1995* (Geneva,WHO).

Whynes, D. (1992) 'The Growth of UK Health Expenditure', *Social Policy and Administration*, 26 (4), 285–95.

Whynes, D. (1997) *Can the NHS Reforms Make GPs into Entrepreneurs?* ESRC Briefing Paper No.3 (Nottingham, ESRC Programme on Economic Beliefs and Behaviour).

Widgery, D. (1988) *The National Health: A Radical Perspective* (London, Hogarth).

Wilding, P. (1982) *Professional Power and Social Welfare* (London, Routledge).

Wiles, R. and Higgins, J. (1992) *Why Do Patients Go Private? A Study of Consumerism and Health Care* (Southampton, Institute for Health Policy Studies).

Wilkinson, R. (1992) 'Income Distribution and Life Expectancy', *British Medical Journal*, 304, 165–8.

Wilkinson, R. (1994) *Unfair Shares* (Ilford, Barnado's).

Wilkinson, R. (1996) *Unhealthy Societies* (London, Routledge).

Wilkinson, S. and Kitzinger, C. (1994) *Women and Health* (London, Taylor & Francis).

Williams, A. (1985) 'The Cost of Coronary Artery Bypass Grafting', *British Medical Journal*, 291, 326–9.

Williams, A. (1988) 'Health Economics: The End of Clinical Freedom?', *British Medical Journal*, 297, 183–8.

Williams, B. and Nicholl, J. (1994) 'Patient Characteristics and Clinical Caseload of Short Stay Independent Hospitals in England and Wales 1992/3', *British Medical Journal*, 308, 1699–1701.

Williams, S. and Calnan, M. (eds) (1996) *Modern Medicine: Lay Perspectives and Experiences* (London, UCL Press).

Williamson, C. (1992) *Whose Standards? Consumer and Professional Standards in Health Care* (Milton Keynes, Open University Press).

Wilsford, D. (1991) *Doctors and the State: The Politics of Health Care in France and the United States* (London, Duke University Press).

Wilson, M. (1975) *Health is for People* (London, Darton, Longman & Todd).

Wilson, R., Buchan, I. and Whalley, T. (1995) 'Alterations in Prescribing by General Practitioner Fundholders: An Observational Study', *British Medical Journal*, 311, 1347–50.

Windsor, P. (1986) *Introducing Körner: A Critical Guide to the Work and Recommendations of the Steering Group on Health Service Information* (Weybridge, British Journal of Health Care Computing).

Winkler, F. (1987) 'Consumerism in Health Care: Beyond the Supermarket Model', *Policy and Politics*, 15 (1), 1–8.

Winslow, C., Kosekoff, J., Chassin, M., Kanouse, D. and Brook, R. (1988) 'The Appropriateness of Performing Coronary Artery Bypass Graft Surgery', *Journal of the American Medical Association*, 260, 505–9.

Wistow, G. (1992) 'The National Health Service', in D. Marsh and R. Rhodes (eds), *Implementing Thatcherite Policies* (Buckingham, Open University Press).

Wistow, G. and Barnes, M. (1993) 'User Involvement in Community Care: Origins, Purpose and Applications', *Public Administration*, 71 (3), 279–99.

Wistow, G., Hardy, B. and Turrell, A. (1990) *Collaboration Under Financial Constraint: Health Authorities' Spending of Joint Finance* (Aldershot, Avebury).

Wistow, G., Knapp, M., Hardy, B. and Allen, C. (1994) *Social Care in a Mixed Economy* (Buckingham, Open University Press).

Witz, A. (1992) *Professions and Patriarchy* (London, Routledge).

Witz, A. (1994) 'The Challenge of Nursing', in Gabe, J., Kelleher, D. and Williams, G. (eds), *Challenging Medicine* (London, Routledge), 23–45.

Wohl, A. S. (1984) *Endangered Lives: Public Health in Victorian Britain* (London, Unwin Methuen).

Woolhandler, S. and Himmelstein, D. U. (1991) 'The Deteriorating Administrative Efficiency of the US Health Care System', *New England Journal of Medicine*, 324, 1253–8.

Worcester, R. (1996) 'Public Has Had Enough of Privatisation', *Independent on Sunday*, 7 April, 8.

Wordsworth, S., Donaldson, C. and Scott, A. (1996) *Can We Afford the NHS?* (London, Institute of Public Policy Research).

Yates, J. (1995) *Private Eye, Heart and Hip* (London, Churchill Livingstone).

Yates, J. R. W. (1996) 'Medical Genetics', *British Medical Journal*, 312, 1021–5.

Young, H. (1991) *One of Us*, final edn (London, Macmillan).

Zola, I. K. (1975) 'Medicine as an Institution of Social Control', in G. Cox and A. Mead (eds), *A Sociology of Medical Practice* (London, Collier Macmillan).

Index